AF838183

Hypovolemic Anemia of Trauma: The Missing Blood Syndrome

Authors

C. Robert Valeri, M.D.
Captain
Medical Corps
United States Navy
Adjunct Research Professor of Medicine
Boston University School of Medicine
Naval Blood Research Laboratory
Boston, Massachusetts

Mark D. Altschule, M.D.
Biomedical Consultant
Office of Naval Research
Honorary Curator of Prints and Photographic Materials
Francis A. Countway Library of Medicine
Harvard Medical School
Boston, Massachusetts

CRC Press, Inc.
Boca Raton, Florida

Library of Congress Cataloging in Publication Data

Valeri, Cesare Robert, 1932-

Hypovolemic anemia of trauma.

Bibliography: p.
Includes index.
1. Anemia, Hypovolemic. 2. Wounds and injuries—Complications and sequelae. I. Altschule, Mark David, joint author. II. Title. [DNLM: 1. Anemia—Prevention and control. 2. Wounds and injuries — Complications. 3. Hypotension—Prevention and control. 4. Shock—Prevention and control. 5. Blood volume. WO149 V163h]
RC641.7.H93V34 617'.2 80-18693
ISBN 0-8493-5389-0

This book represents information obtained from authentic and highly regarded sources. Reprinted material is quoted with permission, and sources are indicated. A wide variety of references are listed. Every reasonable effort has been made to give reliable data and information, but the author and the publisher cannot assume responsibility for the validity of all materials or for the consequences of their use.

All rights reserved. This book, or any parts thereof, may not be reproduced in any form without written consent from the publisher.

Direct all inquiries to CRC Press, Inc., 2000 N.W. 24th Street, Boca Raton, Florida 33431.

© 1981 by CRC Press, Inc.

International Standard Book Number 0-8493-5389-0

Library of Congress Card Number 80-18693
Printed in the United States

PREFACE

This book is written to report on our clinical experiences during the years 1968 to 1972 when we studied over 300 patients who after sustaining war injuries in South Vietnam were transferred to Chelsea Naval Hospital, later named Boston Naval Hospital, Chelsea, Massachusetts. The patients were called to the attention of our research facility when the use of general anesthesia for routine debridement of wounds precipitated a life-threatening state of hypotension. Observations by the clinical staff led to a series of tests which established the presence of chronic hypovolemia.

When washed red blood cells were administered to the patients with this clinical disorder before their surgical procedures, hypotension during operations and post-operatively was eliminated. Determinations of blood volumes were made using ^{51}Cr-labeled red blood cells to measure red blood cell mass and iodinated albumin and iodinated cold agglutinin to measure plasma volume. Cardiac output and the distribution of blood flow had to be measured in these patients to understand how the critical organs such as the heart and brain were protected in spite of a 40% reduction in total blood volume. Peripheral red blood cell levels of 2,3 DPG and creatine were measured to help assess the red cell mass deficits in the patients.

To gain some understanding of the mechanism of the reduced blood volume, we studied the patient's red blood cell production as well as the destruction of the patient's own red blood cells and the donor red blood cells. It became apparent that red blood cell production was impaired and both the patient's and the donor's red blood cells were being destroyed through an alternative pathway producing oxyporphyrin-like substances instead of the usual urobilinogen breakdown product of hemoglobin. The degradation of red blood cell-hemoglobin through the alternative pathway was thought to be responsible for the so-called *missing blood syndrome*.

C. Robert Valeri
Mark D. Altschule

THE AUTHORS

C. Robert Valeri, M.D. is a Captain in the U.S. Navy, assigned to the Naval Blood Research Laboratory at Boston University School of Medicine, Boston, Massachusetts. Dr. Valeri is a graduate of Harvard Medical School, and is currently an Adjunct Research Professor of Medicine at Boston University School of Medicine. Dr. Valeri's previous publications include his book *Blood Banking and the Use of Frozen Blood Products,* CRC Press, Cleveland, Ohio, 1976, as well as contributions to *The Red Blood Cell,* edited by D. M. Surgenor and the Xth edition of *Best and Taylor's Physiological Basis of Medical Practice,* edited by J. R. Brobeck. He has authored more than 200 scientific publications. Dr. Valeri's current research involves simplification of methods to freeze human red cells, platelets, and clotting, oncotic, and opsonic proteins of plasma to support the operational needs of the U.S. Navy.

Mark D. Altschule, M.D. is a biomedical consultant at the Office of Naval Research and honorary curator of prints and photographic materials at the Francis A. Countway Library of Medicine, Harvard Medical School, Boston, Massachusetts. Dr. Altschule received his B.S. from the College of the City of New York and his M.D. from Harvard Medical School. He is a member of ten scientific and professional organizations and is on the editorial board of several journals. He has published 12 books, 400 scientific papers, and 200 editorials and book reviews. Dr. Altschule's current research interests emphasize lipofuscin metabolism in reactions to various stresses.

DEDICATION

This book is dedicated to the Men of the United States Armed Forces wounded in action in Vietnam.

ACKNOWLEDGMENTS

The authors would like to acknowledge the assistance provided by the staff of doctors, nurses, and corpsmen of the Chelsea Naval Hospital's Orthopedic Service and the Naval Blood Research Laboratory during the period of these studies. Of paramount significance, of course, was the attitude and demeanor of the patients who participated not as subjects in a research project but rather as enthusiastically interested participants; they realized that all the tests made on them had the sole aim of defining a treatment for their refractory condition. This was clinical medicine at its finest.

The generosity of the investigators involved in carrying out the special studies reported here is acknowledged: Dr. Marilyn E. Miller — erythropoietin assays; Drs. Robin Bannerman and Martha Kreimer-Birnbaum — the urinary and fecal dipyrroles; and Dr. Donald Borg — urinary oxyporphyrins. Studies of red cell sensitivity to adrenochrome were performed with the help of Zoltan L. Hegedus. We also acknowledge the cooperation of Dr. Belton R. Burrows and Dr. John Cardarelli who provided us the use of the total body counter at the Boston Veterans Administration Medical Center, Jamaica Plain, Massachusetts and Dr. Scott Kramer, Commanding Officer at the Chelsea Naval Hospital. The data reported in the tables and figures were compiled and statistically analyzed by Linda E. Pivacek. Dr. Pierre Biron, Dr. John Howard, Dr. Irma Szymanski, Dr. Michael Jakubowski, Dr. Michael Wofford, Dr. Amiel Copper, Dr. Charles Zaroulis, and Dr. James Crowley assisted in the clinical studies performed on these patients. The technical assistance of William Raymond, Kenneth Patti, Robert Norton, George Lowrie, Richard Sheibley, William Gillum, and Frank Hawkins is greatly appreciated.

Dr. Charles P. Emerson's critical comments have been of immense value to us. The results of Cynthia A. Valeri's editorial efforts are evident on every page. Marilyn E. Sullivan spent many tireless hours preparing this manuscript for publication. The medical art work was done by William O'Leary and Donald O'Leary.

This work was supported mainly by the Naval Medical Research and Development Command, without whose sustained support this research could not have been accomplished. Some of the work was carried out under the terms of a contract with the Office of Naval Research, and of a grant from the John A. Hartford Foundation.

TABLE OF CONTENTS

Chapter 1

ON THE TRAIL OF A "NEW"SYNDROME, THE CHRONIC HYPOVOLEMIC ANEMIA OF TRAUMA

"How is it that, one fine morning, Duchenne discovered a disease that probably existed in the time of Hippocrates?" asked Charcot. Charcot answered the question himself, saying, "Disease is ancient and nothing about it has changed. It is we who change, as we learn to recognize what was formerly imperceptible." We now know, of course, that Charcot's theory was only partly true and that new diseases do arise: toxic and allergic effects of many new chemicals have been introduced into industry and into daily life during the past 150 years. New diseases may also arise as a result of mutations among microorganisms, particularly viruses. In addition, some old diseases have appeared as new ones, sometimes in modified form under previously nonexistent circumstances. Thus, laborers in the Alps digging the first tunnels displayed unrecognized symptoms of anemia, which later proved to be the same disease as that observed in Egypt and known as hookworm anemia. In any case, completely *new* diseases are indeed rare.

This monograph describes a syndrome only recently defined. That is not to say that it did not exist previously, for observations suggestive of its existence were first recorded over half a century ago. The first of these observations was made by Keith in World War I and reported in 1919. Using a dye method of uncertain accuracy to measure plasma volume and estimate blood volume in wounded men, Keith (1919) made the observation that the decrease in blood volume was often greater than the visible blood loss could explain. Admittedly Keith's patients were in far from optimal conditions when he studied them. They were dehydrated, starved, and half-frozen, and were received at his hospital after many hours of being transported back from the front lines over the deplorable Flanders roads in vehicles that today can only be imagined. Keith recognized the role of hemorrhage in the decrease of blood volume but was unable to define the most important cause of the loss. His method of measurement (his own invention) often produced significant errors, and his findings of decreased blood volume may be open to argument. Nevertheless, during and after World War II a number of physicians reported that trauma victims, both military and civilian, required larger amounts of blood transfusions than expected from the observed or calculated blood loss (Seaman and Ponder, 1943; Richards, 1944a, 1944b; Vaughan et al., 1946; Vaughan, 1948; Grant and Reeve, 1951; Norlander, 1955; Topley and Clarke, 1956). Some physicians found it difficult to reckon the low blood volumes observed after trauma with the calculated or observed blood loss (Emerson and Ebert, 1945; Noble and Gregersen, 1946; Stanton et al., 1949; Clarke et al., 1955). Although some studies made a day or two after trauma showed no discrepancies between reductions in plasma and blood volumes and the calculated or observed blood loss (Evans et al., 1944; Dacie and Homer, 1946), other investigators reported anemia developing a week or more after trauma (Cartwright and Wintrobe, 1952; Gelin, 1956). Undertransfusion has been cited as one reason for the discrepant decrease in blood volume (Grant and Reeve, 1951; Topley and Clarke, 1956; Simmons et al., 1969a).

The mechanisms responsible for unexpectedly low blood volumes after treatment have been discussed by a number of authors. Some thought the mechanism to be deficient hemoglobin synthesis (Seaman and Ponder, 1943; Vaughan et al., 1946; Vaughan, 1948). Cartwright and Wintrobe (1952) ascribed the anemia in their trauma cases to the defective entry of iron into the porphyrin moiety of hemoglobin, basing their conclusion on the similarity between anemia of trauma and the better studied anemia of infection. Norlander (1955) and Gelin (1956) invoked hemolysis as the cause.

Even today the missing blood syndrome is rarely recognized. Conversations with elderly physicians in one place or another have revealed that more than one of them have observed peculiarities in the clinical course of some patient after an accident or an operation. These peculiarities, which revolved about the fact that the patients needed more blood transfusions than the circumstances seemed to warrant (Gardner, 1969), probably were viewed as unusual manifestations by experienced physicians who understood that no two patients are alike and few conform to textbook descriptions.

WORLD WAR II EXPERIENCE

The experiences of World War II led to a considerable body of published works that indicated the existence of a syndrome called *anemia of trauma,* although there was little speculation regarding its cause. Seaman and Ponder (1943) and Vaughan et al. (1946, 1948) suggested bone marrow suppression as the main or perhaps only cause, but were unable to define the depressing factor. Cartwright and Wintrobe (1952) pointed out the ineffectiveness of iron in its treatment. Wound infection as a mechanism and additional transfusion as treatment were both proposed, both with little enthusiasm.

At the time America entered World War II the Committee on Transfusions of the National Research Council, supported by other official bodies, had announced a policy that stated "most instances of shock are associated with hemoconcentration, and a given quantity of plasma is more effective than an equal quantity of whole blood in treatment." The concept was that plasma for the intravascular space and sodium chloride for the interstitial space were therapeutic measures adequate to re-establish equilibrium in a wounded man (Beecher and Burnett, 1944; Beecher, 1945; Beecher and Altschule, 1977). Edwin Cohn's newly developed blood fractionation procedures made it possible to accumulate many thousands of pints of human plasma. Yet there were no facilities for blood transfusions, and when plasma was used in severely wounded men in the North African operations the results were disastrous. Plasma not only was lacking in sustained effectiveness in trauma but actually had deleterious effects in many cases.

At that time Edward D. Churchill was consultant to the U.S. Fifth Army, not a man to tolerate in silence either bad medicine or official obtundity. When he failed to achieve official approval to replace plasma transfusions by blood transfusions, he took the issue before the public via the newspapers. A report on page 4 of the *New York Times* of August 27, 1943 had the effect he desired, and the official position about plasma was revoked (despite the complaints of Edwin Cohn). By the middle of World War II, the treatment of trauma patients (as opposed to burn patients) with plasma alone was thoroughly discredited. Aside from the implications of the role of government agencies in dictating clinical practice, these experiences in World War II taught us that plasma was of limited usefulness in the wounded, a principle still in effect 25 years later. That blood was necessary to treat the wounded was clear, although the magnitude necessary for a therapeutic transfusion was less definitive.

KOREAN EXPERIENCE

Blood transfusions for the wounded again became the subject of extensive study during the Korean military operations. In 1954, Crosby and Howard, then in the United States Army, made the observation that blood volume was not maintained in some patients with wounds of the extremities after blood transfusions, and that the rapid loss of blood observed was not attributable to continued bleeding. Transfusions were given to these patients because of continued low hematocrit values even after the hypovolemia of the acute phase of their injury had been corrected and they were no longer in shock. The transfusions given to correct blood deficits in the acute or subacute stages of trauma produced only transient increases in blood hematocrit levels. This anemia that was difficult to treat and seemed to have a hemolytic component was viewed as a puzzling condition but was not studied intensively, perhaps because it was not seen on any large scale in civilian practice after the war. As a matter of fact, the observations made by Crosby and Howard (1954) were somewhat misleading because they were made only in the acute phase of the trauma and were limited to the effect — or rather the lack of lasting effect — of transfusions in these anemic patients. Since the patients were being given transfusions because they had low hematocrit values, the full implications of the hematologic effects of trauma could not be known at that time.

In the year 1954 another report on blood transfusions in wounded men was published, this one by Prentice's group (which included John Howard). Recognizing by that time that a large amount of data had accumulated on the acute changes induced by trauma and by the resuscitation that followed, these authors decided to study patients during the subsequent period on which the collection of data was scarce, the 6 days after resuscitation and operation. They found that patients with extremity wounds had large requirements for blood, even greater than those of other wounded men, and that they often exhibited persistently large deficits in blood volume despite massive transfusions. Reduced hematocrit levels were seen in the week after resuscitation and operation. These values were misleading inasmuch as blood volume measurements suggested serious deficits both of red blood cell and plasma volumes. Prentice and his co-workers (1954) were surprised to find that these serious deficits of total blood volumes did not cause shock. They concluded that whereas plasma infusions might be essential in patients with abdominal wounds, their patients with wounds of the extremities would not often benefit from this treatment.

Regarding the cause of the blood volume deficits in patients with extremity wounds, Prentice and his co-workers (1954) preferred an explanation based on the possibility that the extensive muscle damage caused by high velocity missiles might have acted to trap blood. However, the discussion also raised the possibility of a hemolytic mechanism, although this was minimized because the authors saw none of the then-recognized evidences of hemolysis, i.e., chills, fever, and jaundice.

The early papers on the chronic anemia of trauma published by Seaman and Ponder (1943) and Vaughan et al. (1946, 1948), suggesting a mysterious depression of bone marrow days after the event, should have stimulated further inquiry, and this applies even more emphatically to the data of Crosby and Howard (1954) and Prentice and his co-workers (1954). Perhaps the fact that their observations were made on patients with war-related injuries accounted for the relative lack of widespread interest. Nevertheless, they deserved better. If only these physicians had studied their patients for a longer period they might have recognized the syndrome that is the subject of the present monograph. Be that as it may, it was not until 15 years had passed and another war developed that the importance of these earlier findings came to be appreciated.

Many of the men with severe extensive trauma studied by us at the Chelsea Naval Hospital survived their injuries primarily because of recent advances in treatment as well as advanced facilities of evacuation from the combat zone. In fact, so many of them did survive that the syndrome to be discussed here proved to be a common occurrence among certain types of them. The grouping of so many of these patients at one Naval Hospital permitted studies to be made which threw some light on the pathologic physiology of the syndrome and the therapeutic course. The etiology of the missing blood syndrome is still not known, but its effective treatment has been established.

EXPERIENCE IN VIETNAM

During the military operations in Vietnam, with the availability of large amounts of antibiotics and of banked blood, with the improvements in surgical and anesthetic techniques, and with the development of procedures for quick evacuation of wounded from the battlefield, many lives were saved that in the other wars would have been lost. However, it soon became clear that after the life-saving treatment, at least some of those with severe wounds of the extremities did not do well. Many of the patients treated at the Chelsea Naval Hospital had a serious chronic illness. These men ate poorly and felt irritable and depressed for weeks or months. Their wounds, although thoroughly debrided before admission and again from time to time after admission, did not heal and, for the most part, showed varying amounts of persistent infection. A number of the patients had to undergo subsequent amputations of one or more extremities or part of them. At best, improvement was incomplete and very slow.

Routine laboratory studies proved to be less than informative since there were no consistently striking abnormalities. The unsatisfactory clinical situation was puzzling and probably would have remained so were it not for a clue afforded by a simple clinical observation. When given an anesthetic in preparation for wound debridement or some other relatively minor procedure, some of the patients developed asystole or severe hypotension. This was unexpected, for by ordinary clinical criteria their circulatory and hematologic status should have been adequate to prevent the complications. The clinical conclusion was that these patients must have some as yet unrecognized disorder of cardiovascular regulation. We recognized that previous studies of the war-wounded had been made only in the acute or subacute phase, that is for periods of less than 2 weeks, and that we were dealing with patients in the chronic phase, that is weeks to months after the traumatic episode. The cardiovascular regulation of our patients with chronic trauma, although seemingly adequate most of the time, was revealed to be extremely fragile by the simple stress of anesthesia.

The possibility that the patients had a markedly decreased blood volume was considered, although on the face of it this seemed unlikely in view of their normal or nearly normal hematocrit values. Nevertheless, measurements made by means of chromium-tagged (Cr-tagged) red blood cells (a method of the highest accuracy) revealed markedly decreased red blood cell volumes. We concluded that we were dealing with a state of both hypovolemia and anemia, i.e., the *hypovolemic anemia of chronic trauma.* It was evident that the condition differed from the ordinary hypovolemia of trauma, a state of shock associated with acute blood loss. The patients studied here were not in shock but clearly had another type of hypovolemia, previously unrecognized as such. It was apparent that the change from the acute phase of trauma into the chronic one involved compensations for decreases in blood volume ordinarily expected with shock, as described by earlier authors (Cournand et al., 1943; Richards, 1944a, 1944b). In fact, in their studies of shock Shoemaker et al. (1973) correlated the fall in cardiac output with the magnitude of the blood volume reduction. We noted, as had Prentice et al. in 1954, that the low blood volume found a week after resuscitation from the effects of acute trauma was not accompanied by signs of shock. Clearly a new equilibrium had been set up, one that had not before been described in any detail. This new equilibrium clearly supported life, but just as clearly it did not support health. Our objective was to study the new, unsatisfactory equilibrium, and, if possible, to devise ways to restore the physiologic state to normal.

CLINICAL EXAMPLES

The clinical picture presented by the patients in this study is exemplified by the following histories.

Case 1

A 22-year-old marine (1A) had been shot through the right hip in Vietnam in 1968. The injury consisted of a through-and-through gunshot wound of the hip that produced comminuted fractures of the femoral neck and head. He was initially treated with resuscitation, debridement of wounds, and traction plus a spica cast.

On August 18, 1968 the patient had a primary delayed closure of his wounds, and was placed in another spica cast and transferred to the Chelsea Naval Hospital, where he arrived 14 days after the injury. There traction was re-instituted and was maintained until November, at which time fluoroscopy revealed nonunion of the femoral neck (Figure 1). Most of the femoral head still appeared to be viable and bone-grafting was considered. Preoperative measurements showed that the red blood cell mass, and the peripheral venous hemoglobin and hematocrit values were normal. Accordingly, bone-grafting was performed 5 days later, and three Hagie pins were inserted for immobilization (Figure 2). This procedure was difficult because scarring was present in the area, and an estimated volume of about 2000 $m\ell$ of blood was lost during the procedure. The patient was given four units of liquid-stored whole blood in the operating room. Postoperatively there was no large hematoma formation at either the graft-donor site or operative site, and no hemovac was used. After the operation the patient was pale, weak, and drowsy, and had persistent tachycardia but no hypotension. At this time, a marked reduction in red cell hemoglobin mass was found. The red cell 2,3 diphosphoglycerate (2,3 DPG) rose from 12 to 19 μmol/g of hemoglobin, and red cell creatine rose from 0.8 to 2.9 μmol/g of hemoglobin. The reticulocyte count was not increased (0.4%). Because of the red cell mass deficit of 400 g of hemoglobin, the patient received five units of washed red blood cells (stored as whole blood at 4°C for approximately 10 days) and quickly experienced excellent clinical improvement. Subsequent measurements revealed first a slight decline and then a gradual increase in red cell mass, together with a gradual restoration toward normal of red cell 2,3 DPG and creatine levels. The patient was maintained in a spica cast for 3½ months. Roentgenographic studies then showed sufficient healing to permit the patient to walk with a three-point gait. The patient eventually progressed to full weight-bearing without support, and the motion of his hip was in the normal range except for a loss of 20° of flexion and abduction. Although it appeared from roentgenograms that a small area of the femoral head was necrotic, the femoral neck went on to heal with only a slightly deformed head.

Case 2

A 23-year-old marine (1B) had been wounded in Vietnam when he stepped on a land mine, sustaining multiple severe compound fractures involving the distal part of the right forearm, wrist, and hand, with loss of the ulnar nerve. He also had an extensively comminuted compound fracture of the right tibia and fibula (Figure 3), an open wound of the left knee joint, and multiple facial wounds.

He was initially treated using plasma expanders and blood; this was followed by debridement of his wounds. He was evacuated by air 8 weeks after injury. On admission to the Chelsea Naval Hospital the left knee wound was closed and the knee was functioning well. The facial wounds were healed. However, the right upper and lower extremity wounds were open and grossly infected. The skin defect over the right fibula was 51 cm long and 8 cm wide.

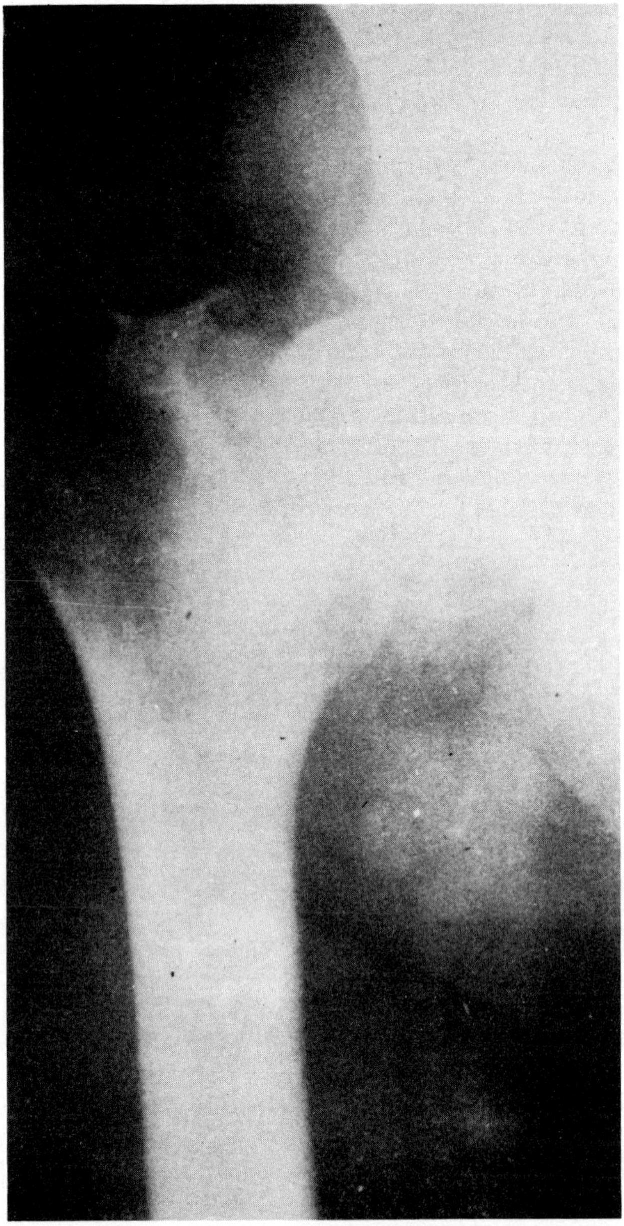

FIGURE 1. Through-and-through gunshot wound of the right hip of Patient 1A that produced comminuted fractures of the femoral neck and head resulting in non-union of the right femoral head.

The initial peripheral venous hematocrit value was 34%, and the hemoglobin concentration was 11 g/100 mℓ. The red blood cell hemoglobin mass was found to be 300 g, when compared with the normal value for this patient's body surface area of 500 g. The patient's 40% loss of the circulating red cell mass evidently caused tissue hypoxia, for the level of 2,3 DPG increased from 12 to 22 μmol/g of hemoglobin, and red cell creatine level increased from 1.2 to 3 μmol/g of hemoglobin. The red blood cell hemoglobin mass was restored toward normal by transfusion of washed previously frozen erythrocytes.

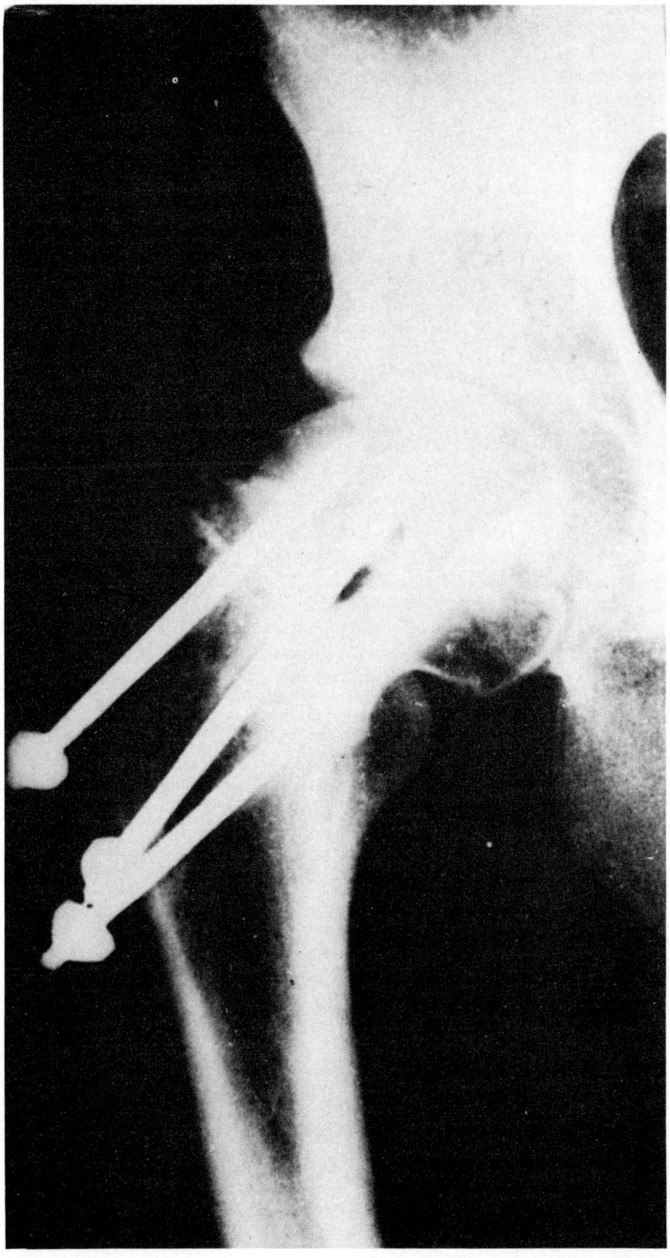

FIGURE 2. The result of bone grafting and insertion of three Hagie pins in the neck and head of the right femur of Patient 1A.

Four days after admission a 10-cm long segment of nonviable tibia was removed, leaving a 10-cm gap between the main tibial fragments. The soft tissues were further debrided, but closure was not attempted. Although the red blood cell hemoglobin mass was still decreased by 10%, the peripheral venous hematocrit value was 47% and the blood hemoglobin concentration was 16.5g/100 mℓ.

Two weeks later a split-thickness skin graft was placed on a bed of good granulation tissue over the right tibial region and over the upper extremity wounds. The granula-

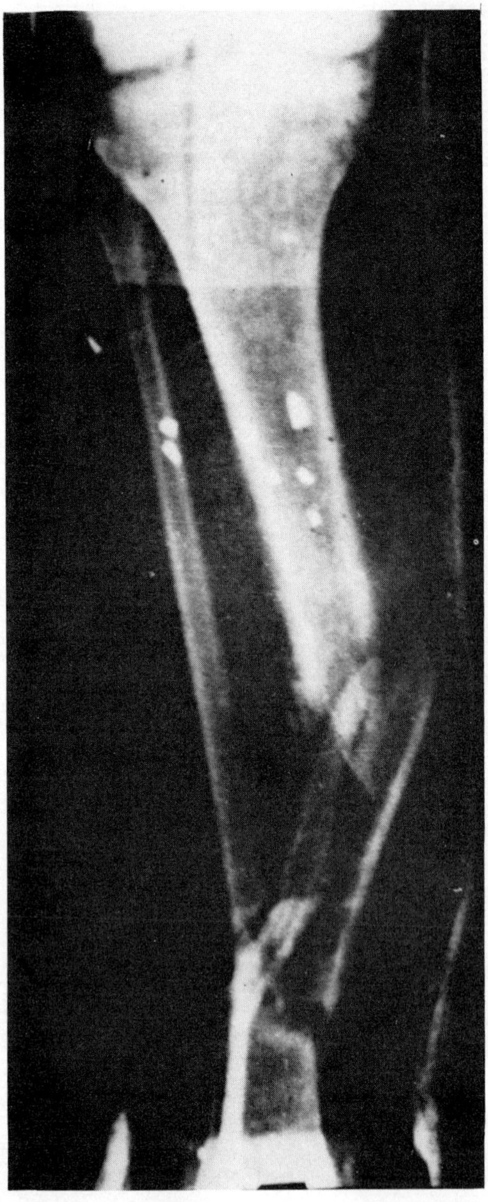

FIGURE 3. Comminuted compound fractures of the right tibia and fibula of Patient 1B.

tion tissue looked healthier than was expected considering the previous septic condition, and it covered most of the exposed bone. Four weeks after admission further skin-grafting of the right forearm was performed. The estimated blood loss during the skin-grafting procedure was only 100 mℓ. Immediately after the operation, the hematocrit value decreased to 36%, the blood hemoglobin concentration was 11.8 g/100 mℓ, and the total circulating red cell hemoglobin mass was 250 g (50% below normal). The red blood cell level of 2,3 DPG, although lower than on admission, was still elevated. The patient was given four units of washed nonfrozen red blood cells. His red cell hemoglobin mass, hematocrit value, and blood hemoglobin concentration all returned toward normal and then fell slightly; 2 years later these measurements were

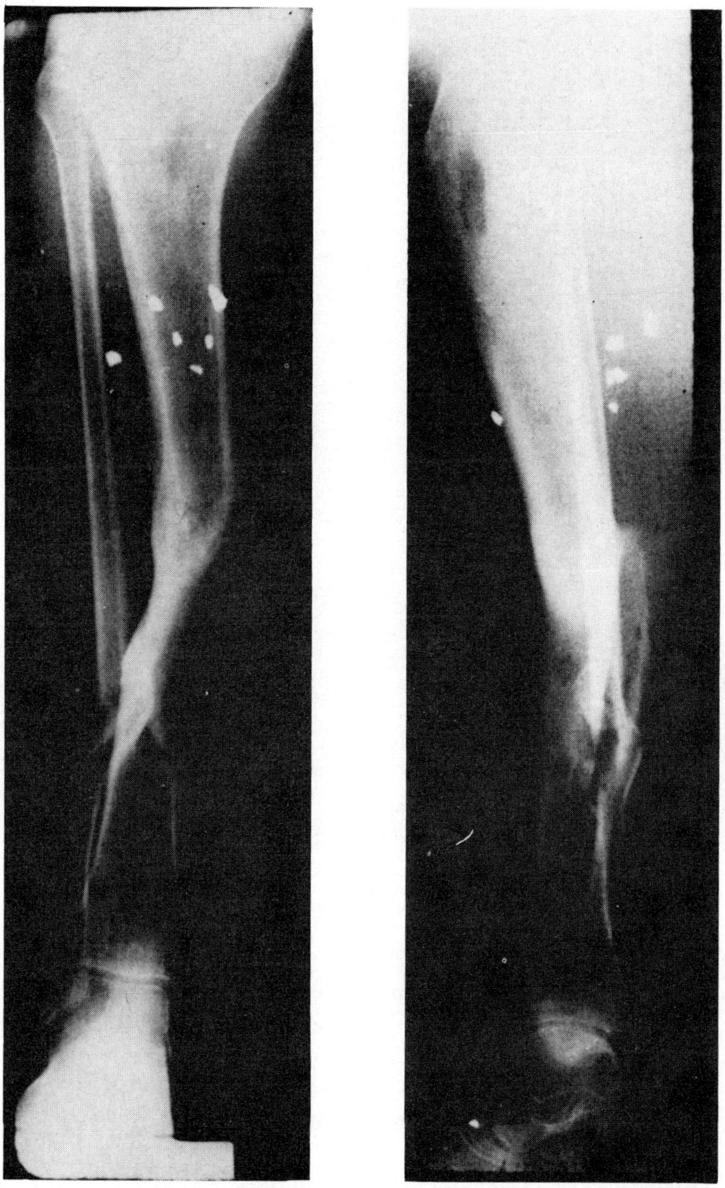

FIGURE 4. Five months after the injury the large gap between the two tibial fragments was found to be bridged by a bar of good bone that had cross-united with the fibula in Patient 1B.

within the normal ranges. Five months after the injury there was good bone ankylosis between the distal end of the radius and the proximal row of carpal bones, and the large gap between the two tibial fragments was found to be bridged by a bar of good bone that had cross-united with the fibula (Figure 4). All the leg wounds were closed and clean. There was no drainage from the leg, and the knee motion rapidly improved.

Case 3

A 19-year-old marine (1C) had been wounded by an exploding mine in Vietnam. He had multiple fragment wounds in the soft tissues of both legs and in the abdomen,

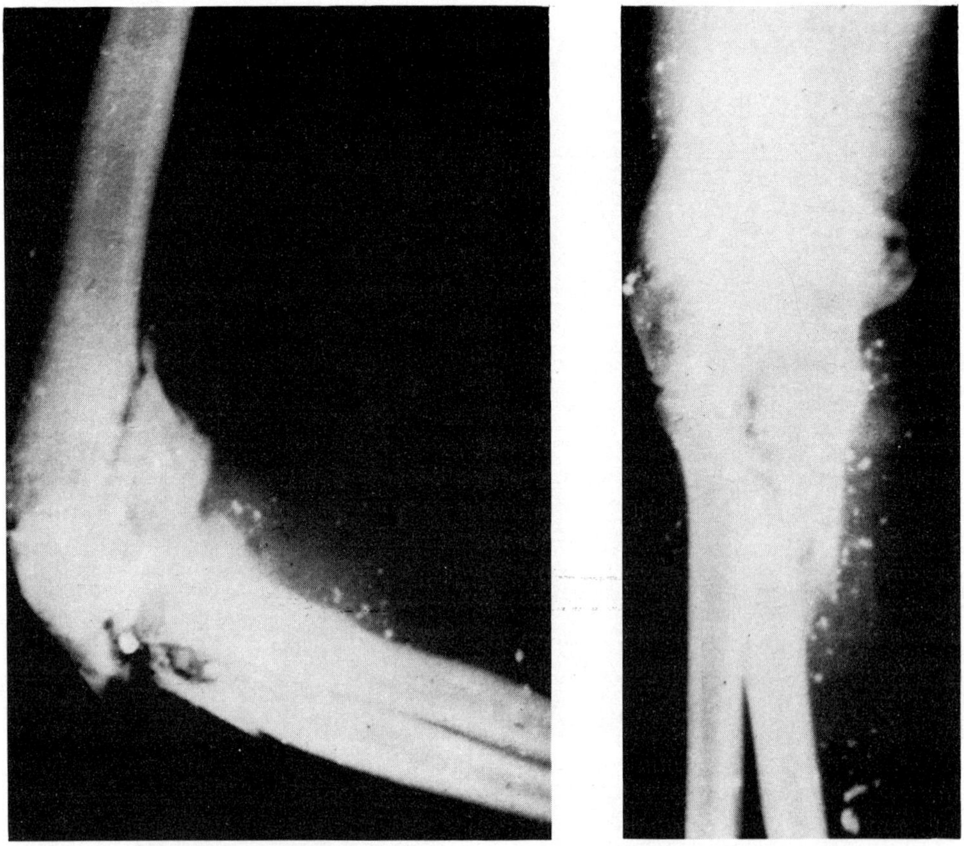

FIGURE 5. Patient 1C had sustained multiple compound fractures of both elbows and loss of both ulna nerves.

together with multiple compound fractures about both elbows and loss of both ulnar nerves (Figure 5). His initial treatment in Vietnam had consisted of transfusion of whole blood for resuscitation, followed by laparotomy and debridement of all wounds.

When he arrived at the Chelsea Naval Hospital 2 weeks after injury, all his extremity wounds were open, and there were large open wounds of the posterior aspects of both elbows.

The total circulating red blood cell hemoglobin mass was 425 g (approximately 35% below the normal value for this patient). The red cell 2,3 DPG level was elevated to 20 μmol/g hemoglobin, and the red cell creatine level was increased to 3.0 μmol/g hemoglobin. After administration of three units of washed erythrocytes, his red cell mass rose to 600 g. Six days after admission, meshed split-thickness skin grafts were placed over both elbow regions. Small openings over both elbow joints could not be skin-grafted because the cartilage was exposed. At this time the peripheral venous hematocrit value was 30%, the hemoglobin concentration was 10 g/100 mℓ, and the red cell hemoglobin mass had fallen to 370 g, lower than on admission. The red blood cell creatine level had increased to 5 μmol/g hemoglobin, and red cell 2,3 DPG concentration had increased to 22 μmol/g of hemoglobin. After transfusion of three units of washed red cells, the red cell hemoglobin mass rose to 570 g. At the time of the survival measurement the reticulocyte count was decreased. The red cell hemoglobin mass again fell, and the red cell concentrations of 2,3 DPG and creatine increased. Three additional units of washed, previously frozen red cells were administered. Throughout the

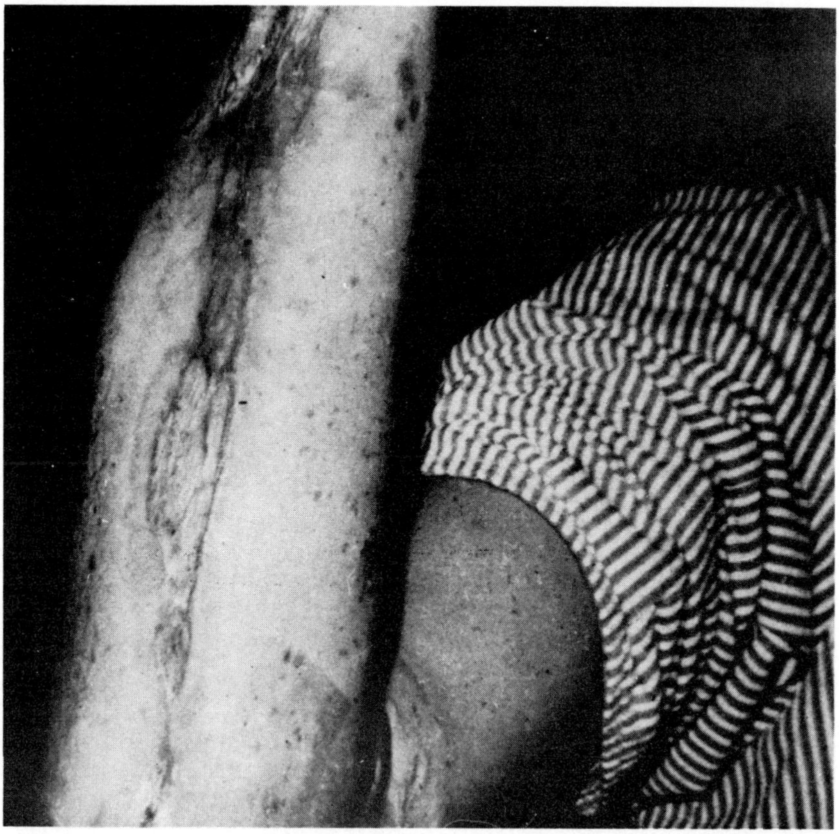

FIGURE 6. Four months after injury to Patient 1C the range of motion of the right elbow was 80 to 120° with 15° of pronation and 10° of supination.

clinical course the decreases in red cell hemoglobin mass were associated with increases in red cell levels of 2,3 DPG and creatine. The peripheral venous hemoglobin and hematocrit levels were not reliable indicators of the red cell mass when the latter had decreased to less than 40% of normal.

The arm casts were left in place for four weeks to allow the skin grafts to mature and to give some stability to the multiple elbow fractures. The grafts took well. Early elbow motion was started despite the fact that the patient still had small open areas on both elbow joints. Four months after injury, drainage of the cloudy synovial fluid from the elbows ceased and motion continued to improve. The range of motion was 80 to 120° on the right, with 15° of pronation and 10° of supination (Figure 6). On the left, the range of elbow motion was from 15 to 90°, supination was normal, and 30° of pronation was present (Figure 7). Limitation of motion was believed to be more a result of poor position of the fracture fragments than of intra-articular scarring.

This patient had four major decreases in red cell mass in spite of the fact that his only operation was one skin-grafting procedure. Despite their severity all the wounds healed well. Although the elbow joints had been open and infected for 12 to 14 weeks, the resultant range of painless motion was remarkable.

Case 4

A 21-year-old marine (1D) had been injured by mortar fire in Vietnam. He sustained the following injuries: compound fracture of the proximal part of the left femur

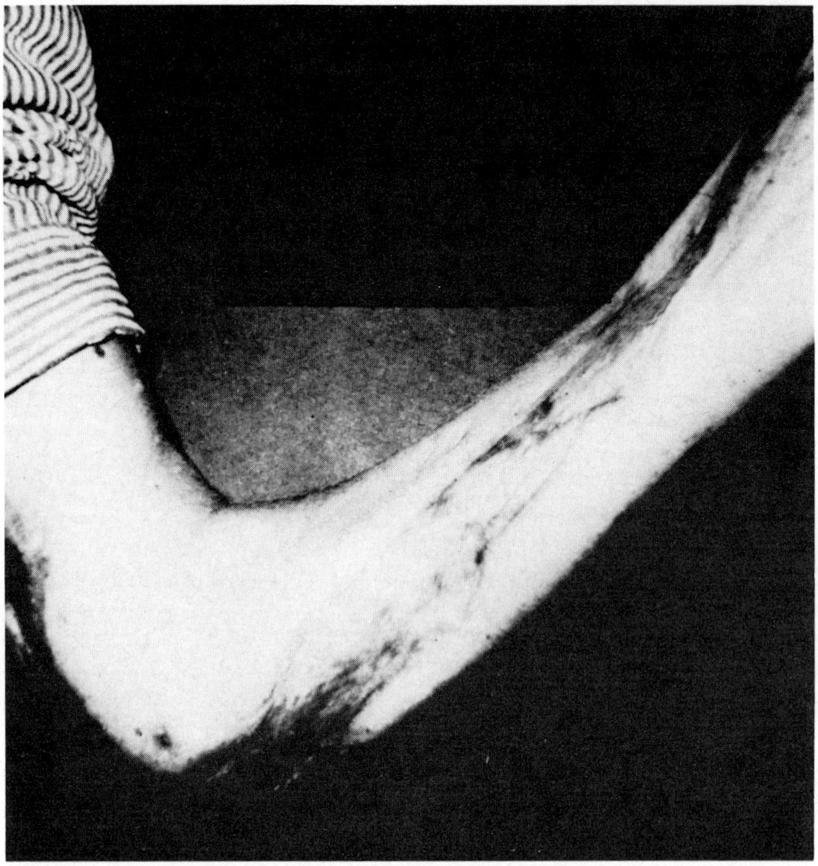

FIGURE 7. Four months after injury to Patient 1C the range of motion of the left elbow was 15 to 90° with normal supination and 30° of pronation. The limitation of motion was thought to be due to poor position of the fracture fragments.

(Figure 8), loss of left nerve function, injured sigmoid colon, severely injured left testicle, and multiple soft-tissue wounds of both legs and the right foot. Initial treatment consisted of resuscitation and debridement, and a colostomy was established. After 2 days and again after 8 days the patient had further debridement of his wounds. Five weeks later a primary delayed closure of most of his wounds was performed. Because of breakdown of the wounds about the left hip and proximal part of the femur, this closure had to be opened.

This patient arrived at the Chelsea Naval Hospital 5 weeks later, where measurements of hematologic parameters revealed a hematocrit value of 40%, and a blood hemoglobin concentration of 13 g/100 mℓ. The circulating red blood cell-hemoglobin mass, however, was only 430 g, a deficit of 250 g from the patient's theoretical normal of 680 g; red blood cell 2,3 DPG and creatine concentrations were elevated. After administration of three units of previously frozen washed red blood cells, his red cell-hemoglobin mass improved, but not quite to his normal value. The transfused red blood cells exhibited shortened survival with a lifespan of about 80 days, and the reticulocyte count was decreased during the time that the survival of the transfused red blood cells was being studied.

Eleven days after admission a split-thickness skin-grafting was done about the left hip. Five weeks later, additional studies showed that although the hematocrit and

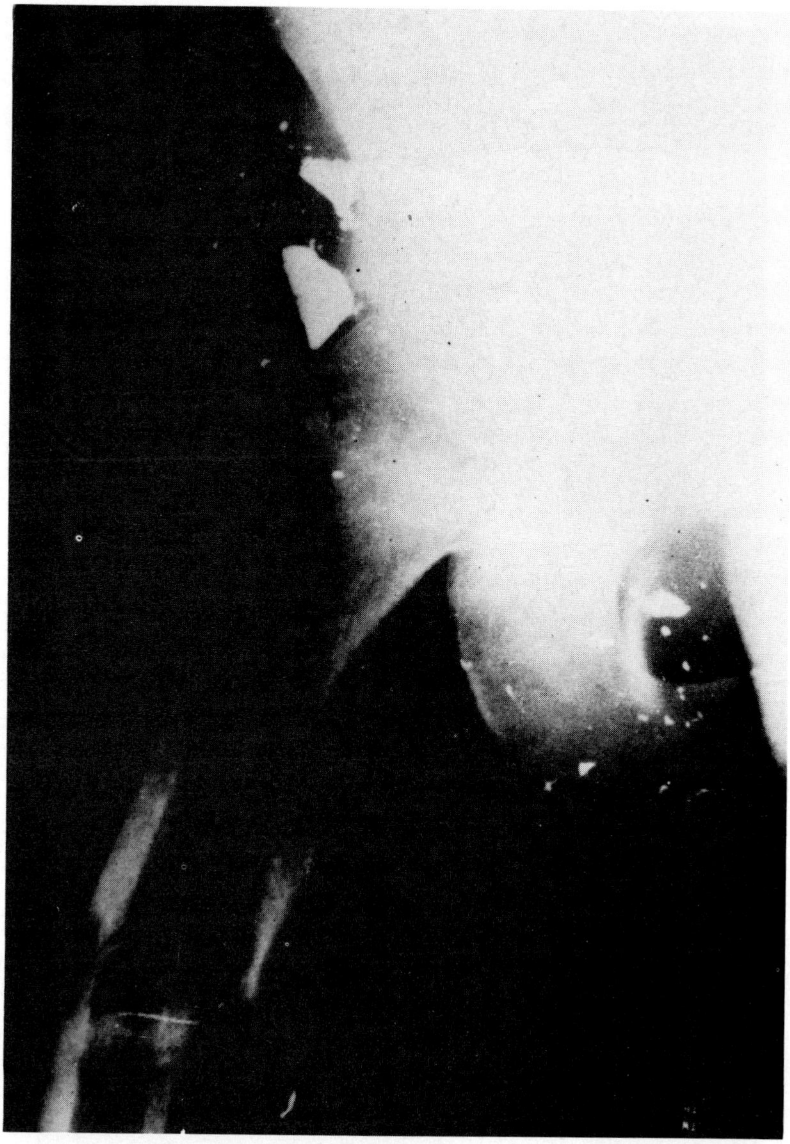

FIGURE 8. Compound fracture of the proximal part of the left femur of Patient 1D.

hemoglobin levels had fallen only slightly, the red blood cell-hemoglobin mass was much decreased, and the red cell 2,3 DPG and creatine levels were both increased. After transfusion of four units of washed red blood cells, the red cell mass increased toward normal. Thereafter, the red cell mass fell but later gradually rose to the theoretical level.

Six weeks after that the patient had further skin-grafting and was placed in Roger Anderson well-leg traction and a Stryker® frame for easier mobilization and treatment of posterior wounds. The hip wounds at first seemed to heal well but within a few weeks some drainage appeared: an abscess about the left hip region developed and the wound was open down to the bone. After traction for 3 months the patient's fractured femur had healed in satisfactory position (Figure 9). His soft-tissue wounds had granulated in. At this time he was ambulatory and was wearing a long brace.

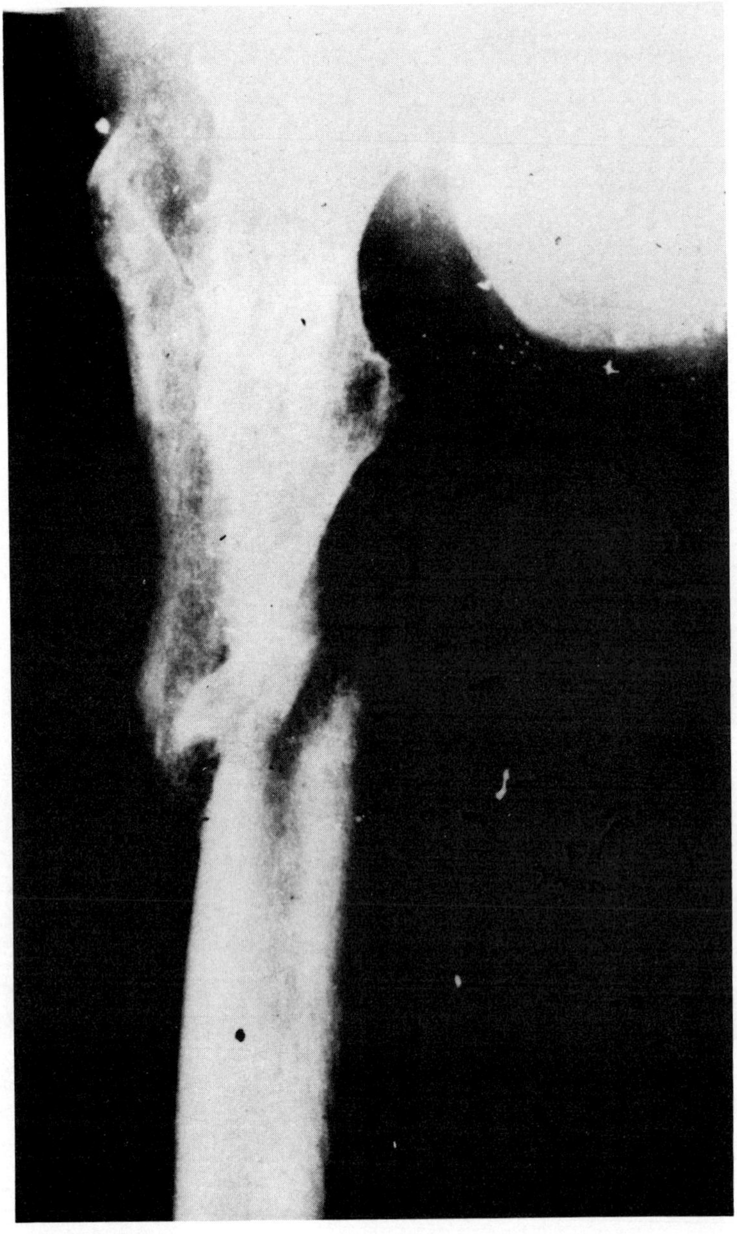

FIGURE 9. Three months after treatment the fractured femur of Patient 1D had healed in a satisfactory position.

Although this patient had open infected intertrochanteric and subtrochanteric fractures of the proximal part of the left femur with penetration of metallic foreign bodies inside the capsule of the hip joint, there was subsequently good motion of the right hip and no joint sepsis or loss of articular cartilage. The hematocrit and hemoglobin measurements were not indicative of the severity of the circulating red cell mass deficit.

Case 5

A 20-year-old marine (1E) had been wounded in Vietnam by a booby-trapped mine.

He sustained severe soft-tissue injury to both buttocks with the loss of some gluteal mass on the right, together with fracture of the proximal end of the right femur, a severely comminuted open fracture of the distal end of the right tibia, and multiple fractures of the right foot with extensive skin loss. Neither peroneal nerve was functioning and the right posterior tibial nerve was destroyed.

On a hospital ship he was initially resuscitated with blood and then his wounds were debrided. The next day he was semicomatose and disoriented, and a diagnosis of fat embolism was made. Two days later gross infection of the wounds was found and they were debrided again. The patient remained febrile and critically ill. Upon arrival at Chelsea Naval Hospital 2 weeks after injury, his spica cast was soaked with purulent material. Pseudomonas organisms were cultured from his wounds, which were further debrided. He continued to be febrile, and pseudomonas organisms were found in cultures of his urine; gram-negative septicemia was diagnosed.

Blood studies revealed a circulating red cell hemoglobin mass of 500 g, a deficit of 320 g from his theoretical normal value of 820 g. The red cell creatine level was increased to 4.2 μmol/g hemoglobin, and the 2,3 DPG concentration was increased to 24 μmol/g hemoglobin. The hematocrit value was 32%, and the blood hemoglobin concentration was 11.5 g/100 mℓ. The next day the red cell hemoglobin mass deficit was corrected by transfusion of five units of washed red blood cells, but no change in the hematocrit or hemoglobin value was noted.

Because of his continued febrile course another exploration of the right lower leg was performed; this demonstrated considerable nonviable fibrotic avascular musculature. Because his foot was without nerve supply and it appeared to be the source of sepsis, a right below-the-knee open amputation was performed. The right lower extremity was maintained with skin traction on the stump and skeletal traction through the distal end of the femur. The stump eventually closed with skin traction.

Despite having received 17 units of whole blood during and after the operation, 2 weeks after the amputation the patient was again found to have a deficit of 320 g of circulating hemoglobin, when the hematocrit value was 35 vol% and blood hemoglobin concentration was 12.5 g/100 mℓ.

The seriousness of the wounds and the poor general condition of the patients described here were typical of what was encountered in this series of cases. The only abnormalities revealed by routine laboratory measurements were a slightly low serum folate concentration, a slightly elevated direct bilirubin level, and a slight increase in serum alkaline phosphatase activity (Chapter 3). All the deviations from the normal were too small to be physiologically significant.

THE CLINICAL PROBLEM

One fact that was especially puzzling throughout the study of these severely wounded men was that they did not maintain a normal blood volume after their initial resuscitation at the time of trauma, but in spite of this did not show the signs of shock evident when their blood volumes were low at the time of the trauma. Although this was a problem in pure physiology, it was not regarded so by us for we had the clinical responsibility of treating patients with a serious chronic illness. We did make physiological studies, but the data derived from these studies were used only as guides to treatment. In this respect, the study was never thought of as a research project but rather a series of tests, each test made in a sequence determined by the results of the previous tests. These tests were carried out with the enthusiastic participation of the patients. The normal subjects serving as controls eagerly volunteered as comrades-in-arms to our patients. Thus, clinical studies aimed at the cure of a demoralizing illness had one immediate effect. It raised morale!

Since at the outset the only definite abnormality we were able to recognize was the decreased blood volume with decreased red blood cell mass, we treated it even though at the time we did not understand its origin or mechanism. In trying to restore the blood volume and its components to normal we chose to use washed red blood cells. The literature contains data on the use of electrolyte solutions in primary resuscitation after trauma severe enough to produce shock (Cournand et al., 1944; Frank et al., 1945; Doyle et al., 1951; Carey et al., 1965; Baue et al., 1967; Coran et al., 1971; Lowery et al., 1971; Hardaway, 1978; Virgilio et al., 1979a, 1979b) but the effects are short-lived (Altschule and Gilligan, 1938; Gilligan et al., 1938; Cournand et al., 1944). Plasma also has been shown to be useful in resuscitation, but its effects are short-lived (Cournand et al., 1944) and the dilution of the already decreased red blood cell mass may produce untoward effects (Beecher, 1945; Beecher and Altschule, 1977). We chose not to use dextran solutions such as had been employed by some in resuscitation (Witham et al., 1951; Carey et al., 1965, 1967, 1969; Shoemaker et al., 1973). In our studies a few observations were made on the use of crystalloid solutions but the results were not especially beneficial, and the red blood cell volumes usually were restored to normal by the transfusion of washed red blood cell concentrates or previously frozen washed red blood cells. Less specific approaches also were used: namely, provision of iron, ascorbic acid, niacin, folate, and hyperalimentation, as well as the use of antibiotics and appetite stimulants. Of all these, only direct restoration of the blood volume had any detectable beneficial effect as evaluated from appetite, feeling of well-being, need for antibiotics and pain medication, the rate of wound healing, and the need for further amputations during the period of treatment.

During the course of these treatments the loss of both red blood cells and plasma was measured as accurately as possible. Red blood cell loss into the wounds, the other tissues, and the gastrointestinal tract was estimated. Red blood cell production was calculated using reticulocyte counts, iron clearance and its incorporation into circulating erythrocytes, and the dilution of the donor's transfused cells by the recipient's newly produced erythrocytes. Concurrently, we studied red blood cell destruction involving both the patient's own cells and the circulating transfused cells, recognizing that two main pathways of hemoglobin degradation were available, one through bilirubin and urobilinogen production and the other through the production of porphyrin compounds. We recognized that both pathways could produce dipyrrols and monopyrrols, the ultimate breakdown products of hemoglobin.

At the end, the syndrome was treated with some degree of success, although we were reminded of the words of John Peters (1948), "The disorders encountered in disease may be regarded as the normal physiologic responses to unusual conditions produced by pathologic processes." In other words, we had no definite idea of what caused the syndrome. Although much suggestive evidence was accumulated, no final decision regarding etiology could be reached. The peculiarities of the regulation of blood volume and cardiovascular function remain unexplained.

Our attempt to analyze a previously undefined clinical syndrome without an adequate body of physiologic and biochemical data suitable for that purpose forced us to follow Sir Thomas Browne's advice of three hundred and fifty years ago, "Let thy studies be free as thy thoughts and contemplates, but fly not only on the wings of imagination" (Finch, 1950).

Chapter 2

BLOOD VOLUME MEASUREMENTS

The blood volume, as depicted in physiology and medicine, has two components, the plasma volume and the red blood cell volume; the volume of leukocytes and platelets, seen as the so-called *buffy layer* when the hematocrit measurement is made, is not included in the measurement of blood volume. Blood volume though often mentioned in clinical practice is rarely measured. Indeed, it is technically difficult to make independent measurements of the two components, plasma volume and red blood cell volume, and simultaneous measurements are not usually feasible (Gregersen, 1953; Serkes et al., 1965; Brozovic et al., 1966; Underwood and Howland, 1966; Hoye, 1967; Swan and Nelson, 1971; Nelson and Swan, 1971; Kelly and Terry, 1973). Accordingly, it has become customary to calculate the blood volume from either the red blood cell volume or the plasma volume and the *total body hematocrit* (Mayerson et al., 1948; Strumia et al., 1968). Such calculations are not ideal, however. Measuring red blood cell volume by radioactive labeling has limitations, the primary one being the use of radioactive materials. Although plasma volume usually is easier to measure, the results may be unreliable and may even be highly erroneous. Moreover, estimation of the total body hematocrit value on which the calculations are based, may be subject to considerable error (Fudenberg et al., 1961; Loria et al., 1962; Mollison, 1972). For these reasons, many physicians in clinical practice have been discouraged from making measurements of the total blood volume, and for the most part have done quite well without such data. However, in the situation that we encountered in our patients with traumatic injuries in which we had to deal with a disorder that appeared to be secondary to a reduced blood volume, it became imperative that specific measurements be made. In fact, as events evolved, it became evident that these measurements were crucial to the understanding and successful treatment of the disorder.

CURRENT BLOOD VOLUME METHODS

When red blood cells are taken from healthy persons and patients with various disorders, tagged with ^{51} Chromium(^{51}Cr) in vitro and then injected intravenously into the original donor, the red blood cell volume is accurately measured by the dilution of the radioactivity in the total circulating red blood cell volume. This value together with the total body hematocrit value is used to calculate the total blood volume. Plasma volume may be measured by the intravenous injection of either radioactive iodinated plasma albumin or of a dye that attaches itself to the patient's own plasma albumin. Hence, methods of this type actually measure the volume in which albumin distributes, which in normal persons includes mainly the plasma volume plus a relatively small volume comprising part of the interstitial and lymphatic fluid volumes. Accordingly, plasma volume measurements made in *normal persons* by these methods are reasonably accurate (Figure 1). However, in *patients* the assessment of plasma volume using Evans® blue dye or iodinated albumin overestimates the plasma volume because of the entry of the Evans® blue and iodinated albumin into an extravascular space during the mixing time (Gibson and Evans, 1937a; Freinkel et al., 1953; Strumia et al., 1968) (Figure 2). This occurs even in the absence of detectable edema or of albuminuria. The injected dye and the iodinated albumin go wherever the plasma albumin goes, and this includes the site of wounds (Mouridsen, 1969), an important consideration to us in our treatment of wounded men. When the iodinated albumin method was first introduced it was said to be more accurate than any dye-injection

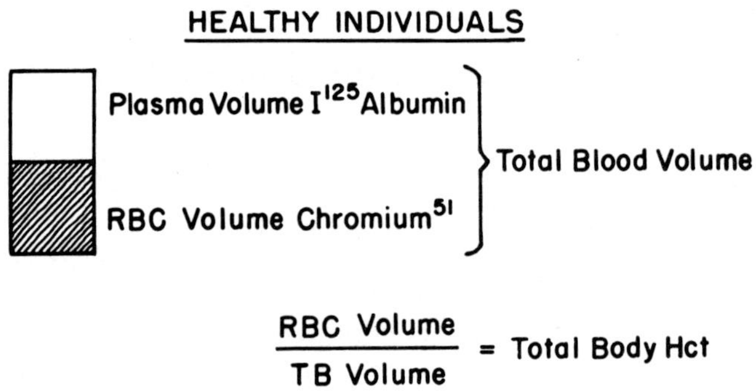

FIGURE 1. Blood volume in normal persons using ^{51}Cr-labeled autologous red blood cells to measure red blood cell volume and ^{125}I albumin to measure the plasma volume. The total body hematocrit was calculated from the ^{51}Cr red blood cell volume divided by the sum of the ^{51}Cr red blood cell volume and the ^{125}I albumin plasma volume. In these healthy persons there was agreement within ± 5 to 8% between the red blood cell volume measured by ^{51}Cr-labeled autologous red blood cells and the red blood cell volume indirectly estimated from the ^{125}I plasma volume and a value for total body hematocrit obtained by multiplying the peripheral venous hematocrit by a standard correction factor (f = 0.90) to compensate for the difference between large and small vessel hematocrits throughout the body. (Adapted from Mollison, 1972.)

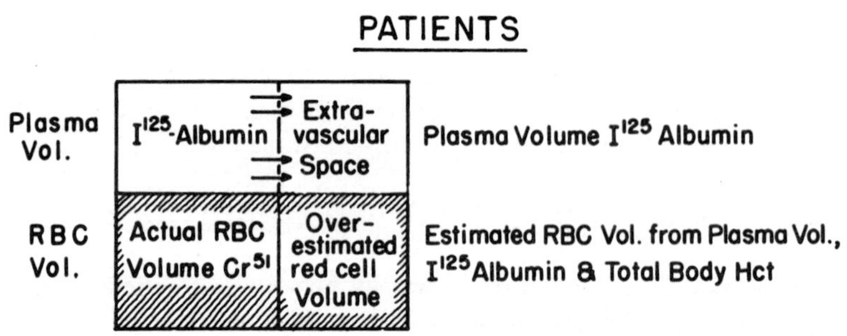

FIGURE 2. Blood volume in patients using ^{51}Cr-labeled autologous red blood cells to measure red blood cell volume and ^{125}I-labeled albumin to measure the plasma volume. ^{125}I-labeled albumin in patients overestimated the plasma volume because the 4S albumin molecule with a molecular weight of 68,000 was distributed into the extravascular space during the mixing period. An overestimation of the red blood cell volume occurred when the red blood cell volume was calculated from the measured ^{125}I albumin plasma volume and the total body hematocrit value (derived from the peripheral venous hematocrit value multiplied by 0.90).

method, and it stimulated considerable interest. However, studies have shown that iodinated albumin, like any dye that becomes bound to albumin, distributes itself during mixing not in the plasma volume but in the total albumin space in animals (Ferrebee et al., 1941; Miller, 1947; Hendley and Schiller, 1954; Huggins et al., 1963; Mouridsen, 1969; Abel and Wolf, 1973) (Figures 3 and 4) and in man (Reeve and Bailey, 1962; Moore et al., 1968; Siggaard-Andersen et al., 1969; Coleman et al., 1970; Hoye et al., 1972; Parving et al., 1974; Smith et al., 1978).

In patients, reliable measurements of red blood cell volume can be made by labeling

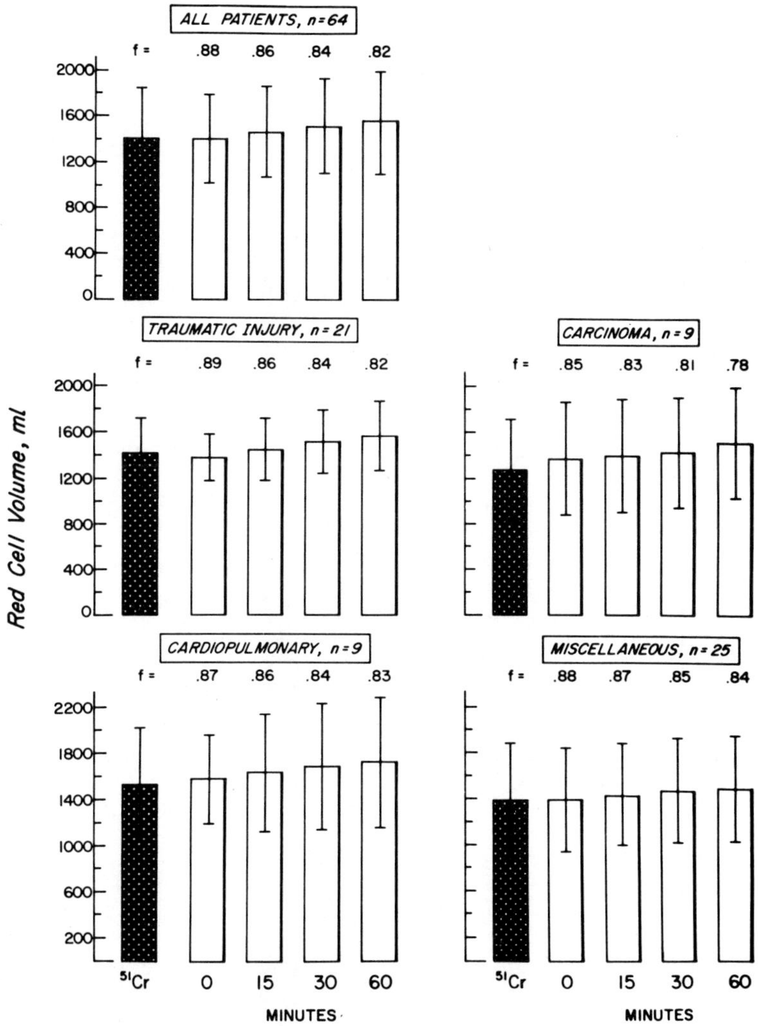

FIGURE 3. The red blood cell volume in 64 patients of various types measured directly with ^{51}Cr-labeled autologous red blood cells (solid bars) and calculated indirectly from the plasma volume measured at 0, 15, 30, and 60 min following infusion of the iodinated albumin together with the total body hematocrit value estimated from the peripheral venous hematocrit multiplied by 0.90 (open bars). The f factor was independently derived from the measured ^{51}Cr red blood cell volume, the measured iodinated plasma volume, and the measured peripheral venous hematocrit.

the patient's red blood cells with ^{51}Cr and autotransfusing them (Figures 5 and 6) (Daane et al., 1969). This procedure requires proper handling during collection and labeling to avoid red blood cell damage before autotransfusion. Heat-treated iodinated albumin, which does not transmit hepatitis and is injected directly, can be used to measure plasma volume (Tullis, 1977a, 1977b). This labeling technique is not difficult, but interpretation of the results is complicated by the fact that in patients the albumin distributes itself immediately from the plasma volume into the extravascular fluid volume. To calculate the blood volume by either of these labeling techniques, ^{51}Cr for red blood cells or iodinated albumin for plasma, one must know the total body hematocrit value. The total body hematocrit is estimated from the measured peripheral ven-

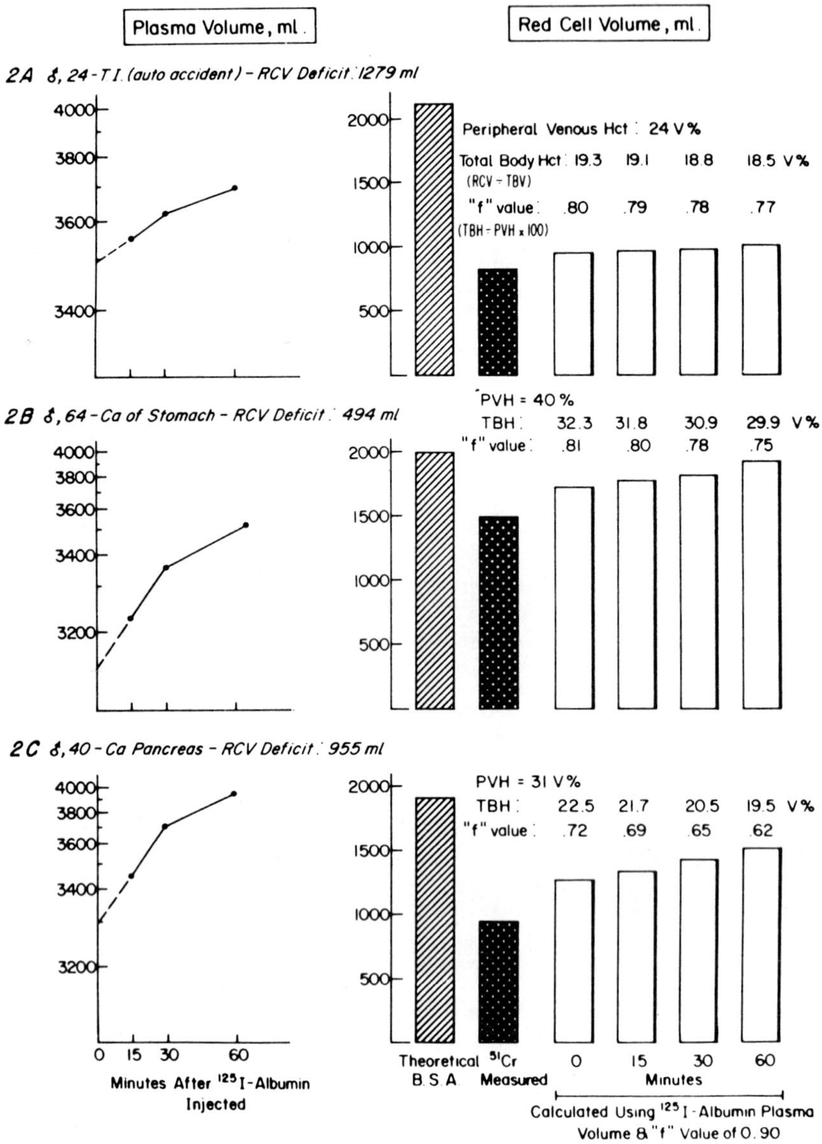

FIGURE 4. The red blood cell volume in three patients measured directly using ^{51}Cr-labeled autologous red blood cells and estimated indirectly from the plasma volume measured at 0, 15, 30, and 60 min after infusion with iodinated albumin together with the total body hematocrit value derived from the peripheral venous hematocrit multiplied by 0.90. The f factor was independently calculated directly from the measured ^{51}Cr-labeled red blood cell volume, the iodinated albumin plasma volume, and the peripheral venous hematocrit. The theoretical red blood cell volume was estimated from the body surface area (BSA) of the individual subjects.

ous hematocrit and a correction factor (Mollison, 1972), and the correction factor varies according to the size of the spleen (Fudenberg et al., 1961; Loria et al., 1962; Mollison, 1972). Usually normal healthy individuals and patients with normal-sized spleens have a correction factor of 0.90 (Strumia et al., 1968; Valeri et al., 1973).

As already noted, when a patient's blood volume is estimated from the measured

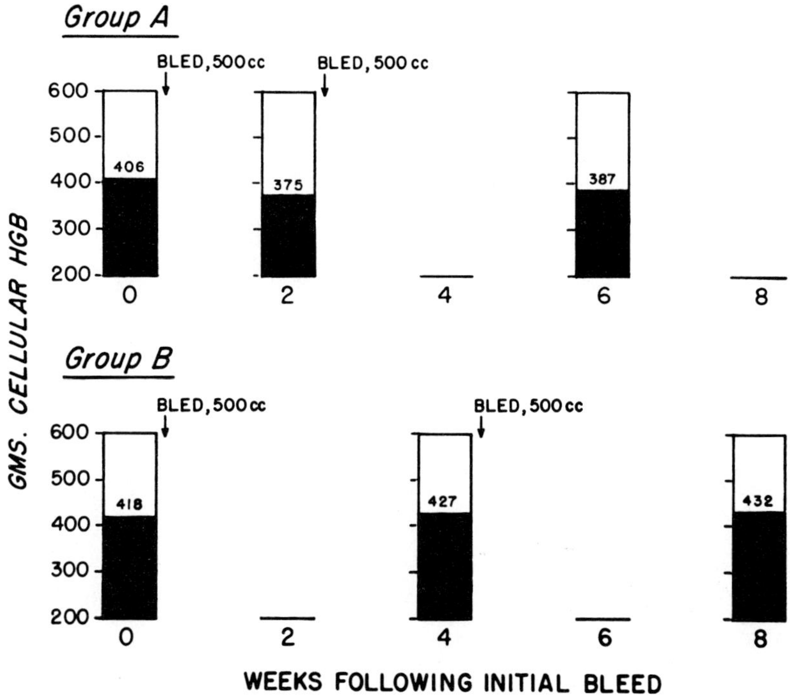

FIGURE 5. Cellular hemoglobin measured using ^{51}Cr-labeled autologous red blood cell volume and the mean corpuscular hemoglobin concentration (MCHC, %) in women bled on two occasions. The second phlebotomy was performed 2 to 4 weeks after the first. Four weeks after the second phlebotomy, the donors underwent elective gynecologic surgery, and their autologous previously frozen red blood cells and fresh frozen plasma were available for reinfusion at the time of operation. (From Daane, T. A., Valeri, C. R., and Barton, R. K., *Am. J. Obstet. Gynecol.*, 105, 394, 1969. With permission.)

plasma volume and an estimated total body hematocrit value, the accuracy of the results may be questionable, especially if the plasma volume is measured with a low molecular weight substance such as albumin or a dye like Evans® blue which binds to albumin after injection (Strumia et al., 1968; Valeri et al., 1973). Moreover, the factor used to correct the peripheral venous hematocrit value to the total body hematocrit value approaches unity as the size of the patient's spleen increases, so estimates may be inaccurate in patients with large spleens (Fudenberg et al., 1961; Loria et al., 1962; Mollison, 1972).

CALCULATING TOTAL BODY HEMATOCRIT

In order to establish a valid correction of the peripheral venous hematocrit value to the total body hematocrit value in *patients,* measurements of red blood cell volume and of plasma volume must be made independently (Figures 7 to 9), although a plasma volume measured with iodinated albumin or Evans® blue dye should not be used to establish the correction factor (Strumia et al., 1968). To ensure accuracy, plasma volume should be measured with a high molecular weight substance like iodinated 19S macroglobulin or fibrinogen (Figure 10) (Waldmann and Strober, 1969; Berlin, 1977; Valeri et al., 1973) although these molecules, unlike albumin, have been implicated in the transmission of hepatitis.

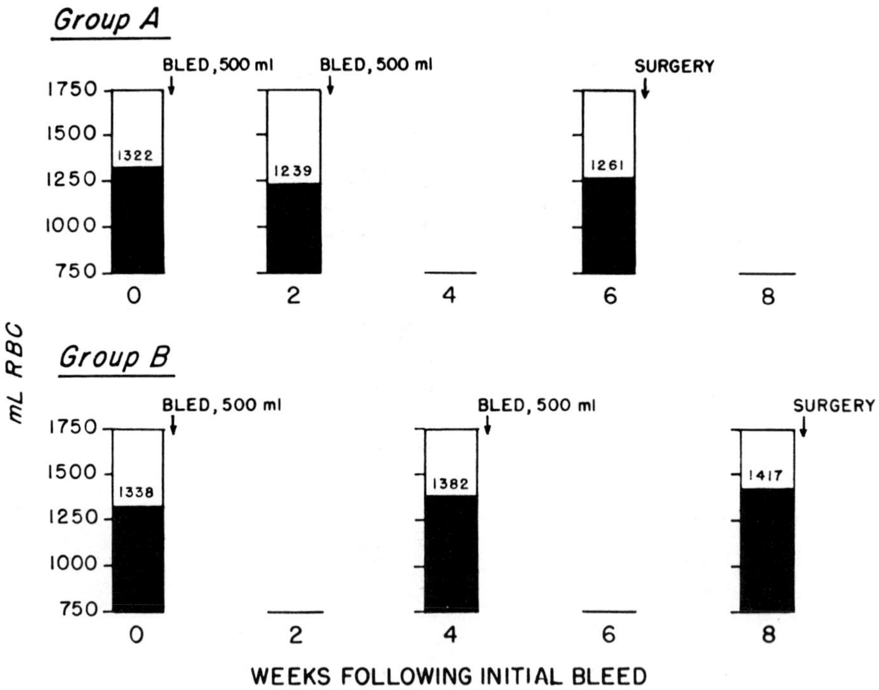

FIGURE 6. Red blood cell volume measured using ^{51}Cr-labeled autologous red blood cells in women bled 500 mℓ of blood on two occasions. The second phlebotomy was performed 2 or 4 weeks after the first. Four weeks after the second phlebotomy the donors underwent gynecologic surgery, and their autologous, previously frozen red blood cells and fresh frozen plasma were available for reinfusion at the time of operation. (From Daane, T. A., Valeri, C. R., and Barton, R. K., *Am. J. Obstet. Gynecol.*, 105, 394, 1969. With permission.)

In our studies the red blood cell volume was measured with ^{51}Cr-labeled autologous red blood cells, and the plasma volume was measured with iodinated 19S macroglobulin obtained from a patient with cold agglutinin disease (Figure 11) (Cooper, 1968; Cooper and Hobbs, 1970; Valeri et al., 1973). The total body hematocrit value calculated from these measurements was compared to the peripheral venous microhematocrit value, and the factor of 0.90 was used to correct the peripheral venous microhematocrit value to the total body hematocrit value (Figure 12).

NORMAL BLOOD VOLUME STANDARDS

For normal healthy men and women, nomograms have been developed to estimate blood volume, red blood cell volume, and plasma volume from body surface area determined from their weight and height (Dubois and Dubois, 1916; Gibson and Evans, 1937b; Sendroy and Cecchini, 1954; Smith, 1958; Nadler et al., 1962; Retzlaff et al., 1969; Feldschuh and Enson, 1977; Szymanski, 1978). A deficit in a patient's red blood cells or plasma may be estimated from a theoretical value derived from a nomogram of a healthy individual with a similar body surface area. Such a theoretical value is influenced by age (Cohn and Shock, 1949; Piomelli et al., 1962), nutritional status (Mikhail et al., 1975; Viart, 1976, 1977; Fondu, 1977; Golden et al., 1977; Waterlow et al., 1977; Fondu et al., 1978), and physical activity (Muldowney et al., 1957; Lamb et al., 1964, 1965; Miller et al., 1964a, 1964b, 1965; Friman, 1979; Remes, 1979), in addition to a variety of environmental factors (Berry, 1974; Kimzey et al., 1976; Pace, 1977).

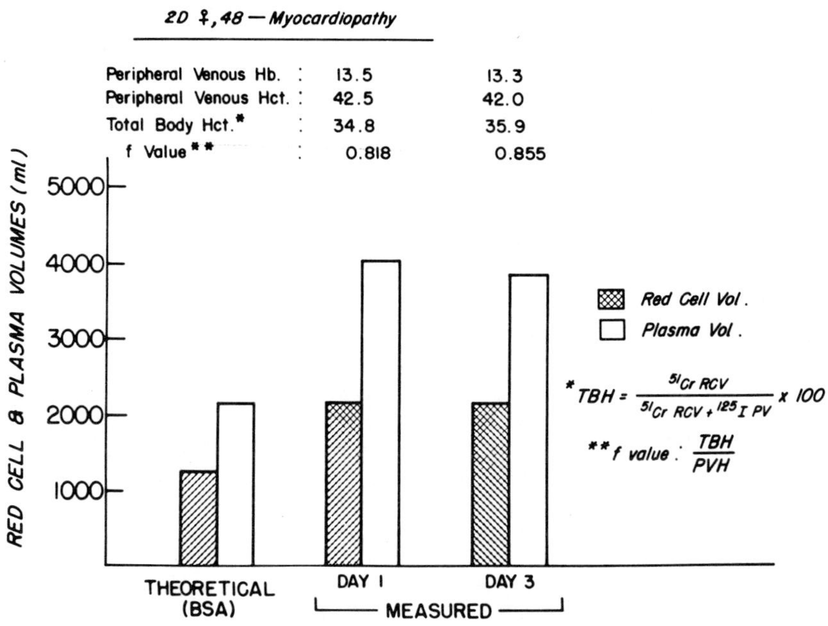

FIGURE 7. ^{51}Cr red blood cell volume and ^{125}I plasma volume measured in a 48-year-old woman (2D) with myocardiopathy. Both values were greater than the theoretical values estimated from the body surface area. The factor used to correct the peripheral venous hematocrit to the total body hematocrit value was calculated from the measured ^{51}Cr red blood cell volume, ^{125}I albumin plasma volume, and peripheral venous hematocrit values. In this patient the factor ranged from 0.82 to 0.86.

To make a reliable assessment of blood volume in a patient, knowledge of the normal values for plasma volume, red blood cell volume, and total blood volume are necessary, and this usually is not available unless, of course, the patient had been studied before the disease condition developed. Generally, this kind of information is available only in patients subjected to certain types of operation, in which case the blood volume measured in the person before the surgical procedure provides accurate estimation of red blood cell and plasma volume space (Valeri and Fortier, 1969a) (Figure 13). Blood volume measurement made on a patient after recovery from the disease state also should establish his normal value (Chapter 6). Thus, the use of nomograms derived from the body surface area, although not always highly accurate, appears to be the only available method for estimating the alterations in blood volume (Figure 14). The potential for error exists in all the approaches listed above. Blood volume measurements usually are not made in clinical medicine. The more common practice is to estimate a red blood cell deficit from the peripheral venous hemoglobin and hematocrit measurements, and these estimates have little validity.

The uncertainties associated with the measurements of blood volume were always uppermost in our minds when treating our patients who, because their peripheral venous hemoglobin and hematocrit levels were only slightly reduced, required direct assessment of blood volume. During the time of our study, the surgical service at the Chelsea Naval Hospital was using the Volemetron® to measure blood volume (Williams and Fine, 1961). This instrument utilized iodinated albumin to measure the blood volume and red blood cell volume from the total body hematocrit value, the latter being estimated from the peripheral venous hematocrit value multiplied by the factor 0.90. We were aware that the use of iodinated albumin to measure blood volume in

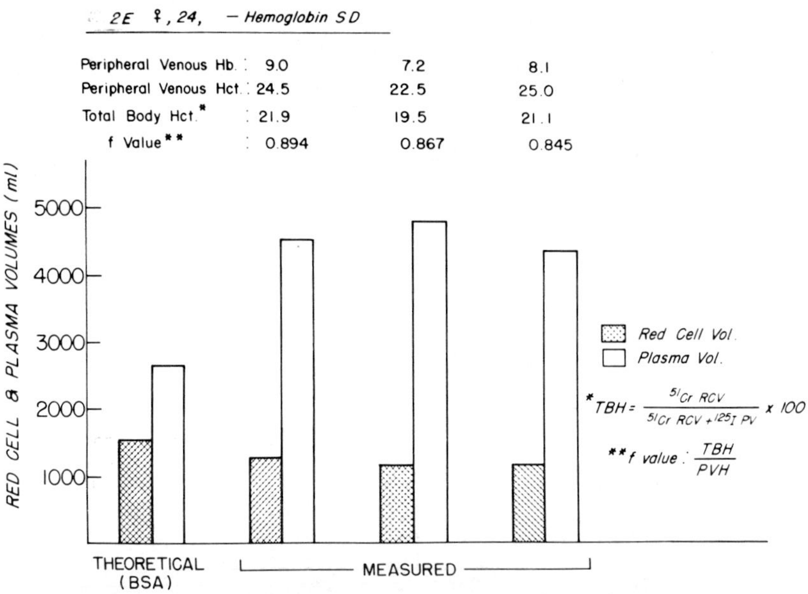

FIGURE 8. ^{51}Cr-labeled red blood cell volume and ^{125}I-labeled plasma volume in a 24-year-old black woman (2E) with SD hemoglobinopathy measured on three separate occasions over a 2-year period. Red blood cell volume was lower than and plasma volume was greater than the theoretical values. The factor correcting the peripheral venous hematocrit value to the total body hematocrit value was calculated from the measured ^{51}Cr red blood cell volume, ^{125}I albumin plasma value, and peripheral venous hematocrit value. In this patient the f factor ranged from 0.85 to 0.89 during the measurements over the 2-year period.

our patients would result in an overestimation of the plasma volume, red blood cell volume, and total blood volume, and so chose another approach. We measured the red blood cell volume with ^{51}Cr-labeled autologous red blood cells, and calculated the blood volume and plasma volume from the total body hematocrit derived from the peripheral venous hematocrit and the factor 0.90.

The orthopedic patients under study exhibited significant decreases in red blood cell volume, plasma volume, and total blood volume, i.e., hypovolemia with reduced red blood cell volume and plasma volume, a condition called *stress anemia* (Biron et al., 1972). The orthopedic physicians caring for these patients at first found it difficult to accept these findings of marked hypovolemia in the face of normal or only slightly reduced peripheral venous hematocrit and hemoglobin levels during the subacute and chronic phases of the patients' traumatic injuries.

Before a deficit in red blood cell and plasma volumes could be demonstrated in these patients, it was necessary to establish normal values for them. Since most of them were still critically injured, our estimations of the theoretical red blood cell volume and plasma volume could only be made from the weight and height of the patient at the time that the red blood cell volume was measured (Dubois and Dubois, 1916). In some instances, weights had to be estimated because the presence of casts precluded accurate measurements. Another complicating factor was decreased physical activity in many of the patients who were at bed rest or had restricted movement. The factors of weight loss, inaccurate weight and height measurements, and restricted ambulation all had some effect on the theoretical values of red blood cell volume and plasma volume estimated from the body surface area nomogram. Because of this we conducted a series

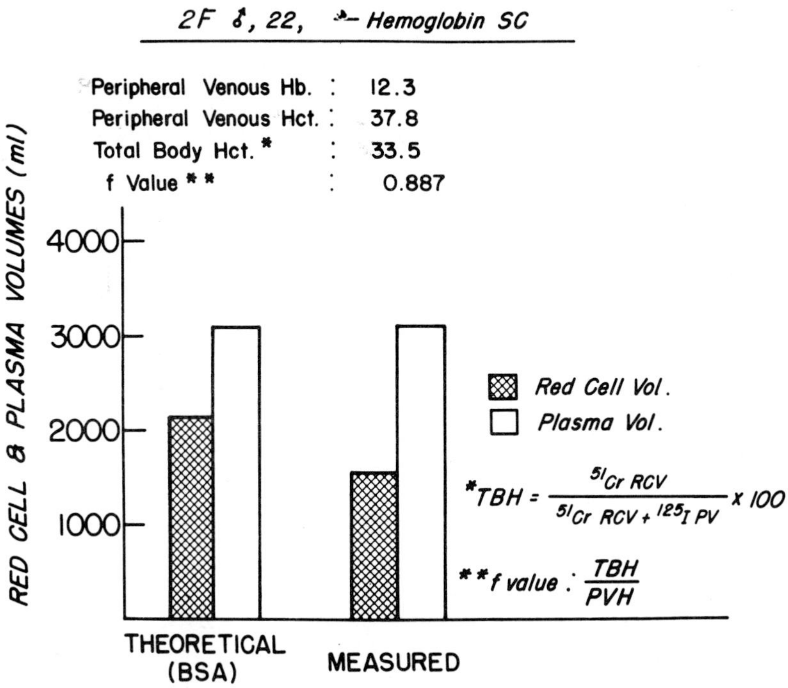

FIGURE 9. The ^{51}Cr-labeled red blood cell volume and the ^{125}I-labeled plasma volume in a 22-year-old black man (2F) with SC hemoglobinopathy. The red blood cell volume was lower than and the plasma volume was similar to the theoretical values. The f value was calculated from the measured ^{51}Cr red blood cell volume, ^{125}I albumin plasma volume, and peripheral venous hematocrit. In this patient the factor was 0.89.

of studies in patients and in normal subjects to validate measurements of red blood cell, plasma, and total blood volumes.

TECHNIQUES OF BLOOD VOLUME MEASUREMENTS MADE ON PATIENTS AT CHELSEA NAVAL HOSPITAL

At the outset of our study, we measured the blood volumes in healthy persons and in patients suffering from different disease states using ^{51}Cr-labeled autologous red blood cells to measure the red blood cell volume and iodinated albumin to measure the plasma volume. The blood volume was calculated from the sum of the ^{51}Cr-labeled red blood cell volume and the ^{125}I albumin-labeled plasma volume. The total body hematocrit value was derived from these measurements and then the factor that corrects the peripheral venous hematocrit to the total body hematocrit was estimated. There was a greater degree of variability in the calculation of the f value in the patients than in the healthy persons (Figure 12).

The radioactive iodinated albumin technique overestimated the plasma volume in *patients,* but was accurate in *healthy persons* (Strumia et al., 1968; Valeri et al., 1973; Parving et al., 1979; Rothschild et al., 1979) (Figure 12). The patients had increased vascular permeability associated with tissue hypoxia or other factors, and the radioactive iodinated albumin spread rapidly into the extravascular space resulting in overestimation in plasma volume. In healthy persons, on the other hand, the albumin distributed itself primarily in the plasma volume during the mixing period.

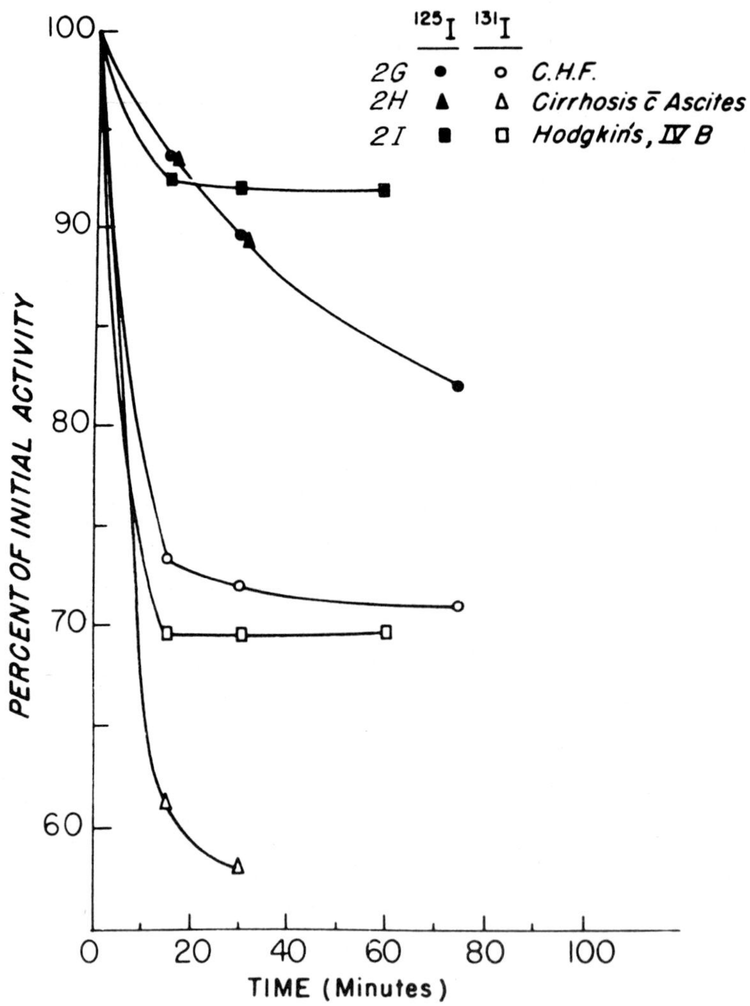

FIGURE 10. The simultaneous dilution of ^{125}I-labeled cold agglutinins (a 19S macroglobulin with a molecular weight of 1.0 million) and ^{131}I-labeled albumin (a 4S molecule with a molecular weight of 68,000) in the blood of three patients. The distribution of the iodinated albumin into a larger volume is apparent during the immediate 20-min postinfusion period. One patient had congestive heart failure, one cirrhosis with ascites, and one had Hodgkin's Disease Class IV, B. These disease states manifest increased vascular permeability; the iodinated albumin molecule distributed immediately into the extravascular space, whereas the large 19S macroglobulin distributed itself within the plasma volume space.

Studies were done to ensure that the albumin was properly iodinated (McFarlane, 1956, 1957) and that the albumin was not denatured (Steinfeld et al., 1958; Freeman, 1959; Cohen et al., 1961). Improper iodination of the albumin would result in infusion of free iodine that would be removed from the blood by the thyroid gland, salivary glands, and by urinary excretion, leaving falsely low levels in the blood and so giving falsely high plasma volume measurements. Greater than 99% of the iodine was associated with the albumin as was shown by the fact that it was precipitated by trichloroacetic acid. Another possible source of error was also investigated, i.e., an overestimation of plasma volume as a result of the rapid removal of denatured albumin from

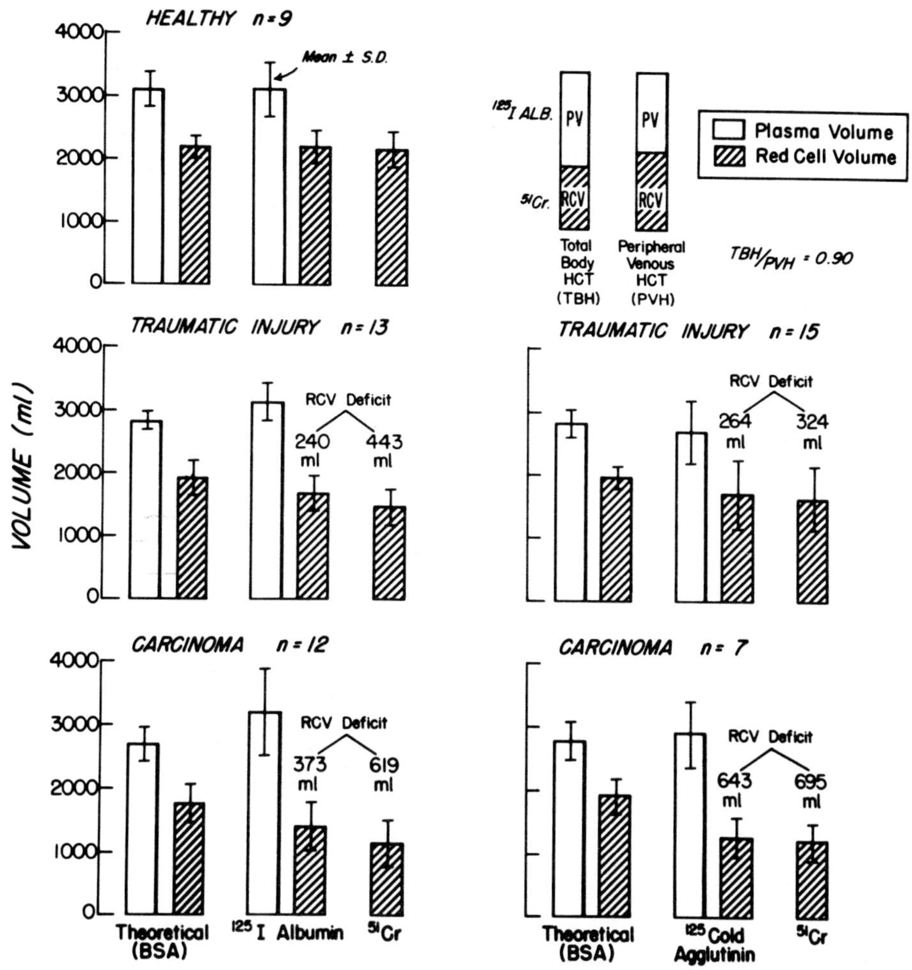

FIGURE 11. The plasma volume measured using ^{125}I-labeled albumin and ^{125}I-labeled cold agglutinin in healthy persons and in patients with traumatic injuries or carcinoma. The theoretical red blood cell volume and plasma volume were estimated from the body surface area. The red blood cell mass deficit was estimated from the theoretical red blood cell volume and the ^{51}Cr measured red blood cell volume. It was also calculated from the indirect estimate of red blood cell volume using the plasma volume measured with iodinated albumin or iodinated cold agglutinin and the total body hematocrit value (calculated from the peripheral venous hematocrit multiplied by 0.90). The estimate of the red blood cell mass deficit measured indirectly with iodinated cold agglutinin was similar to the value observed when the red blood cell volume was measured directly with ^{51}Cr autologous red blood cells. The estimate of the red blood cell mass deficit measured indirectly with iodinated albumin was 60% lower than the deficit observed when the red blood cell volume was measured directly with ^{51}Cr autologous red blood cells. (From Valeri, C. R., Cooper, A. G., and Pivacek, L. E., *Arch. Intern. Med.* 132, 534, © 1973, American Medical Association. With permission.)

the blood. However, acrylamide gel electrophoresis failed to demonstrate any denaturation of the iodinated albumin.

The iodinated albumin method consistently overestimated plasma volume in *patients* with a variety of diseases. The observed increase in vascular permeability was not related to a red blood cell mass deficit (Table 1); correction of the red blood cell mass deficit by a therapeutic transfusion of red blood cells did not reduce vascular permeability (Table 1).

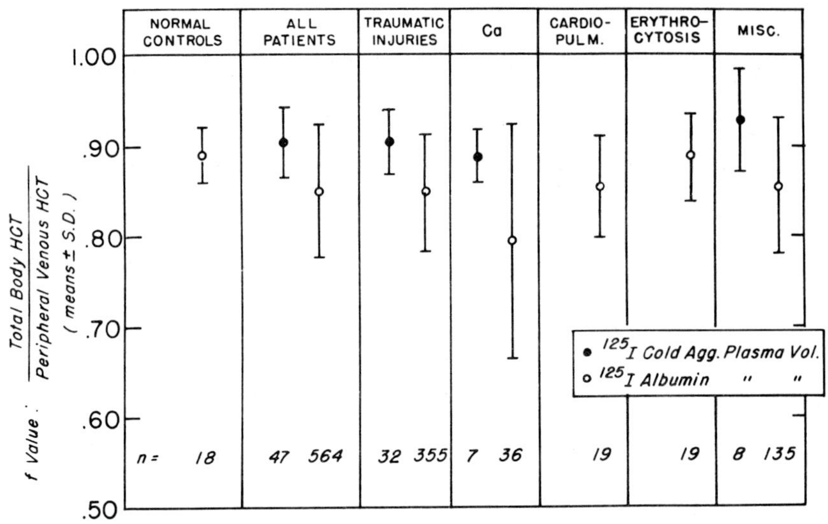

FIGURE 12. The factor used to correct the peripheral venous hematocrit value to estimate the total body hematocrit was calculated from the ^{51}Cr red blood cell volume, the plasma volume measured with iodinated albumin or iodinated cold agglutinin, and the peripheral venous hematocrit value. The factor to correct the peripheral venous hematocrit value to the total body hematocrit value was 0.89 when iodinated albumin was used in normal persons and patients with erythrocytosis. It was 0.85 in patients with traumatic injuries and cardiopulmonary insufficiency, 0.78 in patients with carcinoma, and 0.87 in patients with miscellaneous diagnoses, and 0.90 when iodinated cold agglutinin was used in the same patients. (From Valeri, C. R., Cooper, A. G., and Pivacek, L. E., *Arch. Intern. Med.*, 132, 534, © 1973, American Medical Association. With permission.)

The method using ^{51}Cr-labeled autologous red blood cells gave reliable measurements of red blood cell volume as demonstrated by repeated measurements made on the same person within a seven-day period (Table 2). Steps were taken to minimize cellular damage during collection and labeling of the autologous red blood cells so that measurements would be valid (Figures 5 and 6).

The f value was established from measurements of red blood cell volume made with ^{51} Cr and of plasma volume using an iodinated 19S macroglobulin and the peripheral venous hematocrit. Iodinated 19S macroglobulin, unlike the 4S 68,000 molecular weight iodinated albumin molecule, has a potential for hepatitis (Tullis, 1977a, 1977b). For this we took the precaution of obtaining the 19S macroglobulin from a hepatitis antigen negative person who had a high titer of cold agglutinin. The cold agglutinin, 19S macroglobulin, was labeled with ^{125}I or ^{131}I. Patients were studied using ^{51}Cr autologous red blood cells and ^{125}I-labeled cold agglutinin. The f value, derived from the measured ^{51}Cr red blood cell volume, ^{125}I-labeled cold agglutinin plasma volume, and the peripheral venous hematocrit for patients without splenomegaly, was 0.90 (Valeri et al., 1973) (Figure 12). When iodinated albumin was used to measure plasma volume in the normal healthy persons, the plasma volume was found to be 5 to 10% larger than when iodinated cold agglutinin was used.

We next undertook to establish the accuracy of our estimations of normal red blood cell volume, plasma volume, and total blood volume values for each patient. The possibility was considered that the reductions in plasma volume, red blood cell volume, and total blood volume in the patients represented adaptive decreases related to immobilization and weight loss (Deitrick et al., 1948; Lamb et al., 1964, 1965; Miller et

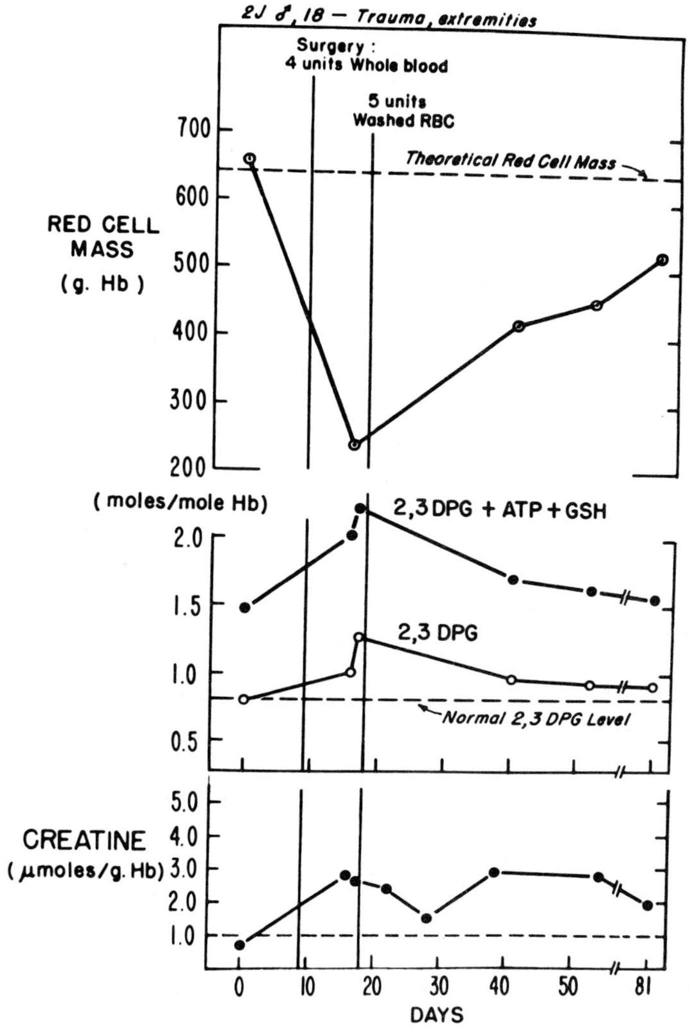

FIGURE 13. Red blood cell mass (g Hb), red blood cell 2,3 DPG and creatine levels, and the sum of the red blood cell 2,3 DPG, ATP, and glutathione (GSH) levels in an 18-year-old white man with traumatic injuries (2J). Measurements were made prior to operation and again following the surgical procedure. The patient received four units of whole blood intraoperatively and five units of washed red blood cells during the postoperative period. The patient had a normal red blood cell mass, and normal red blood cell levels of 2,3 DPG, creatine, ATP, and GSH prior to operation. Although four units of whole blood were transfused intraoperatively, 7 days postoperatively the red blood cell mass was decreased to 35% of normal and the levels of red blood cell 2,3 DPG, creatine, and the sum of the 2,3 DPG, ATP, and GSH levels were increased significantly. With restoration of the red blood cell mass towards normal, the red blood cell levels of 2,3 DPG and the sum of 2,3 DPG, ATP, and GSH returned towards normal.

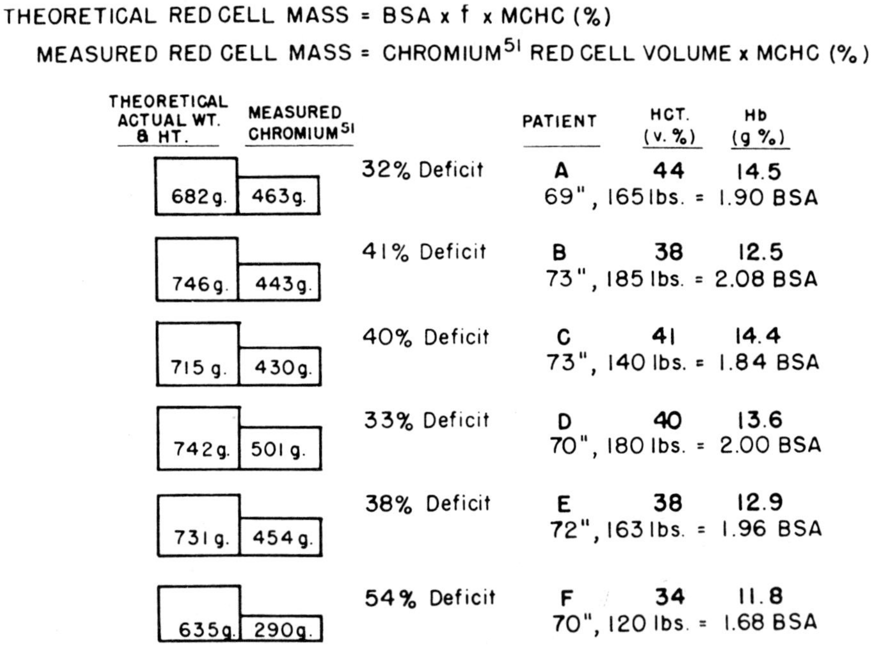

FIGURE 14. The theoretical red blood cell mass of cellular hemoglobin estimated from the body surface area (BSA) multiplied by the mean corpuscular hemoglobin concentration (MCHC, %) and a factor that was different for men and women, and the red blood cell mass measured using the ^{51}Cr red blood cell volume × MCHC, %. A red blood cell mass deficit of less than 40% was associated with only slight decreases in hemoglobin and hematocrit levels in patients with traumatic injuries.

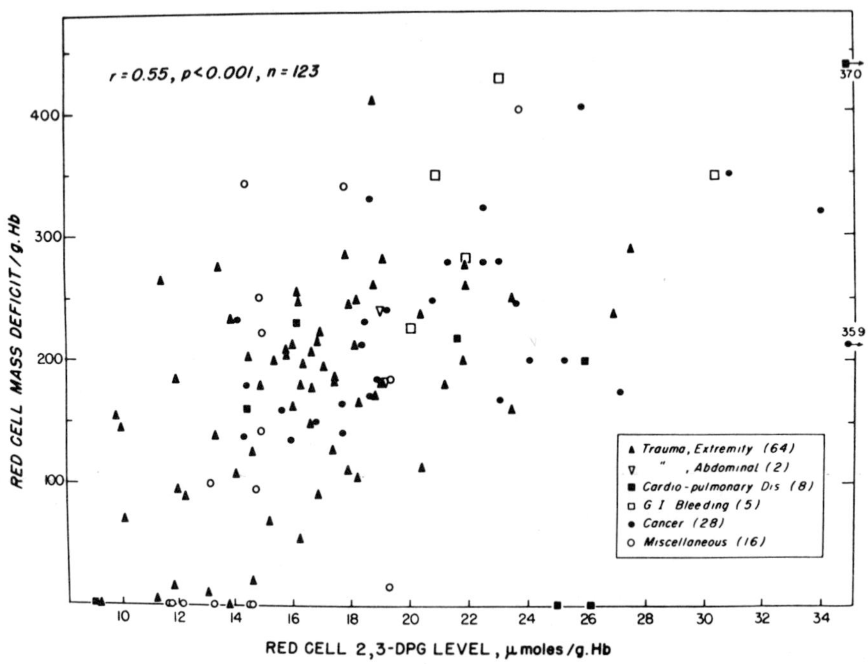

FIGURE 15. The relation between red blood cell 2,3 DPG level and the red blood cell mass deficit in 123 patients with traumatic injuries, cardiopulmonary disease, gastrointestinal bleeding, cancer, or miscellaneous diagnoses. (From Valeri, C. R. and Fortier, N. L., *N. Engl. J. Med.*, 281, 1452, 1969. With permission.)

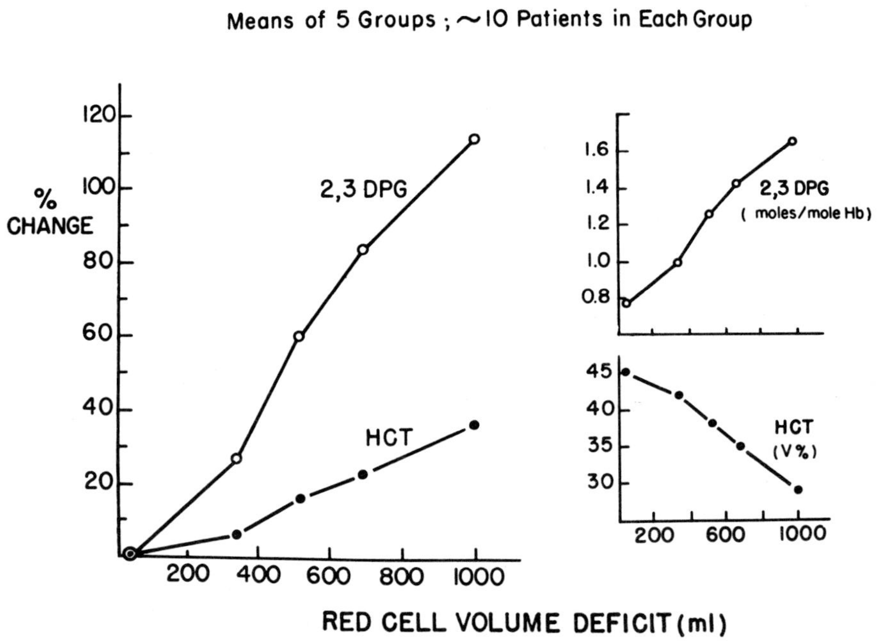

FIGURE 16. Percentage changes in hematocrit value and red blood cell 2,3 DPG level related to the red blood cell volume deficit. A 400 mℓ deficit in red blood cell volume produced a 10% decrease in hematocrit and a 40% increase in the red blood cell 2,3 DPG level. A 600 mℓ deficit in the red blood cell volume produced a 20% decrease in hematocrit and a 70% increase in the red blood cell 2,3 DPG level. A 1000 mℓ deficit in red blood cell volume produced a 35% decrease in hematocrit and a 115% increase in the red blood cell 2,3 DPG level; a red blood cell volume deficit of 1000 mℓ was associated with a hematocrit of 30 vol% and a red blood cell 2,3 DPG level of two times normal.

al., 1964a, 1964b, 1965). However, the observation that hypotension developed during general anesthesia argued against this. Moreover, the ability to detect decreases in red blood cell volume and total blood volume preoperatively and to restore the red blood cell deficit by transfusion of washed red blood cells eliminated the occurrence of intraoperative and postoperative hypotension in these patients (Biron et al., 1972). Furthermore, increases in red blood cell 2,3 DPG levels in these patients suggested that a compensatory mechanism had developed to facilitate oxygen transport to the tissues (Valeri and Fortier, 1967a, 1967b) (Figure 15). This compensatory change indicated that there was a need for more red blood cells than were present.

Our estimates of the theoretical values of red blood cell volume and plasma volume calculated from the body surface area were confirmed by studying patients throughout their period of treatment. Most of the patients in our study had been severely injured, and we followed them during their period of treatment and convalescence which extended for as long as 1 to 2 years (Chapter 6). Some patients had normal blood volumes when we first studied them but subsequently developed decreases in red blood cell volume during the postoperative periods (Figure 13). When the red blood cell volume in patients was measured by ^{51}Cr labeling of autologous red blood cells, significant deficits were detected. However, when the red blood cell volume was estimated from the hematocrit or the total hemoglobin concentration in peripheral venous blood, a red blood cell mass deficit was not apparent because both the red blood cell volume and plasma volume were decreased almost equally (Figures 16 to 20). It was evident

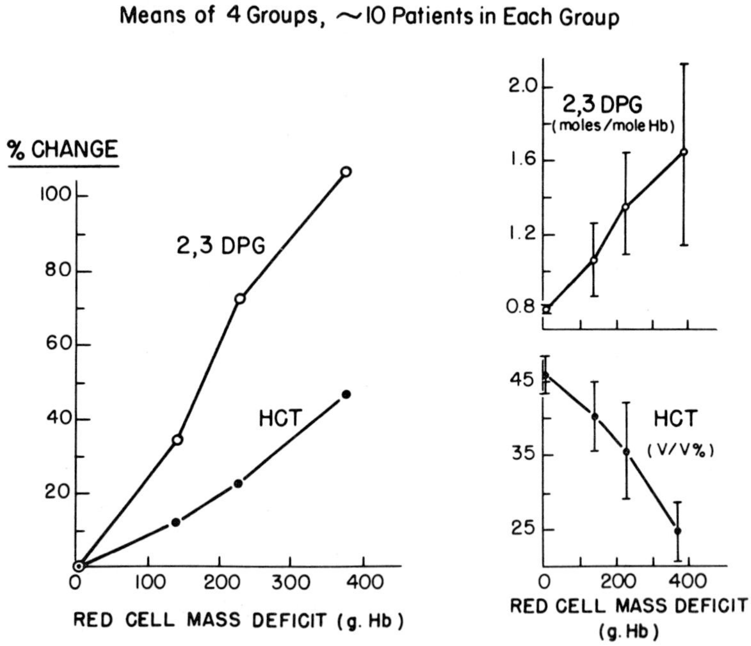

FIGURE 17. Percentage changes in the hematocrit value and red blood cell 2,3 DPG level related to the red blood cell mass deficit. A red blood cell mass deficit of 100 g of cellular hemoglobin was associated with an 8% decrease in hematocrit and a 30% increase in the red blood cell 2,3 DPG level. A 200 g deficit of cellular hemoglobin was associated with a 20% decrease in hematocrit and a 60% increase in the red blood cell 2,3 DPG level. A deficit of 380 g of cellular hemoglobin was associated with a 50% decrease in hematocrit and a 120% increase in the red blood cell 2,3 DPG level. A deficit of 380 g of cellular hemoglobin was associated with a hematocrit of 25% and a red blood cell 2,3 DPG level of two times normal. (From Valeri, C. R. and Fortier, N. L., *Forsvarsmedicin*, 5, 212, 1969. With permission.)

that the usual plasma volume expansion that occurs with anemia had not occurred in these patients with traumatic injuries. Patients with traumatic injuries involving the head, thoracic-abdominal area, and the thoracic-abdominal-pelvic area exhibited slightly lower peripheral hematocrit values than did patients with traumatic injuries involving only the extremities. The patients with traumatic injuries involving the extremities had red blood volume deficits of 800 mℓ and peripheral venous hematocrit values of 38 vol% (Figures 19 and 20). Patients with traumatic injuries involving the head, thoracic-abdominal area, and the thoracic-abdominal-pelvic area exhibited the deficit of 800 mℓ but showed peripheral hematocrit values of 35 vol% instead of the 38 vol% (Figures 21 and 22). It was apparent that the red blood cell mass deficit was not related to the presence or absence of infection nor to whether or not the injury was acute, subacute, or chronic (Figures 20 to 24). The degree of reduction in the peripheral venous hematocrit was influenced by the site of injury (Figure 25).

Simultaneous reductions in red blood cell volume and plasma volume suggest an adaptive anemia such as that noted in panhypopituitarism (Carfts and Meineke, 1959; Rodriguez and Shahidi, 1971). However, the reduction in the total number of red blood cells in our patients accompanied by compensatory increases in red blood cell 2,3 DPG pointed to the activation of a mechanism to improve tissue oxygenation (Valeri and Fortier, 1969a, 1969b; Biron et al., 1972) (Figures 13, 15, 16, and 17). The

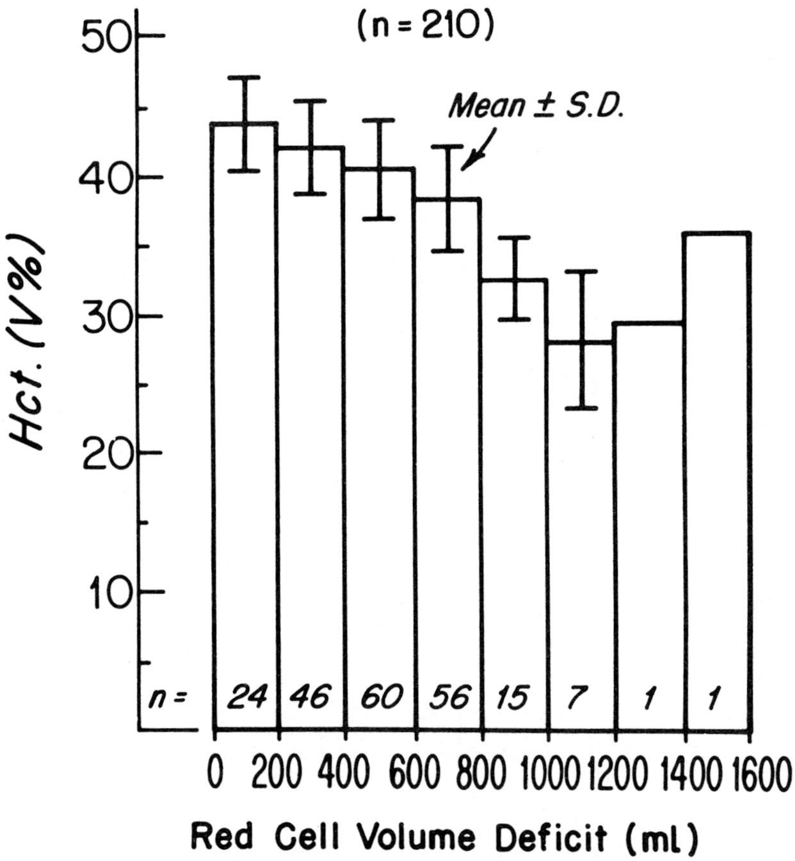

FIGURE 18. Relation between red blood cell volume deficit and the peripheral venous hematocrit levels in 210 patients with traumatic injuries of all types. A deficit of 800 mℓ of red blood cells was associated with a hematocrit value of 38 vol%.

consistent finding of compensatory increases in red blood cell 2,3 DPG supported the conclusion that inadequate numbers of red blood cells were circulating and that the anemia was not adaptive.

In summary, our patients with traumatic injuries usually had significant decreases in both red blood cell volume and plasma volume, normal or slightly reduced peripheral hemoglobin and hematocrit values, increased vascular permeability, increased red blood cell 2,3 DPG levels and, related to the last factor, red blood cells with improved capacity to deliver oxygen.

It should be emphasized that the peripheral hemoglobin and hematocrit levels did not reveal the deficits in red blood cell volume and plasma volume in these patients (Figures 16 to 19), and did not reflect the clinically significant hypovolemia. Moreover, plasma volume was overestimated when iodinated albumin was used to measure blood volume, and this overestimation resulted in falsely high calculated values of red blood cell volume and total blood volume (Figure 10). Only when the red blood cell volume was measured using ^{51}Cr-labeled autologous red blood cells was the hypovolemia apparent. This precise measurement, when used in conjunction with the total body hematocrit value (peripheral venous hematocrit value multiplied by 0.90), gave a reliable measurement of plasma volume and total blood volume. Our estimates of the theoret-

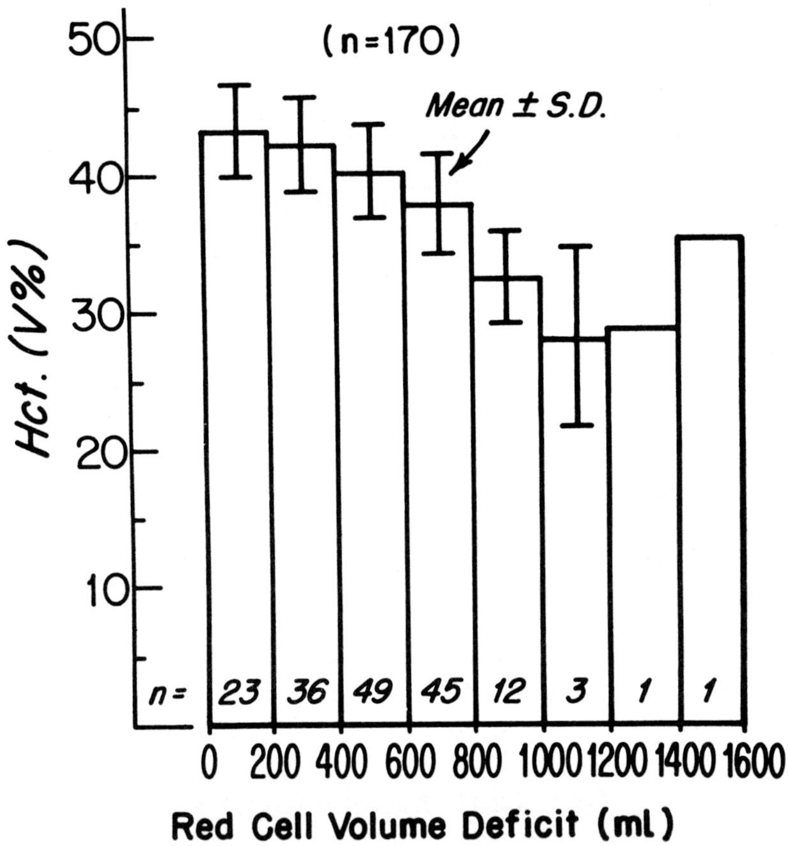

FIGURE 19. Relation between red blood cell volume deficit and the peripheral venous hematocrit levels in 170 patients with traumatic injuries involving the extremities only. A deficit of 800 mℓ of red blood cells was associated with a hematocrit value of 38 vol%.

ical red blood cell volume, plasma volume, and total blood volume in these patients were confirmed as valid in other patients who were studied before and after orthopedic operations. These latter patients had normal blood volumes before operation but developed hypovolemia postoperatively and recovered over a 3-month period of convalescence. The majority of our war-wounded patients had significant hypovolemia at the time of our initial evaluation of them, and over the 6- to 12-month period of convalescence the red blood cell, plasma, and total blood volumes were restored to the theoretical values, estimated from the body surface area nomogram (Chapter 6).

The reduced red blood cell volume clearly was not an adaptive anemia. Although there was a significant reduction in the number of red blood cells, the circulating red blood cells had improved oxygen transport function owing to the increase in the red blood cell 2,3 DPG level from 0.8 moles 2,3 DPG per mole of hemoglobin to 1.6 moles 2,3 DPG per mole of hemoglobin (Figures 16 and 17). The improvement in function compensated for the reduced number, thus eliminating the need for an increase in cardiac output.

Table 1
RELATION BETWEEN RED CELL MASS AND THE f FACTOR IN PATIENTS WITH TRAUMATIC INJURIES

Patient	Date	f Value	Red cell mass (g Hb)
A	12/10/69	0.83	522
	1/7/70	0.87	581
B	3/18/70	0.80	509
	3/27/70	0.82	617
	4/01/70	0.89	604
C	11/12/69	0.83	573
	12/11/69	0.68	401
	12/22/69	0.84	580
D	1/05/70	0.84	483
	1/15/70	0.83	694
E	1/05/70	0.91	452
	1/10/70	0.87	677
F	2/11/70	0.86	423
	2/19/70	0.87	401
G	1/05/70	0.83	481
	1/10/70	0.75	415
	1/19/70	0.78	401
H	12/10/69	0.81	443
	12/22/69	0.93	637
I	12/11/69	0.79	561
	1/20/70	0.86	626
J	12/11/69	0.72	371
	12/22/69	0.75	536
K	12/04/69	0.89	371
	12/10/69	0.84	603
L	2/05/70	0.88	459
	2/27/70	0.90	608

Note: $r = 0.299$, $p > 0.05$, $n = 27$.

MECHANISM OF THE HYPOVOLEMIC ANEMIA

The mechanism of the decrease in plasma volume in our patients is not clear. Plasma volume deficits may occur after operations (Irvin et al., 1972), although one might expect that there would be an increase because extracellular water moves into the circulation after hemorrhage. The changes in plasma volume that occur after hemorrhage are influenced to a minor degree by a shift of water from the intracellular to the interstitial space and then to the circulation (Stewart and Rourke, 1936; Skillman et al., 1967; Shizgal et al., 1972; Watkins et al., 1974b; Byrnes et al., 1978). There is considerable disagreement about the magnitude of these changes, but whatever their size their effects are trivial compared to the effects of fluid administered during resuscitation. It is worth noting that expansion of the plasma volume by intravenous infusion causes a loss of albumin from the circulation (Parving et al., 1974). Be that as it may, the effects of tissue-water shifts were not relevant in our patients since our studies were made weeks after injury.

One factor that theoretically might have been responsible for a low plasma volume was protein deficiency (Blackburn et al., 1973a, 1973b; Greenberg et al., 1976; Free-

Table 2
REPRODUCIBILITY OF THE MEASUREMENTS OF BLOOD VOLUME IN PATIENTS USING ^{51}CR-LABELED AUTOLOGOUS RED CELLS, IODINATED ALBUMIN PLASMA VOLUME, AND THE TOTAL BODY HEMATOCRIT DERIVED FROM THE PERIPHERAL VENOUS HEMATOCRIT MULTIPLIED BY 0.90

		Original blood volume		Repeat blood volume within 7 days of the original	
Patient		^{51}Cr	^{125}I	^{51}Cr	^{125}I
A	RCV	1582	1698	1503	1723
	PV	2136	2332	2030	2327
	TBV	3718	4030	3533	4050
B	RCV	1350	1501	1328	1488
	PV	3000	3350	2965	3322
	TBV	4350	4851	4293	4810
C	RCV	1456	1506	1448	1500
	PV	2811	2909	2797	2909
	TBV	4267	4415	4245	4409
D	RCV	1597	1650	1634	1659
	PV	3059	3162	3128	3178
	TBV	4656	4812	4762	4837
E	RCV	1697	1768	1707	1813
	PV	3172	3307	3189	3388
	TBV	4869	5075	4896	5201
F	RCV	1640	1758	1637	1785
	PV	3241	3460	3224	3517
	TBV	4881	5218	4861	5302

man et al., 1977). Decreases in both red blood cell volume and plasma volume are seen in this condition, and during recovery the plasma volume increases more rapidly than the red blood cell volume and the hematocrit value usually falls (Fondu, 1977; Viart, 1976, 1977). Our patients were not seriously malnourished. A severe protein-calorie deficiency due to causes other than trauma produces a hypovolemic-anemia somewhat like that seen in chronic trauma (Viart, 1976, 1977; Fondu, 1977; Fondu et al., 1978). Plasma protein levels do fall after trauma but there is no net loss of protein from the body (Waterlow et al., 1977; Smith et al., 1978), and if protein-calorie malnutrition was present at all in our patients it was of no great significance.

The hypovolemic-anemia observed in Vitamin A-deficient rats with a decrease in both plasma and red blood cell volumes (Meijia et al., 1979) does not seem to have an exact counterpart in man (Hodges et al., 1978). Other anemias that exhibit approximately equal reductions in red blood cell mass and plasma volume are the anemias of oxygen toxicity (Hyde and Rawson, 1969), of astronauts (Berry, 1974; Kimzey et al., 1976) and of divers (Murray and Jacey, 1977). There also may be unrecognized chem-

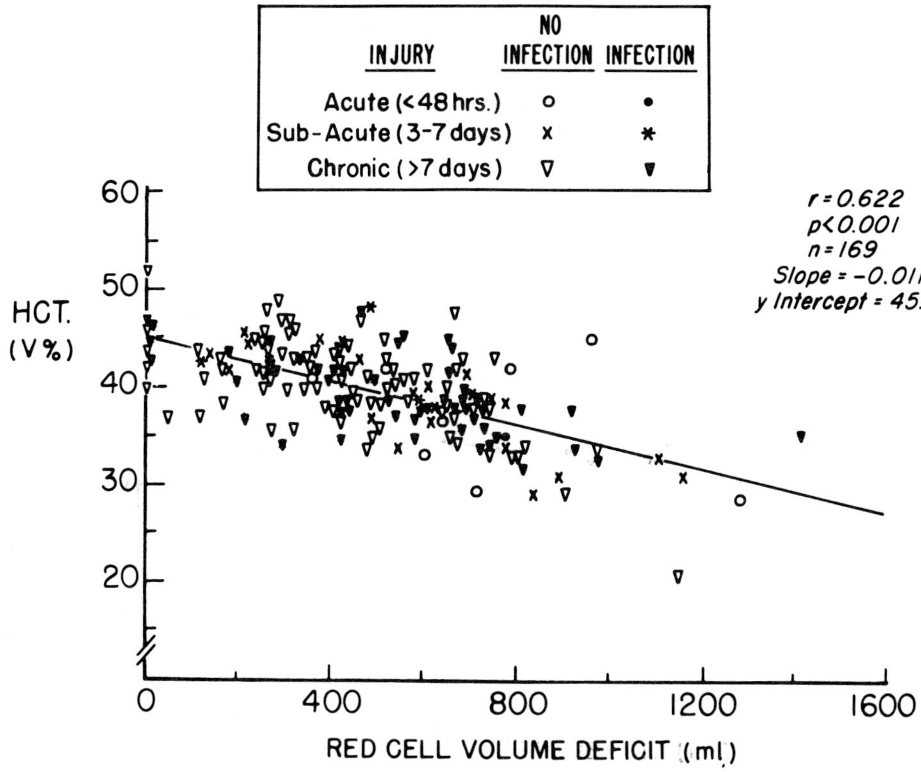

FIGURE 20. Relation between red blood cell volume deficit and the peripheral venous hematocrit levels in 169 patients with traumatic injuries involving the extremities only. Whether the injury was acute, subacute, or chronic and whether or not infection was present are indicated for each of the patients studied.

ical factors operating in these conditions (Murray and Jacey, 1977). The finding that in our patients both components of the blood volume, red blood cell volume and plasma volume, were decreased about equally raised the question of fat embolism, for a similar picture occurs in that condition (Shier et al., 1977). However, this hypothesis was negated by the absence of any clinical, roentgenographic, or laboratory evidence of that disorder (Chapter 1).

Despite numerous reports in the literature suggesting a correlation, the possibility that the decrease in blood volume in our patients was merely an adaptive consequence of prolonged bedrest also was ruled out because of the increase in red blood cell 2,3 DPG which indicated that tissue hypoxia had been present; the anemia was not adaptive but pathological (Finch and Lenfant, 1972). Surprisingly large decreases in blood volume due to decreases in both plasma and red blood cell volumes have been reported following 4 weeks of bedrest or 4 to 10 days of chair rest (Deitrick et al., 1948; Lamb et al., 1964, 1965; Miller et al., 1964a, 1964b, 1965). Average decreases of more than 1 ℓ in blood volume and over 500 mℓ in red blood cell volume after bedrest also have been described (Miller et al., 1965), but since the plasma volumes were measured by a technique using iodinated albumin, their reliability is questionable as are the total blood volumes so calculated. The most recent studies made with more reliable methods show only small changes (Friman, 1979). In any case, our patients were not consistently recumbent and there is no reason to accept bedrest as a major factor in our results.

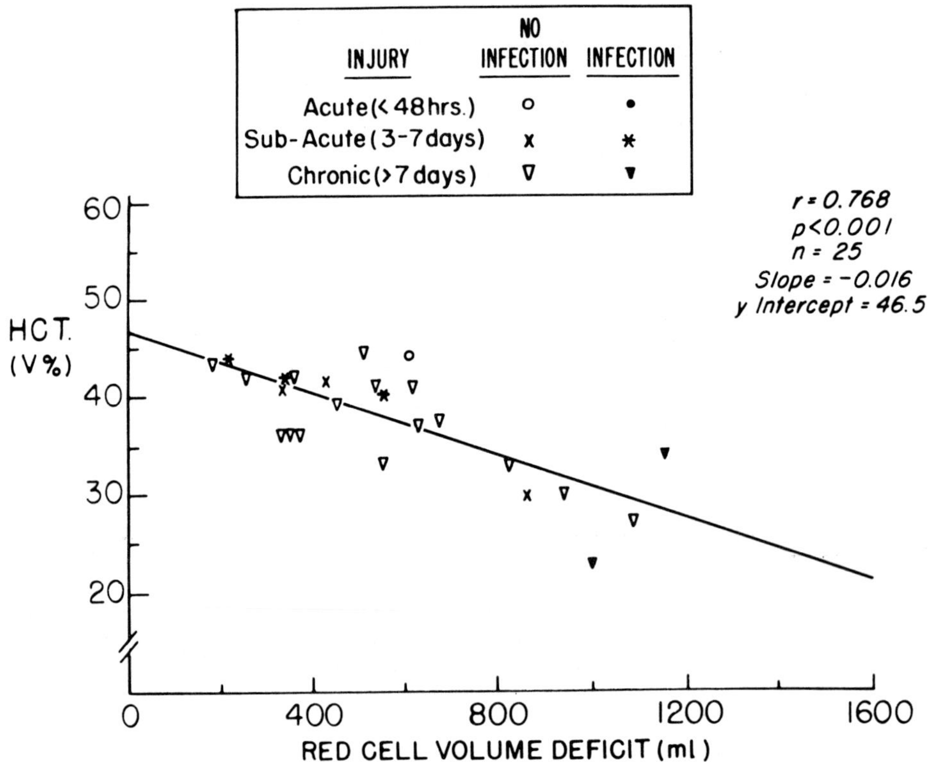

FIGURE 21. Relation between red blood cell volume deficit and the peripheral venous hematocrit value in 25 patients with head injuries. Whether the injury was acute, subacute, or chronic and whether or not infection was present, are indicated for each of the patients studied. A deficit of 800 m*l* of red blood cells was associated with a hematocrit value of 35 vol%.

In stress erythrocytosis there is a reduction in plasma volume (Lawrence and Berlin, 1952; Harris and Kellermeyer, 1970), although red blood cell volume is normal, and this reduction is believed to be secondary to the presence of catecholamines which produce constriction of the vascular bed of the microcirculation (Sutton et al., 1950; Brunjes et al., 1960). We considered these findings of little relevance in our studies since although the plasma catecholamine levels are initially elevated after trauma, they fall rapidly to normal (Benedict and Grahame-Smith, 1978).

Thus, our review of available data on a variety of clinical states offered no clue regarding the origin of the hypovolemic-anemia of trauma, with one possible exception. The work on acute intermittent porphyria (Bloomer et al., 1971), in which condition both red blood cell and plasma volumes are reduced approximately equally, apparently consequent to a moderate suppression of erythropoiesis in the bone marrow, stimulated us to study blood formation in our patients. This is discussed in the next chapter.

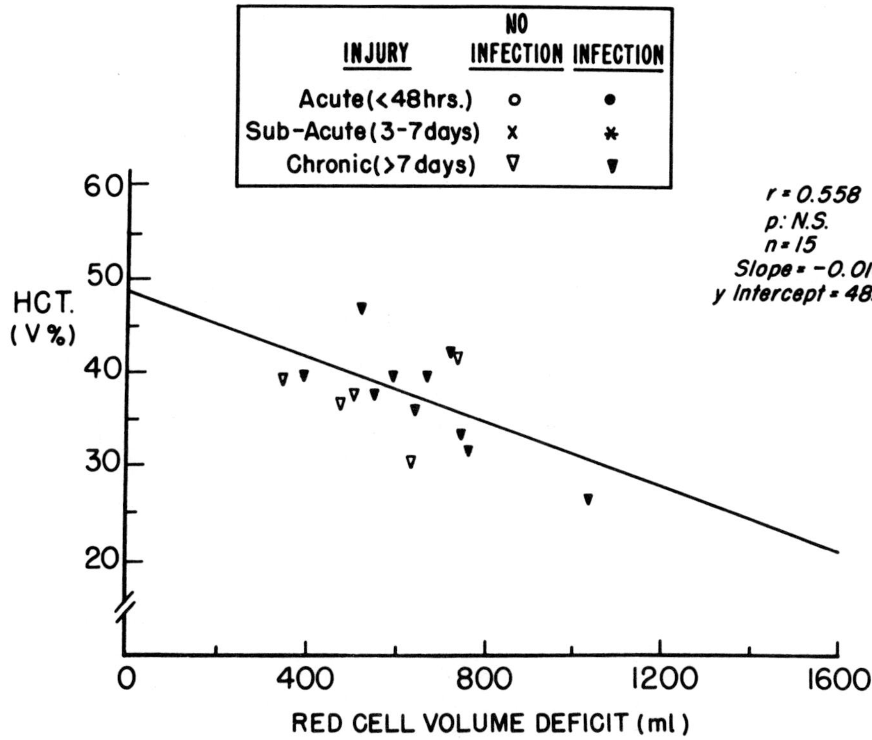

FIGURE 22. Relation between red blood cell volume deficit and the peripheral venous hematocrit value in 15 patients with thoracic-abdominal and thoracic-abdominal-pelvic injuries. Whether the injury was acute, subacute, or chronic and whether or not infection was present are indicated for each of the patients studied. A deficit of 800 mℓ of red blood cells was associated with a hematocrit level of 35 vol%.

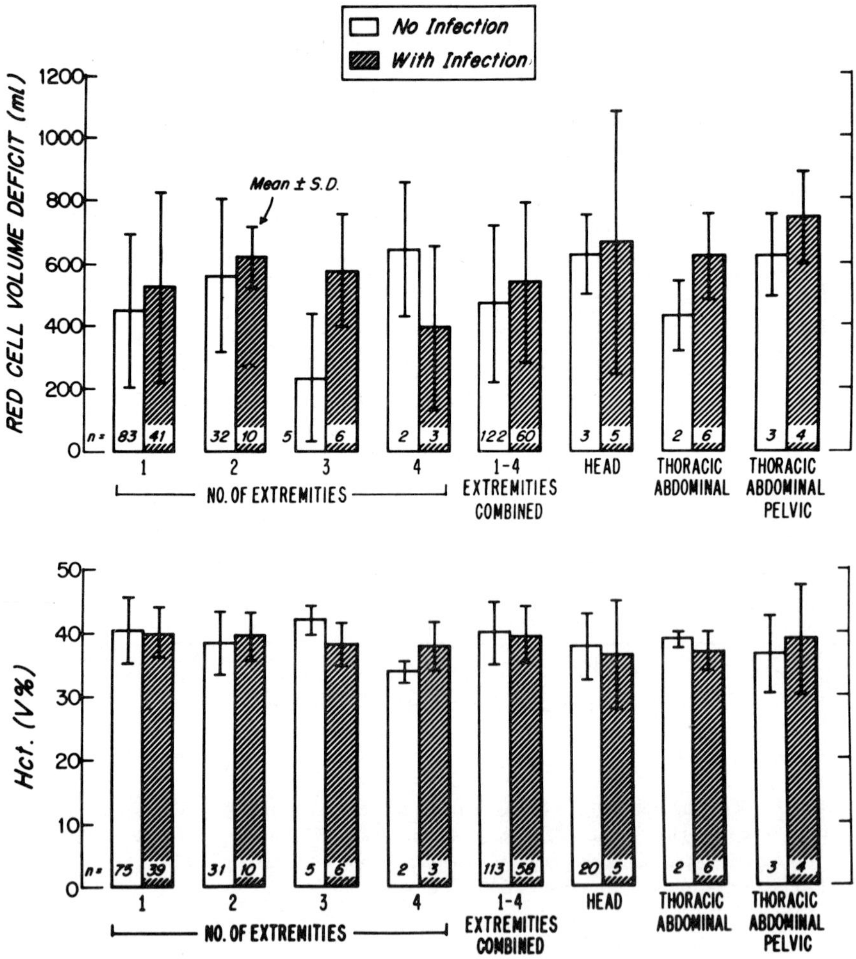

FIGURE 23. Relation between red blood cell volume deficit and peripheral venous hematocrit level in eight groups of 18- to 26-year-old male patients with different types of traumatic injuries. The presence or absence of infection is noted for each group.

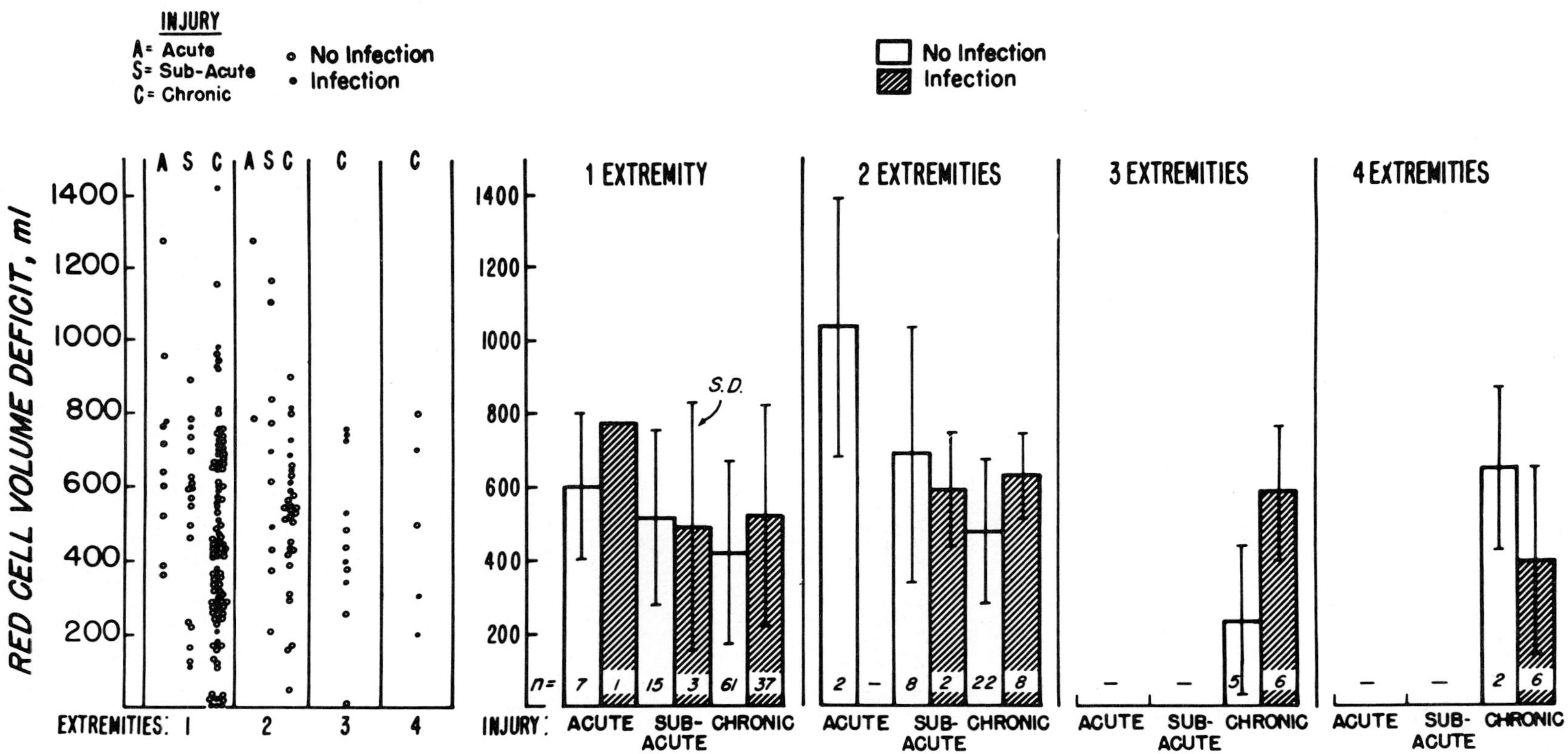

FIGURE 24. Relations between the red blood cell volume deficits and the types of injury sustained by the 18- to 26-year-old men. Whether the injury was acute, subacute, or chronic and whether or not infection was present, are indicated.

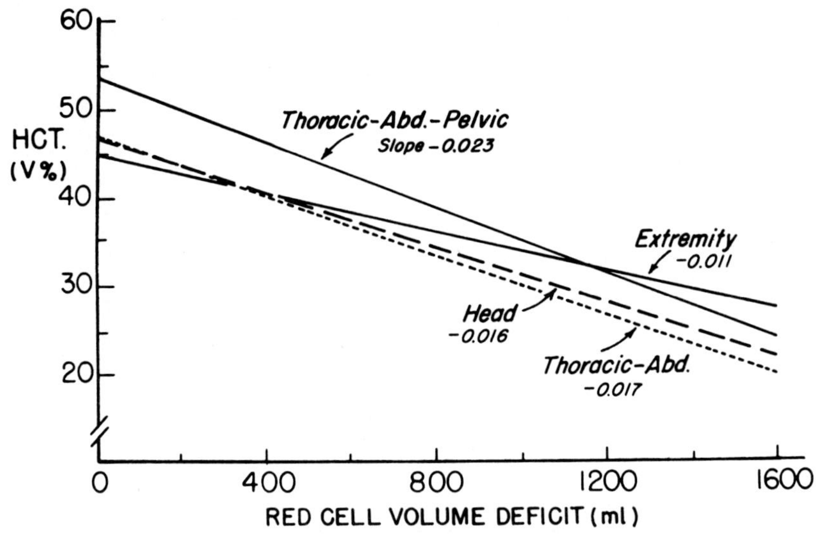

FIGURE 25. A comparison of the relations between peripheral venous hematocrit level and the red blood cell volume deficit in the four groups of patients with extremity injuries only, head injuries, thoracic-abdominal injuries, or thoracic-abdominal-pelvic injuries. Patients with thoracic-abdominal-pelvic injuries had the greatest decrease in hematocrit associated with red blood cell mass deficit, followed by thoracic-abdominal injuries, head injuries, and finally patients with extremity injuries only.

Chapter 3

RED BLOOD CELL PRODUCTION

The observations reported earlier in this monograph show clearly that the patients under study had a pathologic hypovolemic anemia, an anemia that was not an adaptive response to a decrease in oxygen requirement of the body. The finding of elevated 2,3 DPG levels in our patients established the presence of an hypoxic condition, since it is well known that an increase in the 2,3 DPG level is an important body response compensating for tissue hypoxia. The question to be answered was whether the observed red blood cell deficit was caused by impaired red blood cell production, by accelerated destruction of the patients' own cells as well as the transfused red blood cells, or by both impaired production and accelerated destruction.

ROUTINE HEMATOLOGIC FINDINGS

Many authorities have pointed out the importance of assessing red blood cell production in cases of unexplained anemia (Vaughan and Saifi, 1939; Crosby and Akeroyd, 1952; Bush et al., 1956; Bothwell et al., 1957; Stohlman, 1961; Adamson, 1968; Hamstra and Block, 1969; Hillman and Finch, 1969, 1971; Crosby, 1975; Erslev and Silver, 1975; Berlin, 1977; Erslev, 1977; Leite and Hoogstraten, 1977; Werts et al., 1979). Accordingly, studies were made to elucidate the causes of the anemia in our patients so that we might treat them. Before undertaking complicated laboratory studies, we followed the routine clinical course of ascertaining from history, physical findings, and laboratory tests, whether common causes of anemia were present. The routine studies ruled out renal and hepatic diseases as causes (Table 1). Although many of the patients ate poorly, some markedly so, there was no clinical or laboratory evidence of protein or vitamin deficiency. The patients' diets were rich in protein and vitamin supplements. Some but not all of the patients had wound infections, and the lack of uniformity in this regard combined with the fact that the patients with infections were receiving antibiotics convinced us that infection, if it was a factor at all, was at most a secondary and inconsistent one.

Hematologic measurements in our patients showed normal or slightly reduced hemoglobin and hematocrit levels (Chapters 1 and 2) with normal red blood cell morphology, normal red blood cell indices, normal to slightly reduced serum iron and total iron binding capacity (Feldthusen et al., 1953; Feldthusen and Lassen, 1954; Nylander, 1955; Elin et al., 1977), normal serum copper, normal Vitamin B_{12} levels, normal or occasionally slightly low folic acid levels, and normal reticulocyte counts (Hillman and Finch, 1969) (Tables 1 and 2; Chapter 2). The patients had normal white blood cell and differential counts and normal platelet counts. Bone marrow aspiration showed normal red blood cell, white blood cell, and platelet morphology, and the myeloid-to-erythroid ratio was normal or slightly decreased. The bone marrow iron was normal or slightly decreased.

In view of the finding of decreased iron in the bone marrow in some of the patients, all the patients were treated with oral iron or intramuscular (im) iron, but there was no measurable response. Similarly, oral folic acid and pyridoxine were given without effect. In addition, therapeutic doses of niacinamide and Vitamins C and E were given, likewise without response. Inasmuch as all the ordinary clinical approaches tried were unsuccessful, we were obliged to turn to certain of the more highly specialized tests. These tests fell into several categories.

Table 1
HEMATOLOGIC MEASUREMENTS IN PATIENTS WITH TRAUMATIC INJURIES, CARCINOMA, CARDIOPULMONARY DISORDERS, AND MISCELLANEOUS DIAGNOSES

Group	WBC (4—11,000/mm³)	Platelet count (150—350,000/mm³)	Serum iron (60—180 μg%)	TIBC (240—420 μg%)	Vitamin B_{12} (150—710 pg/mℓ)	Folic acid (4—6 ng/mℓ)
I (Traumatic injuries without antibiotics)						
Mean	7,354	292,166	87	264	297	3.8
S.D.	2,276	77,383	57	98	99	1.8
S.E.	402	31,591	10	18	33	0.5
n	32	6	28	29	9	14
II (Traumatic injuries with antibiotics)						
Mean	9,995	327,166	90	288	288	4.5
S.D.	6,354	131,185	42	84	136	3.6
S.E.	1,386	30,920	5	11	25	0.6
n	21	18	62	54	28	36
III (Patients with carcinoma)						
Mean	8,758	238,800	48	164	261	2.7
S.D.	5,672	128,529	16	52	113	1.5
S.E.	1,464	57,479	5	17	40	0.7
n	15	5	11	9	8	4
IV (Patients with cardiopulmonary disease)						
Mean	8,323	188,285	97	214	392	6.2
S.D.	1,742	47,317	70	26	284	4.0
S.E.	551	17,884	20	15	142	2.0
n	10	7	12	3	4	4
V (Miscellaneous diagnoses)						
Mean	7,010	223,857	118	347	337	4.5
S.D.	1,691	107,075	84	88	289	2.4
S.E.	535	40,470	16	31	77	0.5
n	10	7	14	4	7	12

Group	Serum copper (75—160 μg%)	Glucose (70—110 mg%)	Creatinine (0.8—1.5 mg%)	BUN (10—20 mg%)	Bilirubin (total) (0—1.0 mg%)	Bilirubin (direct) 0—0.25 mg%)	MCHC (32—35%)	MCV (75—96 μ^3)
I								
Mean	151	98	1.0	13.8	0.9	0.3	34.4	91.6
S.D.	60	16	0.2	3.3	0.4	0.3	2.3	2.2
S.E.	17	4	0.1	0.8	0.1	0.05	0.9	0.7
n	12	16	14	17	27	24	7	10
II								
Mean	142	90	0.9	12.1	0.8	0.3	33.8	90.3
S.D.	53	29	0.2	3.4	0.4	0.2	1.2	1.5
S.E.	10	3	0.04	0.5	0.05	0.04	0.6	0.7
n	27	59	26	40	63	47	4	4
III								
Mean	146	105	1.2	13.0	0.9	0.3	33.8	94.2
S.D.	12	21	0.4	3.8	0.5	0.1	0.3	1.1
S.E.	5	6	0.1	1.4	0.15	0.02	0.2	0.5
n	5	11	17	8	9	5	4	4
IV								
Mean	144	113	1.4	16.0	1.6	0.4	33.1	91.2
S.D.	53	14	0.7	5.3	0.8	0.1	0.6	2.3
S.E.	23	5	0.2	2.0	0.3	0.04	0.3	1.2
n	5	7	18	7	9	6	4	4
V								
Mean	185	123	0.9	16.9	1.0	0.5	33.4	92.2
S.D.	124	37	0.4	11.4	0.5	0.3	2.0	7.6
S.E.	33	9	0.1	2.8	0.13	0.1	0.5	2.0
n	7	15	22	16	14	13	14	15

Table 1 (continued)
HEMATOLOGIC MEASUREMENTS IN PATIENTS WITH TRAUMATIC INJURIES, CARCINOMA, CARDIOPULMONARY DISORDERS, AND MISCELLANEOUS DIAGNOSES

Group	MCH (27—32 μμg)	RBC pH (7.15—7.20 units)	RBC Na^+ (0.7—0.9 mEq/10^{10} RBC)	RBC K^+ (8—9 mEq/10^{10} RBC)	RBC Cl^- (7.8—8.8 mEq/10^{10} RBC)
I					
Mean	31.7	7.15	0.8	8.9	6.8
S.D.	1.8	0.045	0.1	0.5	1.5
S.E.	0.7	0.014	0.03	0.2	0.5
n	6	9	9	9	9
II					
Mean	30.6	7.17	1.1	8.1	6.8
S.D.	1.1	0.05	0.9	0.5	0.2
S.E.	0.5	0.02	0.45	0.2	0.1
n	4	4	4	4	4
III					
Mean	31.9	7.18	0.7	8.4	7.0
S.D.	0.6	0.03	0.1	0.5	0.3
S.E.	0.3	0.01	0.06	0.3	0.2
n	4	4	4	4	4
IV					
Mean	30.3	7.16	0.7	8.4	7.1
S.D.	1.3	0.00	0.1	0.4	0.1
S.E.	0.7	0.00	0.05	0.2	0.04
n	4	4	4	4	4
V					
Mean	31.1	7.15	1.0	8.7	7.0
S.D.	2.5	0.05	0.3	0.6	0.9
S.E.	0.7	0.01	0.1	0.2	0.2
n	14	15	15	15	14

Table 2
RETICULOCYTE COUNTS IN PATIENTS WITH TRAUMATIC INJURIES, CARCINOMA, CARDIOPULMONARY DISORDERS AND MISCELLANEOUS DIAGNOSES

	Carcinoma	Cardiopulmonary disorders	Miscellaneous diagnoses	Traumatic injuries
Reticulocytes (0.8 ± 1.8)				
No. patients	35	3	41	53
No. observations	207	23	268	333
Mean	0.96	1.62	1.36	0.80
S.D.	0.90	0.72	1.14	0.80
S.E.	0.04	0.11	0.05	0.03
Range	0—4.8	0.6—3.0	0—5.6	0—6.4

SPECIAL STUDIES OF BLOOD FORMATION

The red blood cell production in our patients was measured by two separate procedures: One was the incorporation of ^{59}iron (Fe) into peripheral red blood cells, as discussed below. The other utilized the serial measurement of red blood cell volumes using ^{51}Cr-labeled autologous red blood cells before and after the transfusion of compatible donor red blood cells, a decision that was reached after the attending physician had elected to treat the patients' anemia with red blood cell transfusions before the essential surgical operations. The transfusions consisted of washed previously frozen red blood cells or washed liquid-stored red blood cells. In this procedure compatible donor red blood cells were selected with ABO or RH antigens differing from the patient's so that following transfusion the donor red blood cells were identified and quantitated using an automated differential agglutination procedure.

The transfusion of compatible and identifiable washed red blood cells permitted us to do repeat red blood cell volumes with ^{51}Cr-labeled autologous red blood cells and simultaneously to measure the survival of compatible and identifiable donor red blood cells using the automated differential agglutination procedure (Figures 1 and 2). These repeated measurements of the red blood cell volume following transfusion and simultaneous measurements of the percentage of donor red blood cells made it possible for us to calculate the number of red blood cells produced by the patient (Figures 1 and 2), and demonstrated the extent of the patient's bone marrow depression.

INCORPORATION OF IRON INTO RED BLOOD CELLS

Another method used to measure bone marrow function and related phenomena involved observations made after the intravenous injection of ^{59}Fe citrate and its incorporation into the red blood cells taken from peripheral veins at intervals. The incorporation of the ^{59}Fe into peripheral circulating red blood cells in our patients was found to be similar to that seen in two normal persons whom we studied and also similar to values reported in the literature. One evident difference, however, was that the ^{59}Fe citrate injected into the blood of our patients was removed at a rapid rate compared to rates observed in the two normal persons mentioned and in the persons noted in the literature (Dubach et al., 1946; Finch et al., 1949a, 1949b, 1965, 1970; Huff et al., 1950; Finch and Loden, 1959; Hosain et al., 1967; Morgan et al., 1967; Cook et al., 1970; Mortensen and Eurenius, 1974; Cavill et al., 1979) (Figures 3 and 4). However,

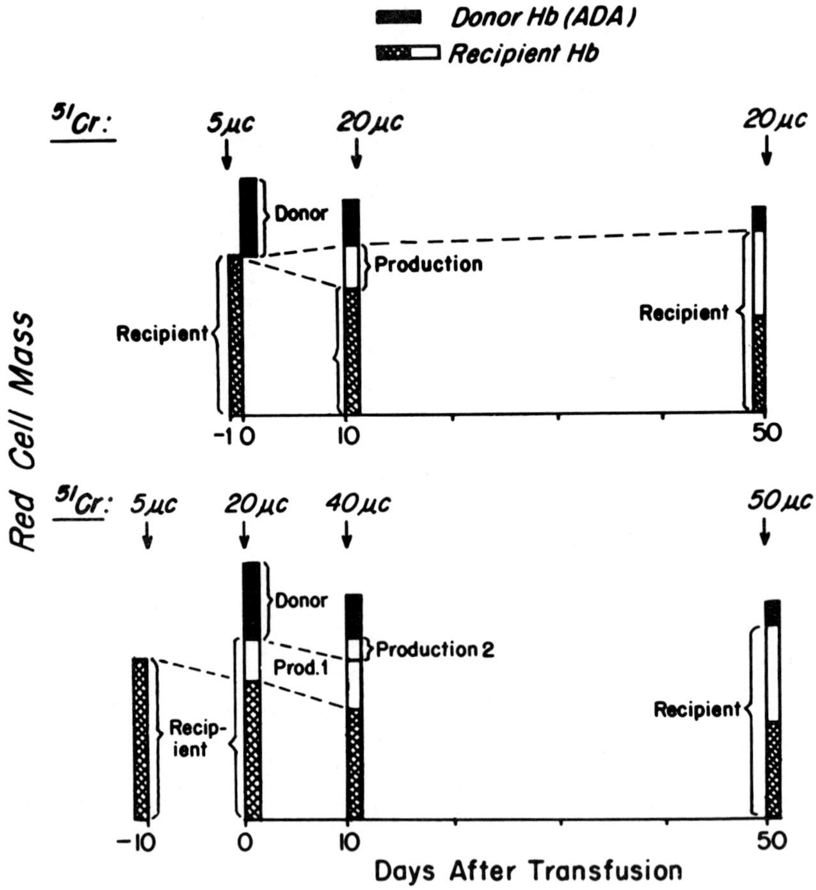

FIGURE 1. Red blood cell production in two patients, estimated from serial red blood cell mass measurements and the survival values of donor red blood cells. Red blood cell mass was measured on three or four occasions with increasing amounts of ^{51}Cr. The transfused compatible donor red blood cells were identified and quantitated by the automated differential agglutination procedure. Following transfusion, the patients' red blood cell production was calculated from measurements of the red blood cell mass and quantitation of the donor red blood cells present in the circulation. The loss of the recipient's own red blood cells was determined by the ^{51}Cr labeling procedure.

the rapid rate of ^{59}Fe removal in our patients was secondary to their reduced plasma volumes (Chapter 2): the plasma iron turnover rate (PITR, mg/kg/day) in the patients was similar to the values observed in the normal persons and in the persons reported elsewhere in the literature (Figures 3, 4, 5A, 5B, and 6 and Table 3).

In eight of the patients in our study, the ^{59}Fe removal from the plasma showed a biphasic exponential disappearance curve over an 8-hr postinfusion period, a rapid initial disappearance followed by a slower rate of disappearance. This suggested initial rapid disappearance from the plasma volume into the erythroid-reticuloendothelial circuit and the interstitial-lymphatic space and then reappearance of the ^{59}Fe from the interstitial-lymphatic space into the plasma volume (Finch et al., 1965; Morgan et al., 1967; Alfrey et al., 1969; Berlin, 1977). The iron binds to the β globulin transferrin which has a molecular weight of only 80,000. The iron-bound transferrin, like albumin, distributed itself rapidly into the extravascular space in our patients and reap-

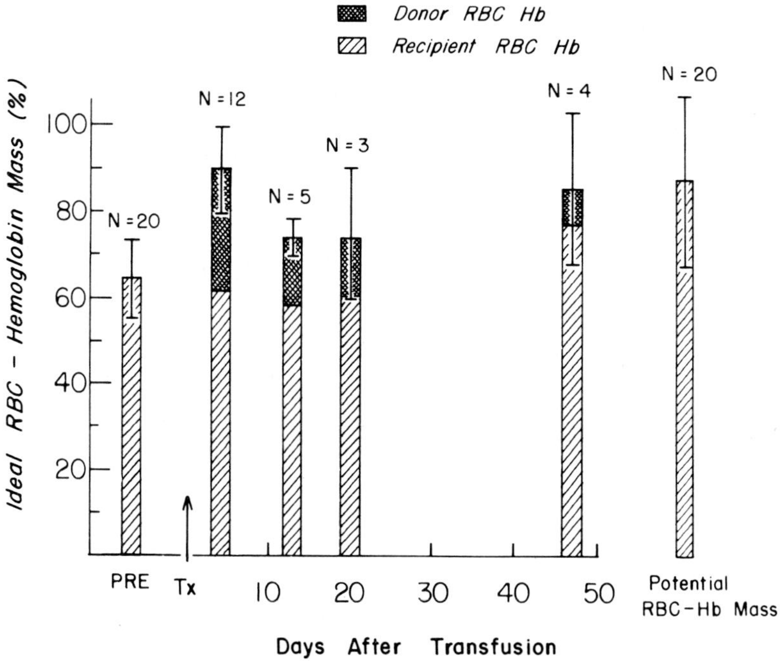

FIGURE 2. The red blood cell-hemoglobin mass in 20 patients with traumatic injuries. Each patient's red blood cell-hemoglobin value was about 35% lower than the ideal value, and red blood cell products were transfused to restore this deficit. Autologous ^{51}Cr-labeled red blood cells were used to measure the red blood cell-hemoglobin mass on five separate occasions before and after transfusion of the compatible donor red blood cells identified and quantitated by the automated differential agglutination procedure. The recipient red blood cell production was calculated from the total red blood cell-hemoglobin measured using ^{51}Cr-labeled autologous red blood cells and the percent of donor red blood cells in the circulation at the time of the red blood cell mass measurement.

peared in the plasma volume during the 8-hr postinfusion period (Figures 5A, 5B, and 6). The clearance of iron from the plasma and its appearance in peripheral red blood cells was normal in absolute terms, but was abnormally low for patients with the measured red blood cell mass deficits reported in Table 3.

Since many of the patients with traumatic injuries had low-grade infection of the wounds, anemia that accompanies chronic infection was considered a possible explanation for the finding of reduced serum iron and total iron binding capacity in a few of the patients (Cartwright and Wintrobe, 1952) (Table 3). In order to test this theory we studied the reutilization of iron from senescent red blood cells in three patients (Figures 7, 8, and 9). These patients had received ^{59}Fe citrate intravenously to study the clearance of ^{59}Fe from the plasma and its incorporation into the peripheral red blood cells. Reutilization of ^{59}Fe from senescent red blood cells was observed in three patients studied, indicating that the impairment of red blood cell production was not secondary to the anemia of infection (Freireich et al., 1957; Haurani et al., 1965; Werts et al., 1979) because the anemia of infection is characterized by the failure of the body to reutilize the iron from senescent red blood cells. In addition, the survival of the red blood cells as measured by ^{59}Fe showed marked shortening, indicating ineffective erythropoiesis (Chapter 4).

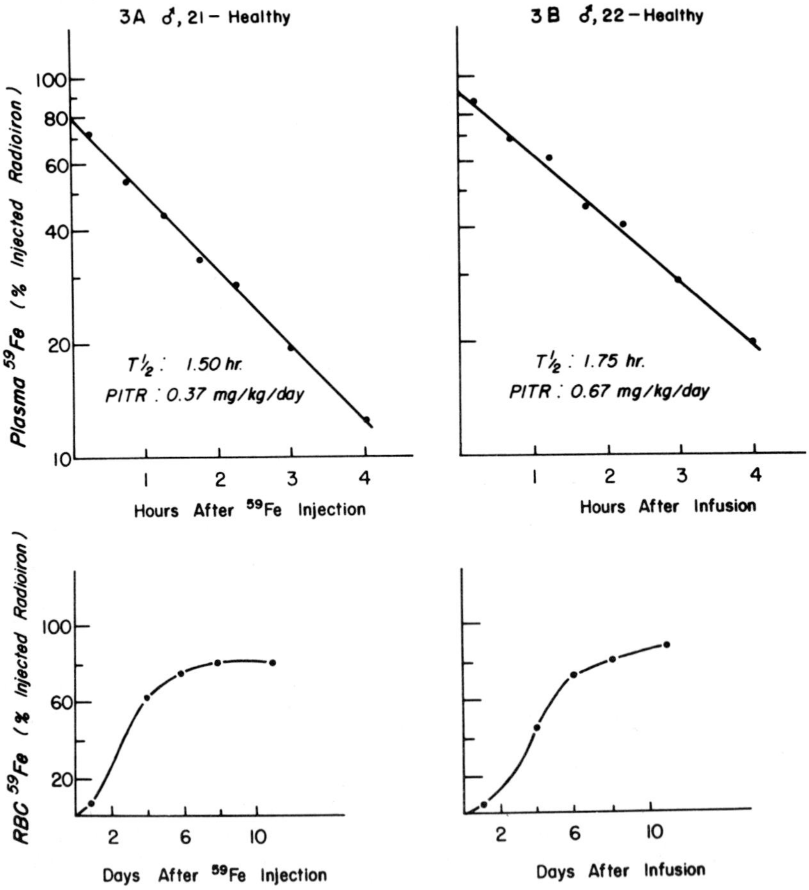

FIGURE 3. The clearance of ^{59}Fe from the plasma and its incorporation into the peripheral red blood cells of two healthy volunteers. The ^{59}Fe disappeared from the plasma at a single exponential clearance rate during the 4-hr postinfusion period.

OTHER STUDIES OF FERROKINETICS IN TRAUMA

In any discussion of iron metabolism, the fall in serum iron level that occurs with any form of trauma in man must be taken into account (Feldthusen et al., 1953; Feldthusen and Lassen, 1954; Nylander, 1955; Baar and Topley, 1956). The low values quickly return to normal except in some patients who might not have had adequate blood replacement after hemorrhage (Baar and Topley, 1956). However, the majority of our patients had normal serum iron levels at the time they were studied weeks after the injury, and all had received large blood transfusions in the acute period. More relevant to the status of our patients were the findings of O'Shaughnessy et al. (1966), who concluded that patients with severe fractures, and presumably with large hematomas in these sites had a storage form of iron that differed from the ferritin/hemosiderin form that in normal physiologic states constitutes the only type of storage iron. These authors determined, albeit inferentially, that this form of iron was localized only to the fracture area, and that it represented iron released from the porphyrin moiety of hemoglobin in the (presumed) hematomas themselves. The persistence of this proc-

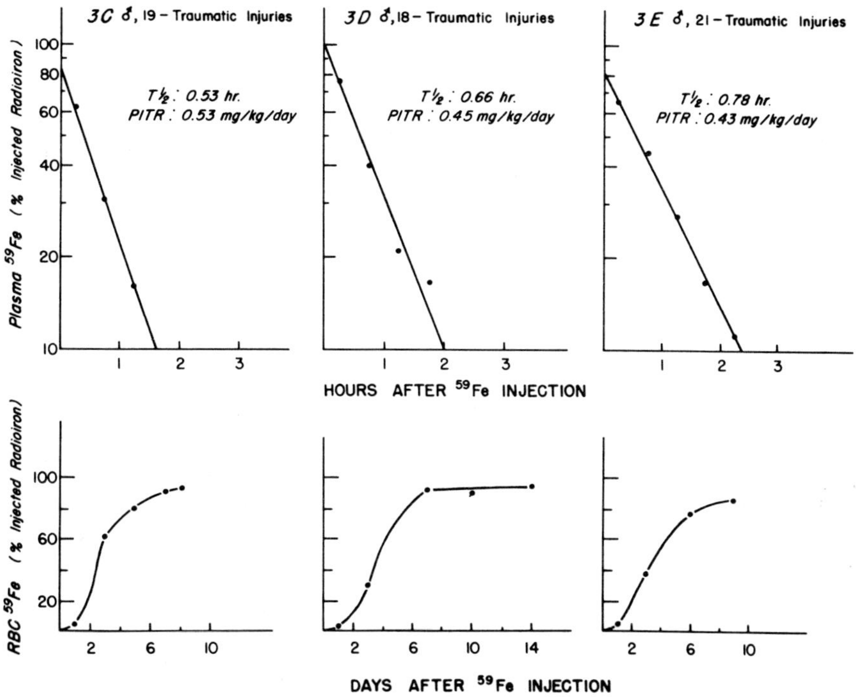

FIGURE 4. The clearance of ^{59}Fe from the plasma and its incorporation into the peripheral red blood cells of three patients with traumatic injuries. The ^{59}Fe disappeared from the plasma at a single exponential clearance rate during the 2½-hr postinfusion period.

Table 3
RED BLOOD CELL VOLUME DEFICIT (mℓ), ^{59}Fe PLASMA CLEARANCE T-½ (HR), THE RED BLOOD CELL ^{59}Fe REAPPEARANCE (%), PLASMA TURNOVER RATE (mg/kg/day), SERUM IRON (μg%), AND IRON BINDING CAPACITY (μg%) IN 2 HEALTHY VOLUNTEERS AND 14 PATIENTS WITH TRAUMATIC INJURIES, AND THE NORMAL VALUES REPORTED IN THE LITERATURE

Patient	^{51}Cr red cell volume deficit (mℓ)	^{59}Fe plasma clearance T—½ (hr)	RBC ^{59}Fe reappearance (%)	Plasma iron turnover rate (mg/kg/day)	Serum iron (μg%)	Iron binding capacity (μg%)
3C	702	0.534	93.7	0.53	50.8	350
3N	690	0.900	80.0	0.51	110.0	384
30	644	0.824	86.2	0.47	69.4	230
3D	611	0.663	94.8	0.45	48.7	455
3P	600	0.950	81.5	0.40	90.0	170
3J	591	0.947	76.8	0.42	54.1	330
3E	583	0.780	86.9	0.43	58.0	265
3K	576	0.855	88.6	0.89	83.8	352
3M	533	1.183	76.4	0.40	76.4	274
3I	421	0.700	87.4	0.51	71.0	176
3Q	417	0.800	84.0	0.33	60.0	—
3R	272	1.150	75.0	0.34	86.0	208
3S	235	0.750	86.9	0.66	73.6	170
3L	181	0.867	90.0	0.60	76.1	300
Healthy						
3A	0	1.500	80.0	0.37	80.0	270
3B	0	1.750	86.0	0.67	120.0	324
Reported normal values		1—2		0.37—0.75	60—180	240—420

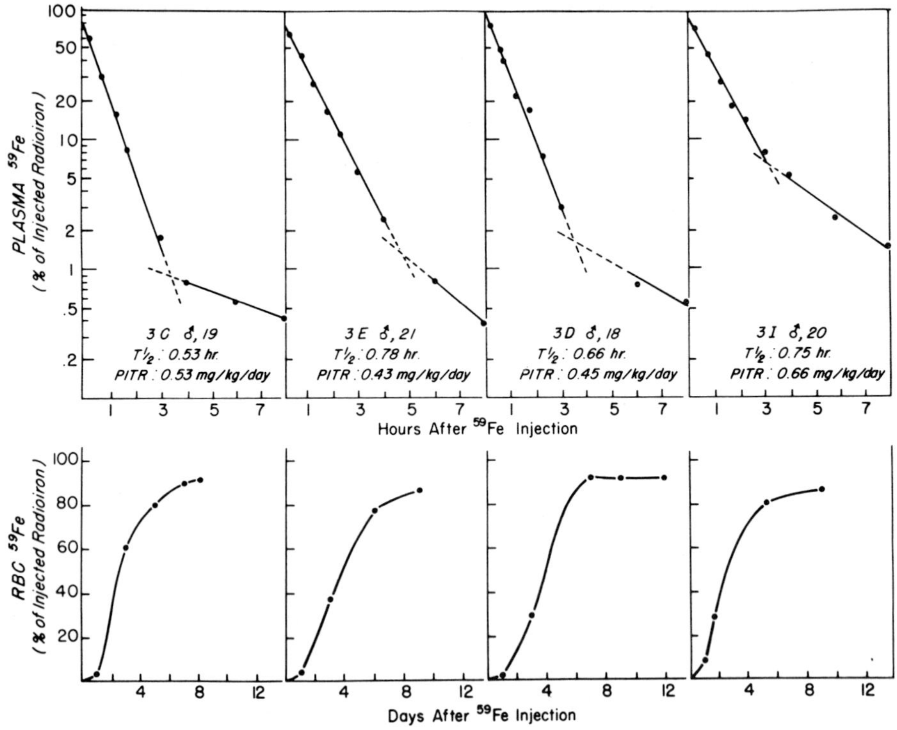

FIGURE 5A. The clearance of ^{59}Fe from the plasma and its incorporation into the peripheral red blood cells in four patients with traumatic injuries. The ^{59}Fe was removed from the plasma by a biphasic exponential clearance mechanism during the 8-hr postinfusion period.

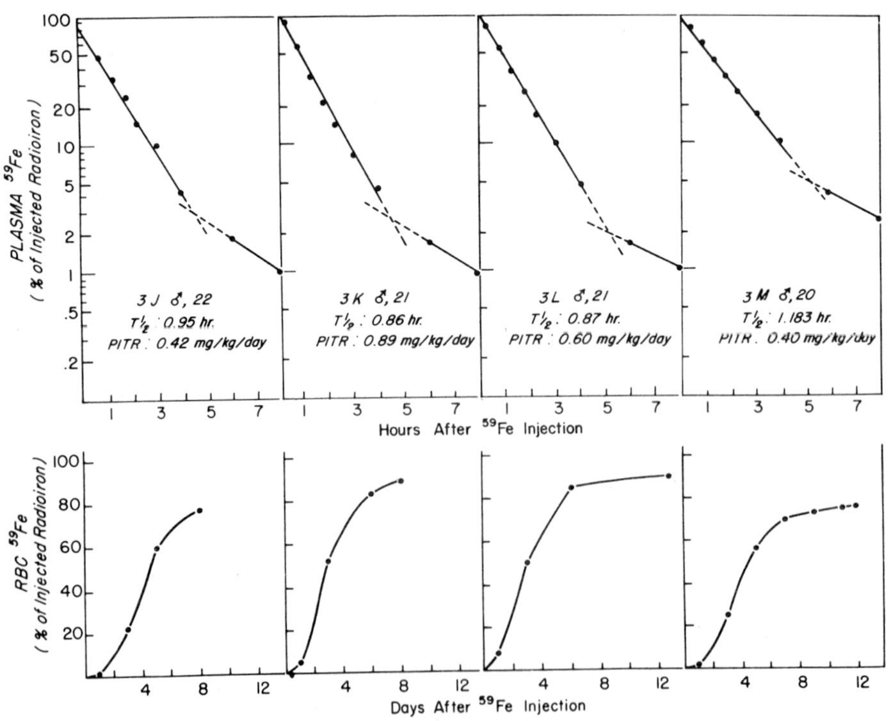

FIGURE 5B. The clearance of ^{59}Fe from the plasma and its incorporation into the peripheral red blood cells in four patients with traumatic injuries. The ^{59}Fe was removed from the plasma by a biphasic exponential clearance mechanism during the 8-hr postinfusion period.

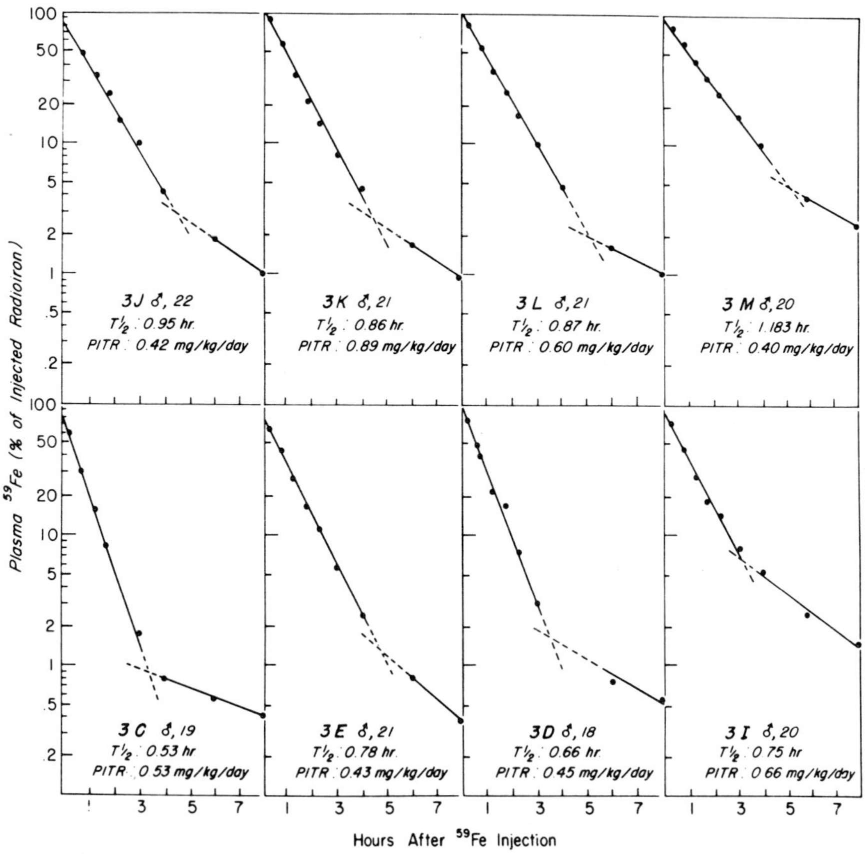

FIGURE 6. The clearance of ^{59}Fe from the plasma of eight patients with traumatic injuries. The ^{59}Fe was removed from the plasma by a biphasic exponential clearance mechanism during the 8-hr postinfusion period.

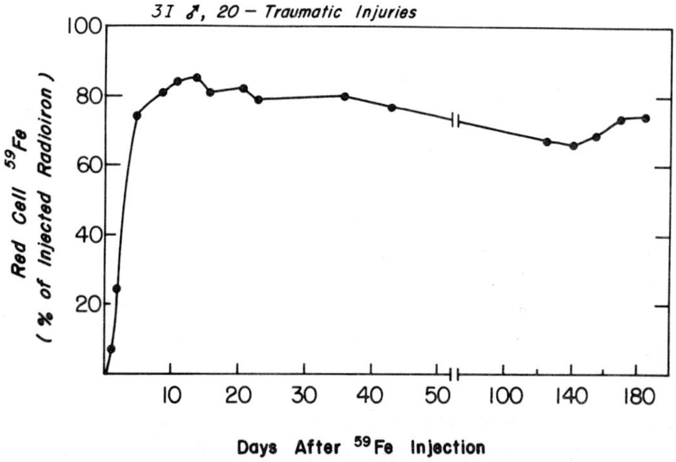

FIGURE 7. The incorporation of ^{59}Fe into the peripheral red blood cells of Patient 31, a 20-year-old male with traumatic injuries. The reutilization of the ^{59}Fe from senescent red blood cells was studied over the 6-month period after its injection.

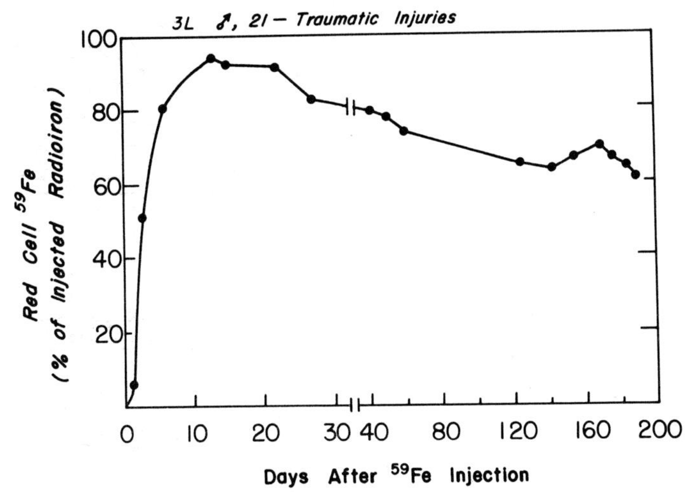

FIGURE 8. The incorporation of ^{59}Fe into the peripheral red blood cells of Patient 3L, a 21-year-old male with traumatic injuries. The reutilization of the ^{59}Fe from senescent red blood cells was studied over the 6-month period after its injection.

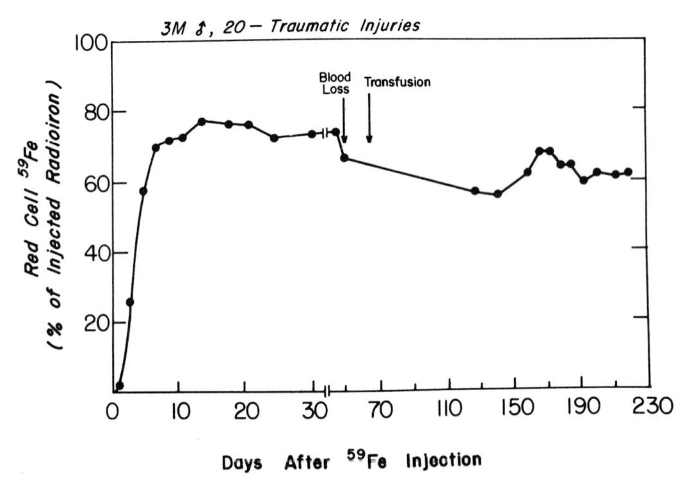

FIGURE 9. The incorporation of ^{59}Fe into the peripheral red blood cells of Patient 3M, a 20-year-old male with traumatic injuries. The reutilization of ^{59}Fe from senescent red blood cells was studied over a 7-month period after its injection. About 50 days after the injection of ^{59}Fe, the patient required red blood cell transfusion because of blood loss.

ess was unlikely in our patients whose fractures had occurred weeks or months earlier, and whose fracture sites had been subjected to repeated debridement. However, it may be that this process is not dependent on the presence of hematomas, but rather occurs in granulation tissue itself (Chapter 4). The significance of the finding of low serum iron levels in some of our patients remains unclear, since its mechanism has not been established and its possible role as a cause of the anemia in our patients is negated by the fact that iron given orally or parenterally did not affect the anemia.

Table 4
ERYTHROPOIETIN (EP) ASSAY IN HYPERTRANSFUSED RATS[a]

Test substance	24-hr ^{59}Fe incorporation	Hematocrit
Saline	0.02 ± 0.01	69.0 ± 0.5
EP (0.25 U)	7.88 ± 0.49	69.2 ± 0.6
EP (0.50 U)	10.50 ± 0.84	69.0 ± 0.7
EP (1.00 U)	12.20 ± 1.49	69.0 ± 0.8
Normal volunteers		
1	0.02 ± 0	68.8 ± 1.7
2	0.01 ± 0	68.0 ± 0.7
Patients		
1	0.002 ± 0	69.0 ± 1.2
2	0.03 ± 0.02	70.2 ± 1.1
3	0.0002 ± 0	70.2 ± 1.2
4	0.01 ± 0	70.2 ± 1.9
5	0.01 ± 0	68.5 ± 1.4

Note: The 24-hr ^{59}Fe incorporation is reported for the controls (saline and EP-treated hypertransfused rats), two normal volunteers, and five patients.

[a] Performed by Dr. Marilyn E. Miller with our great appreciation.

ERYTHROPOIETIN STUDIES

In order to gain additional information on the bone marrow depression found in our patients, urine samples were assayed for erythropoietin activity by Dr. Marilyn E. Miller, using a hypertransfused rat in which the 24-hr ^{59}Fe incorporation into the peripheral red blood cells was measured (Mirand et al., 1965; Gordon, 1973; Miller, 1975; Peschle, 1975). The assays showed a normal or slightly reduced erythropoietin activity in the urine of our patients with traumatic injuries, whereas anemia should cause increased production (Table 4). The relatively decreased erythropoietin excretion could not be explained by protein deficiency or by malnutrition or infection (Schade and Fried, 1976; Sanders et al., 1977), since all patients studied had normal total protein and albumin concentrations in the blood and were eating nutritious diets, although some of the patients did have poor appetite (Heath and Taylor, 1936; Baar and Topley, 1956; Mikhail et al., 1975).

Erythropoietin excretion, hence, by implication, erythropoietin production, is known to be related to the red blood cell affinity for oxygen; decreased red blood cell affinity for oxygen reduces erythropoietin excretion whereas an increase in red blood cell affinity for oxygen increases erythropoietin excretion (Faura et al., 1968; Edwards and Canon, 1972; Jaskunas et al., 1973; Miller et al., 1973, 1974, 1976; Robinson et al., 1973; Shahidi, 1973; Rorth, 1974; Miller, 1975; Schooley and Mahlmann, 1975; Peschle et al., 1978; Miller and Howard, 1979).

As noted in Chapter 2, patients with reduced red blood cell masses were able to compensate for their reduced total number of red blood cells by improving the oxygen transport function of their circulating red blood cells, the compensatory mechanism being an increase in red blood cell 2,3 DPG to 1½ to 2 times normal which, in turn, decreases the red blood cell affinity for oxygen. Ordinarily, one would expect elevated erythropoietin activity in the urine of anemic persons; the absence of increased activity in our patients may have been due in part to the reduced oxygen affinity of the red blood cells. In the anemia associated with burns, as in adaptation to the hypoxia of altitude, impairment in red blood cell production is accompanied by a reduction in red blood cell affinity for oxygen and a decrease in production of erythropoietin. The relations among the number of red blood cells, the red blood cell affinity state for oxygen, and erhtyropoietin production is complex. At the moment, cause and effect cannot be distinguished with any certainty. Nevertheless, we must remember that in our studies it was the activity of the erythropoietin in the urine that was measured and not erythropoietin as a substance. We cannot exclude the possibility that some of the erythropoietin made was clinically undetectable because it was abnormal and hence physiologically inactive.

In summary, the normal reticulocyte counts, normal bone marrow morphology with only slight erythroid hyperplasia, normal to slightly reduced bone marrow iron, and normal or decreased erythropoietin excretion, in our patients indicate that their bone marrow was not responding normally to a reduction in red blood cell volume of as much as 40%.

MECHANISMS OF DEPRESSED MARROW FUNCTION

The decrease in the total number of circulating red blood cells in our patients was not due to renal insufficiency, hepatic insufficiency, infection, or lack of substrate, i.e., iron, Vitamin B_{12}, folate, or copper (Table 1). In contrast to our patients, patients with hereditary hemolytic anemias show increases in red blood cell production of eight to ten times normal (Crosby and Akeroyd, 1952). Measurements of red blood cell production by the ferrokinetic procedure and by serial red blood cell volume measurements before and after transfusion of compatible identifiable donor red blood cells, showed that our patients were not producing red blood cells at a rate appropriate to the red blood cell mass deficit. Two different methods were used to study red blood cell production: one measured the incorporation of ^{59}Fe into the cells, and the other was based on an automated differential agglutination procedure combined with serial red blood cell volume measurements using ^{51}Cr. Both methods gave the same results (Table 5) and showed only slight increases in red blood cell production in the patients, rather than the expected significant increases.

The depression of red blood cell production may have been related to the presence of a toxic substance produced after injury. For example, products derived from catecholamines have been shown to suppress hemoglobin synthesis in chick blastoderm (Prasad and Seale, 1969). Toxic substances produced from catecholamines during traumatic injuries might have been responsible for the suppression of erythropoiesis or for the ineffective erythropoiesis observed in studies on the survival of ^{59}Fe-labeled autologous red blood cells (Chapter 4).

One important clinical observation was that the repeated transfusions given to restore the red blood cell mass to normal corrected the hypovolemic state and gradually restored the red blood cell mass to normal. It may be that repeated red blood cell transfusions remove one or more toxic substances involved in the suppression of effective erythropoiesis and in that way lead to restoration of the total number of red blood cells to normal.

Table 5
RED BLOOD CELL PRODUCTION IN NORMAL VOLUNTEERS AND IN PATIENTS WITH CHRONIC TRAUMATIC INJURIES[a]

RBC production		Normals		Chronic injury patients	
		^{59}Fe n = 2	ADA-^{51}Cr n = 0	^{59}Fe n = 12	ADA-^{51}Cr n = 25
g Hb/day	Mean	8.0	—	9.0	8.6
	Range	(8.0—8.1)	—	(5.7—14.5)	(4.5—16.6)
g Hb/kg/day	Mean	0.098	—	0.142	0.133
	Range	(0.097—0.099)	—	(0.086—0.246)	(0.068—0.261)

These values were estimated from the ^{59}Fe incorporation into peripheral red blood cells and from the survival of donor red blood cells and serial ^{51}Cr red blood cell volume measurements. The donor red blood cells were identified and quantitated by the automated differential agglutination procedure.

Chapter 4

RED BLOOD CELL DESTRUCTION

Our patients with traumatic injuries exhibited such marked decreases in red blood cell mass that it was clear that our investigation must include assessment of red blood cell production and destruction. The previous chapter presented evidence of a decrease in red blood cell production, evidently owing to some type of depression of bone marrow function in our patients. The question that immediately arose was whether the red blood cell destruction was normal or abnormal. Hence, it was essential that we study the survivals of both the patient's own red blood cells and the transfused compatible donor red blood cells (Garby and Groth, 1970; International Committee for Standardization in Hematology, 1971; Cooper, 1977).

RED BLOOD CELL SURVIVAL STUDIES

The survival values of the transfused compatible donor red blood cells were found to vary from patient to patient, ranging from normal to slightly, moderately, and occasionally markedly reduced. In 85 to 90% of the patients with traumatic injuries, red blood cell survival curves were monophasic linear or exponential (Figure 1). To measure the patient's red blood cell mass and red blood cell survival, autologous red blood cells were labeled with ^{51}Cr. Measurements were made of the percentage of compatible donor red blood cells in the circulation after transfusion as well as the total amount of donor hemoglobin (Figure 2). The red blood cell mass, measured using ^{51}Cr-labeled autologous red blood cells, and the percentage of donor red blood cells, measured by the automated differential agglutination procedure, were used to calculate red blood cell destruction. This procedure is referred to as the "ADA-^{51}Cr procedure".

The lifespan of the donor red blood cells was measured after transfusion by the automated differential agglutination procedure, and values ranged from 20 to 130 days (Figure 3). Five of 44 patients (11%) studied had donor red blood cell lifespans after transfusion of less than 50 days. Eleven of the 44 patients (25%) had lifespans of 60 to 90 days, 19 (43%) had lifespans of 90 to 110 days, and 9 (20%) had lifespans of 110 to 130 days (Szymanski and Valeri, 1971). In short, it was clear that in some of our patients the transfused red blood cells were being destroyed at an abnormally rapid rate. Three of the patients studied (Figure 1) received two different donor red blood cell populations in a transfusion, each population containing one to four units of ABO and Rh identical and compatible red blood cells. As a rule, two different donor red blood cell populations will have identical lifespans after transfusion (Szymanski and Valeri, 1971). For example, in Case 4F the lifespan of the two compatible-identifiable red blood cell populations had similar lifespans of 104 and 108 days (Figure 1). Also in Patient 4G, the lifespans of the two compatible-identifiable red blood cell populations after transfusion were similar, 106 and 101 days (Figure 1). The values seen in these two patients were close to normal. However, in the case of Patient 4E two identifiable red blood cell populations compatible by the routine in vitro tests had significantly different in vivo survival values: one red blood cell population had a normal lifespan of 127 days and the other a shortened lifespan of 93 days after transfusion (Figure 1). We did not rule out the possibility that the different rates of red blood cell destruction in this particular patient might have been due to the presence of unrecognized incompatible red blood cells in one of the pooled transfusions (Mollison, 1972).

In a group of 11 patients with traumatic injuries, the survivals of autologous ^{51}Cr-

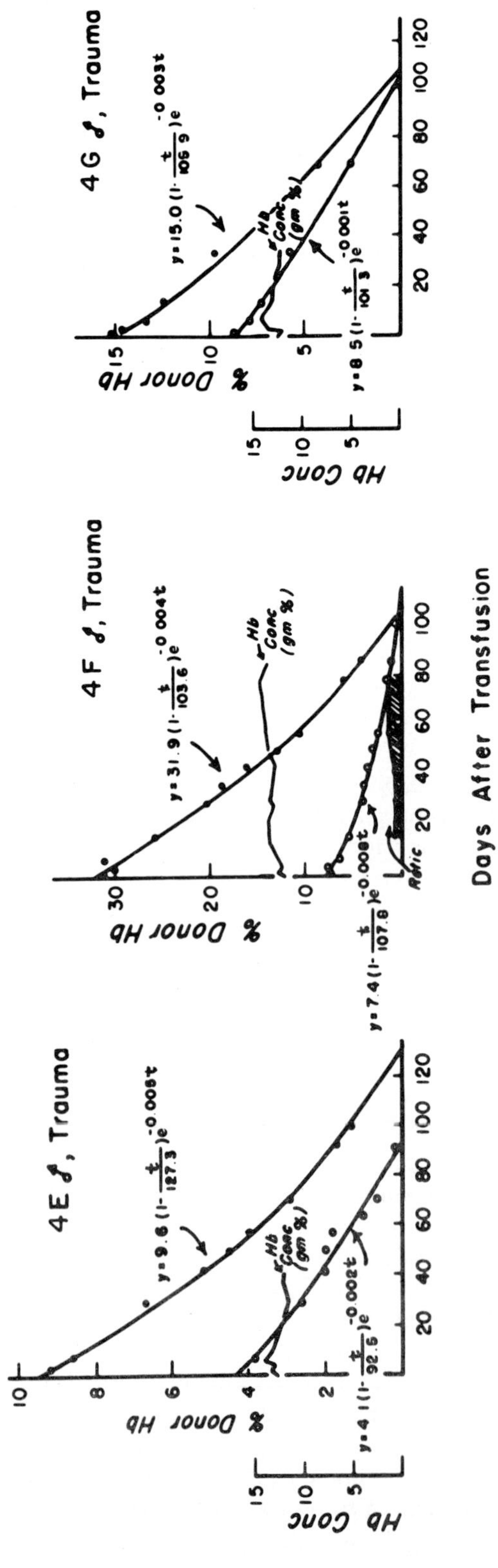

FIGURE 1. The survival of two donor red blood cell populations in each of three patients with traumatic injuries. Each patient was transfused with two populations of donor red blood cells, each population consisting of one to four units of identical red blood cells. The two populations of red blood cells were identified and quantitated by the automated differential agglutination procedure. Reticulocyte counts and hemoglobin concentrations are also reported. (From Szymanski, I. O. and Valeri, C. R., *Vox Sang.*, 21, 97, 1971. With permission of S. Karger AG, Basel.)

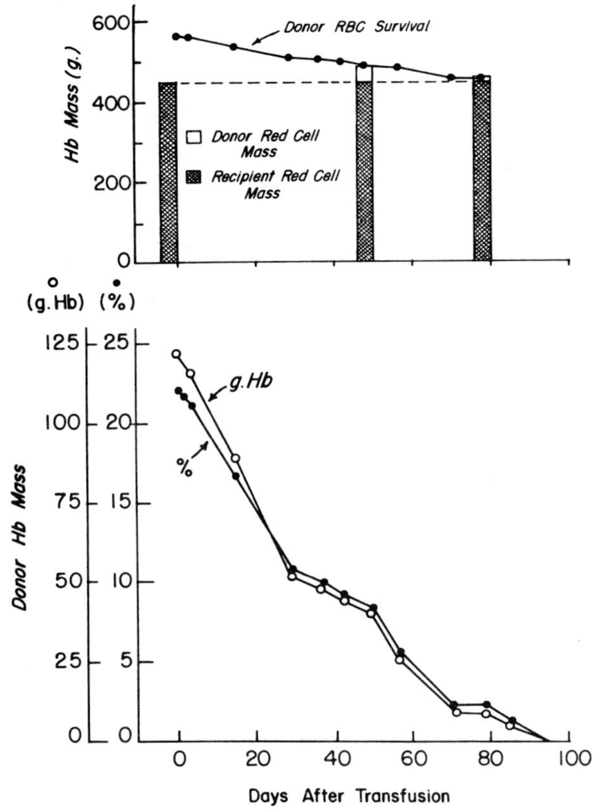

FIGURE 2. The survival of compatible donor red blood cells in a patient with traumatic injuries. The total amount of donor red blood cell-hemoglobin, the percentage of donor hemoglobin, and the total hemoglobin mass consisting of the recipient's red blood cells and the donor red blood cells, are reported during the 3-month posttransfusion period.

labeled red blood cells were within normal limits, with a ^{51}Cr T-½ value of 29.4 days (Figure 4). Survivals of the donor red blood cells in the same 11 patients, measured by the automated differential agglutination procedure, were only slightly reduced, with a lifespan of 95 days (Figure 5).

SIGNIFICANCE OF BIPHASIC RED BLOOD CELL SURVIVAL CURVES

In another group of our patients, survival curves of the donor red blood cells after transfusion were distinguished by being biphasic, suggesting that these patients initially may have possessed a plasma factor that was damaging to the donor red blood cells. This occurred in 10 to 15% of the patients studied by the automated differential agglutination procedure. For example, Figure 6 shows that of three patients, two had biphasic linear survival curves and one patient had a biphasic exponential curve.

In one patient (4A) survival measurements were made of two different populations of transfused donor red blood cells using the automated differential agglutination procedure, and of the patient's own red blood cells labeled with ^{51}Cr. This A-positive patient with traumatic injuries and pneumonia (Figure 7) had received two units of O-

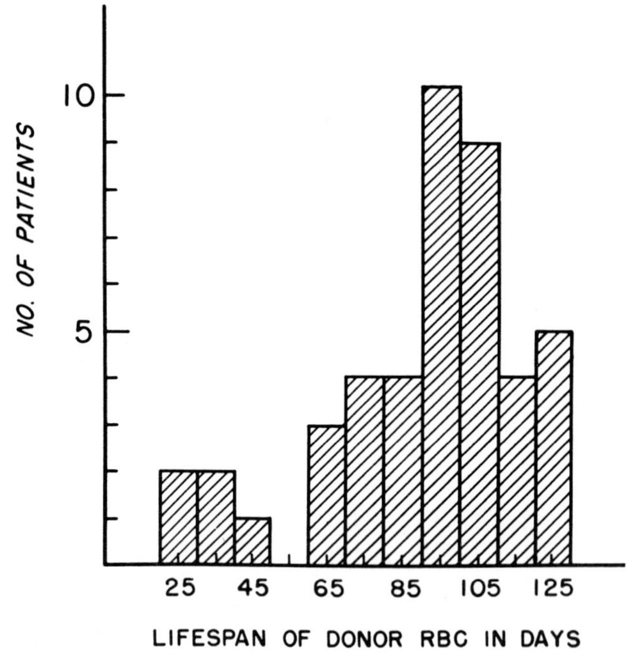

FIGURE 3. Frequency distribution of the red blood cell lifespan in patients with traumatic injuries. (From Szymanski, I. O. and Valeri, C. R., *Vox Sang.*, 21, 97, 1971. With permission of S. Karger AG, Basel.)

positive and two units of O-negative compatible donor red blood cells. The survivals of the two donor red blood cell populations followed biphasic linear curves: in the initial linear phase of the curves, red blood cell survival values were 73 and 79 days, whereas in the second linear phase values were 103 and 109 days. A computer analysis of the data showed that the patient's own ^{51}Cr-labeled red blood cells had a survival of 76 days, a value similar to those in the initial linear phase of each of the two different donor populations (Szymanski and Valeri, 1970). The patient's hemoglobin level increased from 11 to 15 g/100 mℓ of blood following transfusion. His reticulocyte count increased from 1 to 3% during the course of the observations. Between the 20th and 40th day after transfusion, this reticulocytosis was associated with rapid removal of the two transfused donor red blood cell populations that had lifespan values of 73 and 79 days. Between the 40th and 60th day after transfusion, the reticulocyte count decreased from 3 to 1% at the time when the survivals of the two donor red blood cell populations were found to be increased, with linear lifespan values of 103 and 109 days.

In another patient (4B) the lifespan of the transfused donor red blood cell population in the initial phase was 38 days, whereas in the second phase it was 78 days; both components of the biphasic survival curve were linear (Figure 6). In this patient the reticulocyte count increased between the 10th and 50th day of the study, and was the highest when the rate of loss of the donor red blood cells was the greatest.

Although a reduction in the measured survival of transfused red blood cells might be the result of simple dilution of the donor red blood cells with the patient's red blood cells produced at an increased rate, this alone would not explain the observed biphasic survival curves of the two donor red blood cell populations. The observation of bi-

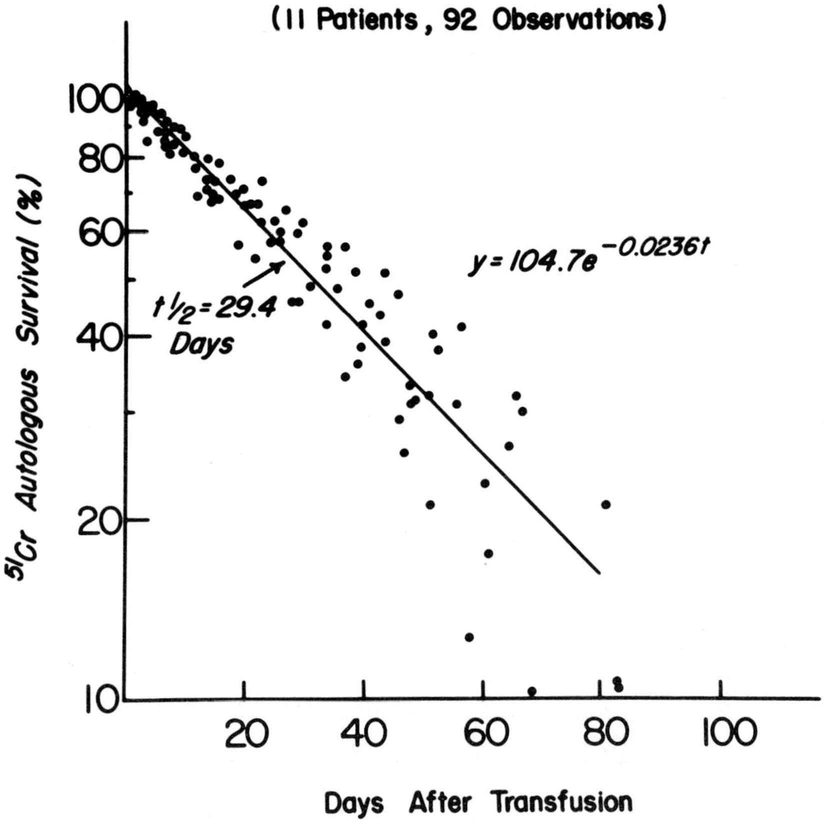

FIGURE 4. The survival of ^{51}Cr-labeled autologous red blood cells in patients with traumatic injuries.

phasic survival curves suggested the removal from the patient's circulation of a toxic substance which had adversely affected the lifespan of the two donor red blood cell populations and of the patient's own red blood cells as well. Our hypothesis is that the presumed toxic substance had two adverse effects — it decreased the survival of the transfused donor red blood cells and impaired erythropoiesis. The disappearance of the presumed toxic substance was accompanied by improvement in the survival of the two donor red blood cell populations as shown by the biphasic survival curves, and by improvement in the patient's red blood cell production as manifested by an increase in the reticulocyte count in peripheral blood. In the three patients reported in Figure 6 with biphasic linear and biphasic exponential red blood cell survival curves, the lifespan in the initial phase ranged from 38 to 60 days, and in the second phase from 78 to 113 days. This would appear to suggest that it took 30 to 40 days after transfusion for the "toxic substance" to be removed from the circulation and for the lifespan to increase.

STUDIES WITH ^{59}Fe-LABELED RED BLOOD CELLS

We also used ^{59}Fe labeling of autologous red blood cells to measure red blood cell destruction. The ^{59}Fe labeling method measures the survival of the patient's newly produced cells, whereas the ADA-^{51}Cr procedure measures the survival of the compatible donor red blood cells which is influenced by the preservation method and by the recipient's state of health (Szymanski and Valeri, 1971).

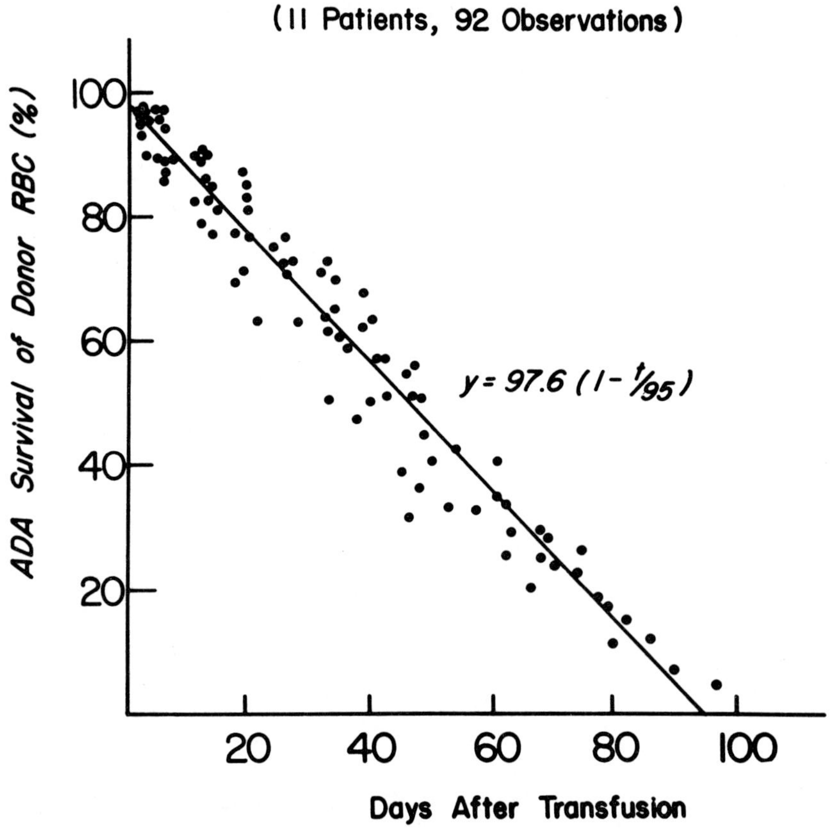

FIGURE 5. Survival of donor red blood cells in patients with traumatic injuries. The survival of compatible donor red blood cells was measured by the automated differential agglutination procedure.

In the normal volunteers, red blood cell destruction measured by the ^{59}Fe method showed 1.02% of red blood cells destroyed per day, whereas the ADA-^{51}Cr method showed 1.06% per day (Table 1); red blood cell lifespan was 98 days with the ^{59}Fe procedure and 94 days with the ADA-^{51}Cr procedure. Thus, in the normal volunteers there were no discrepancies in measurements of red blood cell destruction and lifespan with the two techniques (Table 1). In our patients with traumatic injuries, however, these measurements differed markedly between the two techniques. For instance, in the patients, red blood cell destruction by the ^{59}Fe technique was 1.9%/day compared with 1.14%/day with the ADA-^{51}Cr procedure, and lifespan was 57 days with ^{59}Fe compared with 88 days for the ADA-^{51}Cr procedure (Table 1).

The findings in our patients of normal survivals of ^{51}Cr-labeled autologous red blood cells and of only slightly reduced survivals of compatible homologous red blood cells with the ADA-^{51}Cr technique were not truly indicative of what was going on in these patients (Table 1 and Figures 4 and 5). The ^{59}Fe data gave a more accurate picture, showing that the patient's newly produced red blood cells or some part of them were being destroyed shortly after they reached the peripheral blood. The patients were destroying their own newly-produced red blood cells at a greater rate than they were destroying the compatible donor red blood cells or their own circulating red blood cells. It became evident that at least one of the causes of the reduced red blood cell volume was the presence of ineffective erythropoiesis in our patients.

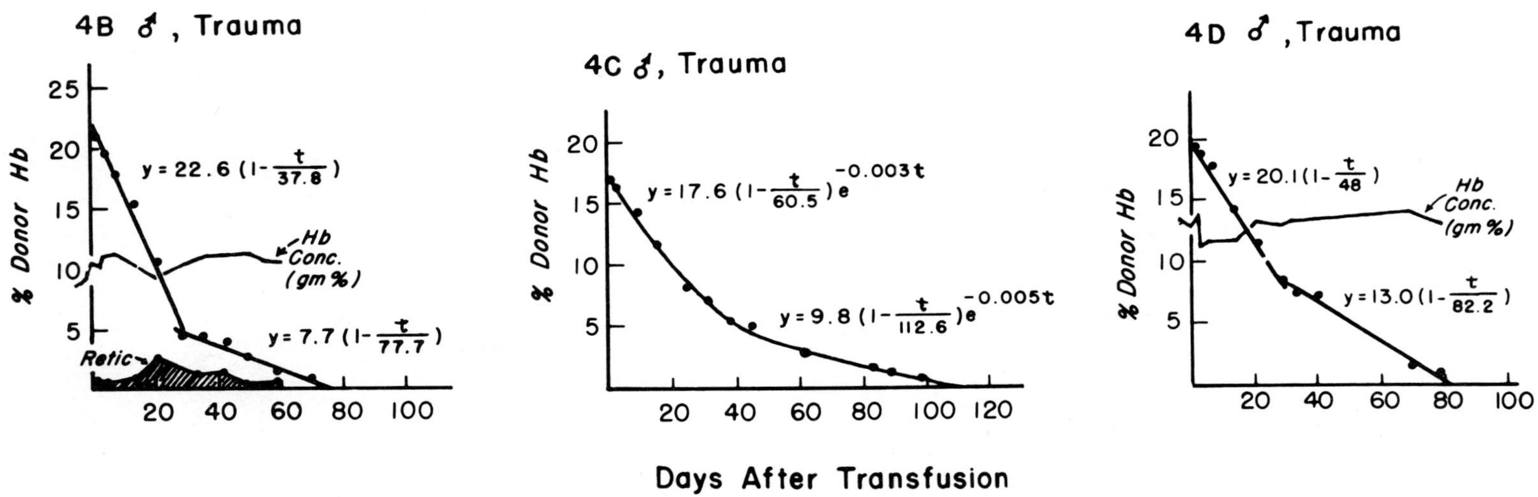

FIGURE 6. The survival of compatible donor red blood cells in each of three patients with traumatic injuries. Compatible donor red blood cells were transfused and the survival of the donor red blood cells reported as percent donor hemoglobin. The reticulocyte counts and the hemoglobin concentrations are also reported. (From Szymanski, I. O. and Valeri, C. R., *Vox Sang.*, 21, 97, 1971. With permission of S. Karger AG, Basel.)

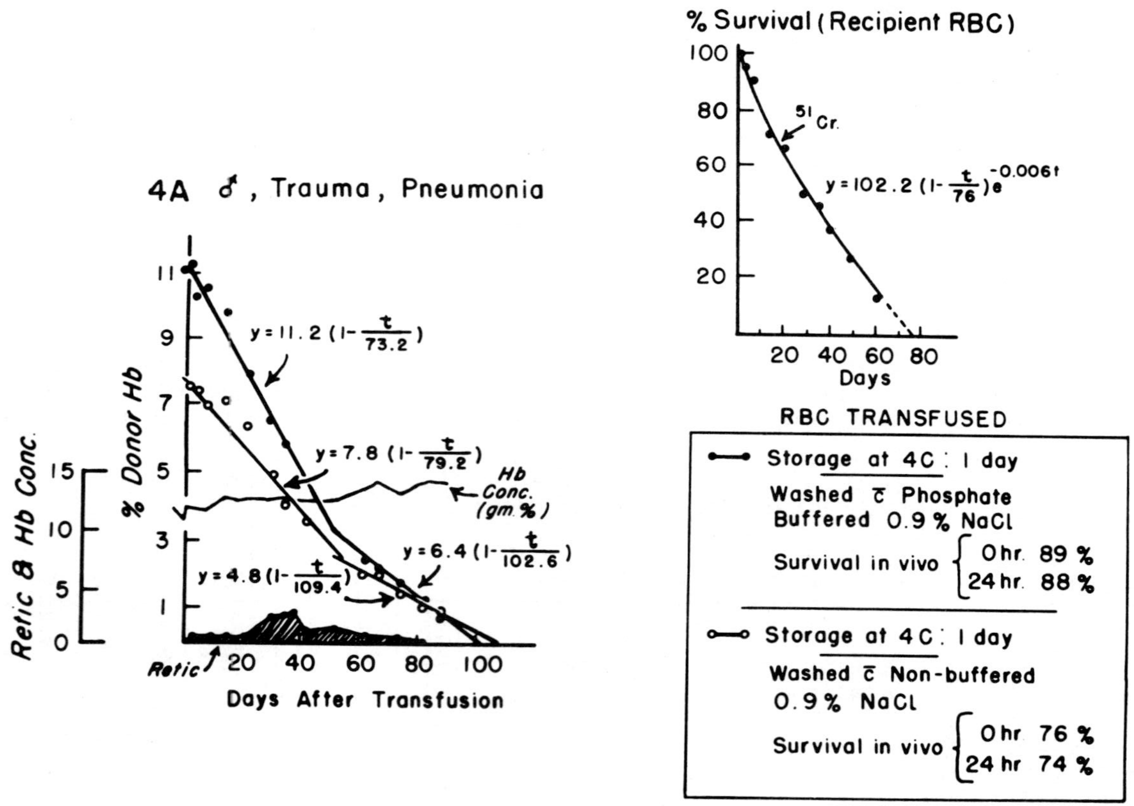

FIGURE 7. The survival of two pooled populations of compatible and identifiable donor red blood cells measured using the automated differential agglutination procedure and the measurement of the patient's red blood cells using the ^{51}Cr labeling procedure. The patient, 4A, was A-positive and received two units of O-positive and two units of O-negative. Red blood cells were identified and quantitated in his circulation using the automated differential agglutination procedure. The reticulocyte count was measured during the 80-day posttransfusion period. (From Szymanski, I. O. and Valeri, C. R., *Vox Sang.*, 21, 97, 1971. With permission of S. Karger AG, Basel.)

Table 1
RED BLOOD CELL DESTRUCTION MEASURED IN NORMAL VOLUNTEERS AND IN PATIENTS WITH CHRONIC TRAUMATIC INJURIES

		Normal volunteers		Chronic injury patients	
		^{59}Fe	ADA-^{51}Cr	^{59}Fe	ADA-^{51}Cr
% RBC/day	Mean	1.02	1.06	1.903	1.14
	Range	(0.99—1.04)	(0.93—1.20)	(1.26—3.4)	(0.91—2.86)
	N	2	6	12	25
Lifespan (days)	Mean	98	94	57	88
	Range	(96—100)	(83—108)	(41—82)	(35—110)
	N	2	6	12	25

Note: Destruction of autologous ^{59}Fe-labeled red blood cells was measured. Destruction of donor red blood cells was estimated from measurements of the recipient's ^{51}Cr red blood cell mass and the survival of the donor red blood cells measured by the automated differential agglutination procedure.

We have already discussed the clinical observation that the blood loss in hemorrhagic shock usually is not as great as the volume of red blood cells required to restore the red blood cell volume to normal. Although there is general agreement among physicians that the blood replacement should be several times greater than the observed blood loss, the nature of this discrepancy still is not fully understood. Suzuki and his associates (1964, 1965) reported that the low red blood cell mass in patients undergoing extensive surgical procedures can be explained by the presence of a noncirculating red blood cell volume, i.e., a sequestered red blood cell volume in the peripheral circulation. These investigators described a rapidly circulating red blood cell volume, a slowly circulating red blood cell volume, and a noncirculating red blood cell volume, in patients following extensive surgical procedures. In addition, they reported that the noncirculating red blood cell volume could be mobilized by low viscosity dextran infusions (Suzuki et al., 1965). In our patients with traumatic injuries, studies made before and after surgical procedures revealed no evidence of a noncirculating red blood cell volume. Rather, some of the patients appeared to be destroying both their own and the transfused compatible donor red blood cells, usually at an accelerated rate. Nevertheless, we decided to make additional studies to investigate whether the transfused blood was being trapped in the wounds and to establish the degree of destruction and of sequestration.

STUDIES OF RED BLOOD CELLS LABELED WITH ^{59}Fe AND ^{51}CR

The patient's own red blood cells were labeled in vivo by infusion of ^{59}Fe citrate. Eight days after infusion 80 to 90% of the ^{59}Fe was incorporated into the peripheral blood cells (the rest of the tagged iron was presumably incorporated into such ferroenzymes as might be made rapidly, e.g., the lining cells of the intestine which have a lifespan of 48 to 72 hr. The ^{59}Fe-labeled red blood cells were collected, labeled in vitro with disodium ^{51}chromate, and reinfused into the patients. Stools, wound dressings, and urine samples were collected prior to and for up to 30 days after infusion of these doubly-labeled red blood cells. The radioactivity in the stools, wounds, and urine samples on each patient was measured in a shielded total body scintillation counter with two 8 × 4 in. NaI crystals, one above and one below each sample. In each patient the same standards were counted first with the blood samples in a well counter and then with the stools, wound dressings, and urine samples in a total body counter. Ratios of ^{59}Fe to ^{51}Cr in the blood samples were calculated and compared to those in the stools, wound dressings, and urine samples. The calculations of the ^{59}Fe to ^{51}Cr ratios were made as follows:

1. Standards and blood samples were counted together in a gamma well counter system with a 3-in. well-type scintillation detector.
2. The same standards, and the stool, wound dressing, and urine samples were counted together in a total body counter in order to correct for counting efficiency and decay rates of ^{59}Fe and ^{51}Cr.
3. Ratios of ^{59}Fe to ^{51}Cr were established in the blood samples.
4. Two different correction factors, one for ^{59}Fe and the other for ^{51}Cr, were established.
5. Stool, wound dressing, and urine samples were counted, and the ratios were calculated and compared to that observed in the blood.

The data showed that in five of the six patients with traumatic injuries studied, a greater excess of ^{51}Cr was found in the stool samples than in the blood samples (Figure 8), indicating that red blood cells were lysed in the gastrointestinal tract. Evidently the ^{59}Fe released by lysis of the red blood cells was reutilized and did not reach the stool. The result was a very low ^{59}Fe to ^{51}Cr ratio in the stool compared to the blood, a finding previously discussed by others (Holt, 1960; Pierson et al., 1961). In all six patients ^{51}Cr alone was found in the urine, a finding attesting to the destruction of the ^{51}Cr-tagged red blood cells (Figure 8). An absence of tagged iron in the urine indicated that the release of ^{59}Fe during hemolysis was followed by major reutilization as well as by excretion of a small portion of it in the stool. The presence of chromium in the urine indicated that the portion of the hemoglobin molecule to which it was bound, the globin, was degraded and its fragments metabolized.

In four of the six patients studied, only ^{59}Fe was present in the wound dressings (Figure 8), suggesting that the ^{59}Fe was preferentially deposited in granulation tissue. Since the ^{59}Fe isotope labels the heme portion of hemoglobin and the ^{51}Cr isotope labels the globin portion of hemoglobin, the data suggest that the red blood cells in the wounds were lysed and degraded, leaving behind heme or porphyrin labeled with ^{59}Fe, while the ^{51}Cr-labeled globin was metabolized and ^{51}Cr excreted in the urine.

FECAL UROBILINOGEN MEASUREMENTS

In short, these studies showed that radionuclide-labeled red blood cells were actually destroyed. Some of the iron was reutilized and some was deposited in the wounds, and the chromium was excreted in the urine and stool. No red blood cells were trapped in the wounds, although heme or porphyrin, or both, derived from red blood cell-hemoglobin, was found there.

We attempted to calculate the amount of red blood cell destruction by measuring the breakdown products of these cells. The catabolism of red blood cell-hemoglobin usually occurs with the opening of the alpha-methene bridge of protoporphyrin. This releases equimolar quantities of carbon monoxide and unfolds the porphyrin molecule so that it produces bilirubin and urobilinogen (Mann et al., 1926; Wasserman et al., 1942; Flink and Skubi, 1946; London, 1950; London et al., 1950; Watson, 1965; Robinson et al., 1967; Barrett et al., 1968; Coburn and Kane, 1968; Bernstein et al., 1969; Landaw et al., 1970; Robinson and Tsong, 1970; Lightner and Quistad, 1971; Ostrow, 1971; Schmid, 1972; Komazawa et al., 1975; Bergan et al., 1977; White, 1977; Smith

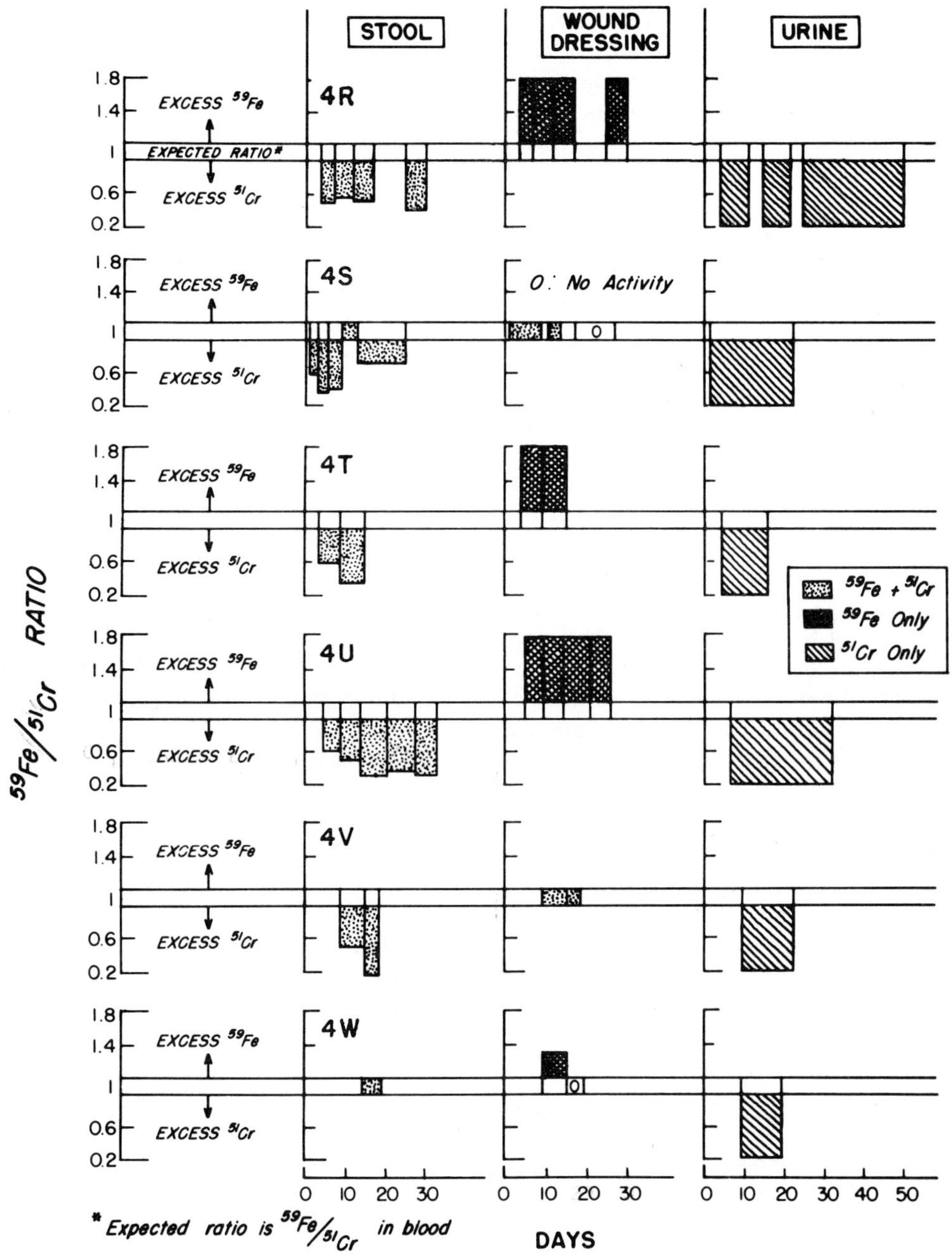

FIGURE 8. The distribution of ^{59}Fe and ^{51}Cr in the stool, wound dressings, and urine of patients who received ^{59}Fe citrate intravenously to study red blood cell production. The ^{59}Fe red blood cells of these patients were labeled in vitro with ^{51}Cr to measure the red blood cell volume and the survival of their own red blood cells. The ratio of ^{59}Fe to ^{51}Cr in the blood was compared to the ratio found in the stools, wound dressings, and urine in the six patients with traumatic injuries.

et al., 1979). This pathway of hemoglobin degradation is usually referred to as the classic pathway. The calculation of red blood cell destruction from measurements of the degradation of hemoglobin into fecal urobilinogen is based on the assumption that for each gram of red blood cell-hemoglobin destroyed, 35 mg of fecal urobilinogen are produced. Thus, fecal urobilinogen output has been used to assess red blood cell destruction in hereditary hemolytic anemia (Crosby and Akeroyd, 1952). However, this test underestimates the hemoglobin degradation and even under the best of circumstances, as in animal experiments for example, the measurement of urobilinogen output accounts for only 70% of hemoglobin degradation. Accordingly, the validity of this approach was examined as part of our investigations.

In Case 4H an incompatible blood transfusion was accompanied by the excretion of increased amounts of fecal urobilinogen during the 48-hr posttransfusion period (Figure 9). In Case 4I, who had received four units of 3-week-old red blood cells, the 260 g of compatible red blood cell-hemoglobin contained 78 g of hemoglobin from nonviable red blood cells (Figure 9), and the breakdown products of the nonviable donor red blood cells were detected 7 days after the transfusion (Figure 9). In both these cases, the amount of measured fecal urobilinogen would account for only about 40% of the estimated loss of red blood cell-hemoglobin. Studies also were made during a time when the normal healthy volunteers and the patients with traumatic injuries were not receiving red blood cell transfusions to assess the destruction of red blood cell-hemoglobin from measurements of fecal urobilinogen. These tests showed that the *normal volunteers* excreted larger amounts of fecal urobilinogen and destroyed larger amounts of hemoglobin per day than did the *nontransfused patients* (Table 2). The nontransfused patients who were on systemic antibiotic therapy excreted smaller amounts of fecal urobilinogen than patients not receiving antibiotics (Table 3). There have been reports in the literature to suggest that nonabsorbable antibiotics reduce the bacterial flora of the gastrointestinal tract and thereby impair the degradation of bilirubin to fecal urobilinogen. Our data tend to support this theory (Table 3).

In our attempts to quantitate the compatible nonviable red blood cells removed from the circulation following transfusion, measurements were made of fecal urobilinogen excretion in three patients who were receiving systemic antibiotics and five patients who were not so treated (Figure 10). In the three patients receiving systemic antibiotics, no fecal urobilinogen was detected during the 3- to 6-day period following the transfusion, and donor red blood cell-hemoglobin removed during the 3-day posttransfusion period and measured by the automated differential agglutination procedure ranged from 20 to 57 g. In the five patients not receiving antibiotics, the amount of fecal urobilinogen detected from the destruction of transfused red blood cell-hemoglobin during the 3- to 6-day posttransfusion period ranged from 11 to 38% of what it should theoretically have been; 12 to 61 g of red blood cell-hemoglobin was removed from the circulation (Figure 10).

It was clear that the products of red blood cell-hemoglobin degradation in the form of fecal urobilinogen could not account for the loss of red blood cell-hemoglobin seen in our patients with traumatic injuries. The patients on systemic antibiotic therapy excreted very little fecal urobilinogen, and those not on antibiotic therapy excreted only about 25% of the expected value (Figure 10). In addition, there was no increase in plasma hemoglobin or bilirubin and no decrease in serum haptoglobin level in our patients (Brus and Lewis, 1959; Langley et al., 1962; Shinton et al., 1965; Sears, 1970). These findings suggested to us that perhaps an alternate pathway of hemoglobin degradation was involved, one that did not produce fecal urobilinogen degradation products (Tables 2 and 3).

CARBON MONOXIDE PRODUCTION

Carbon monoxide production was another measurement we made in an attempt to estimate the degradation of red blood cell-hemoglobin in our patients. In the catabo-

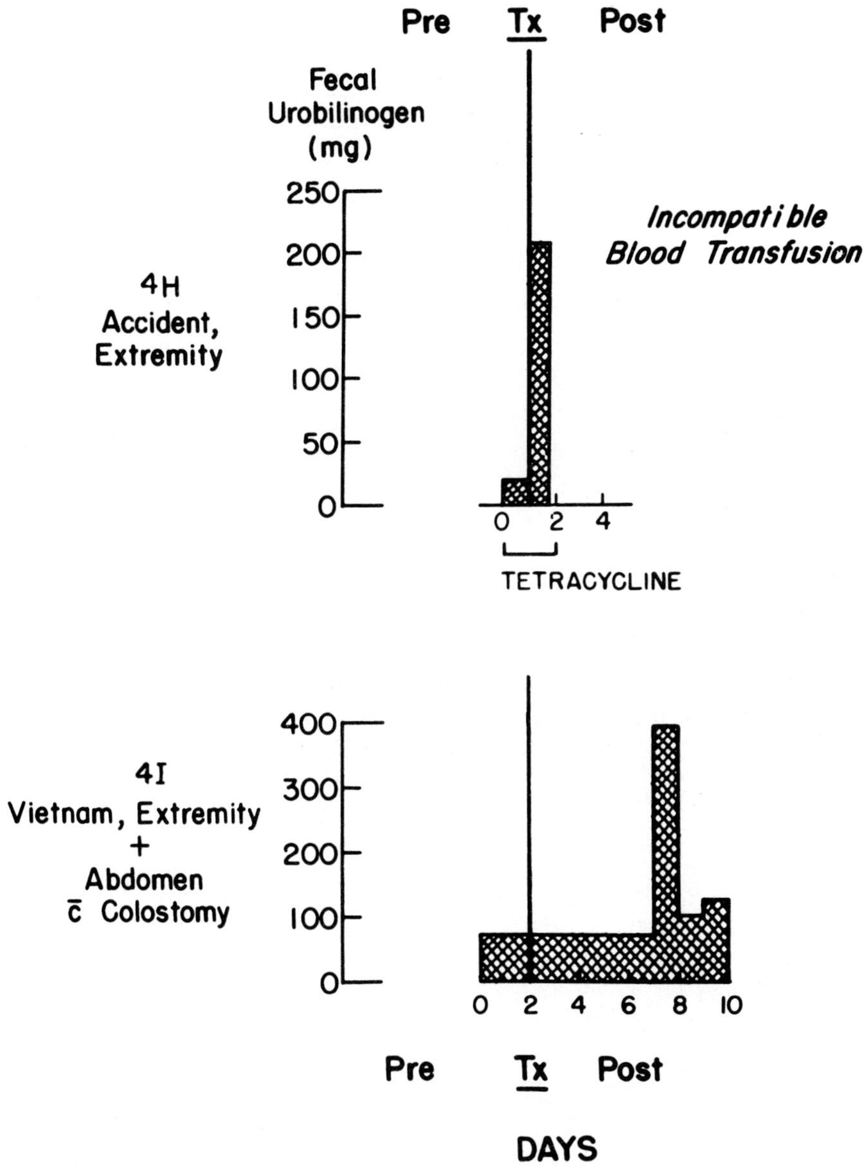

FIGURE 9. The fecal urobilinogen excretion following red blood cell transfusions is shown. Patient 4H had an incompatible red blood cell transfusion reaction, and Patient 4I with a colostomy received four units of red blood cell concentrates stored at 4°C for 3 weeks.

lism of the iron-protoporphyrin of hemoglobin, the opening of the protoporphyrin ring at the alpha-methene bridge releases a molecule of carbon monoxide. The carbon monoxide is released from the alpha-methene bridge carbon atom of heme (Ayres et al., 1965, 1966; Coburn et al., 1966, 1967; White et al., 1967; Coltman et al., 1969; Engel et al., 1969; Rodkey et al., 1969; Logue et al., 1971; Lynch and Moede, 1972; White, 1977; Clark et al., 1978; Werner, 1978). Hence, the degradation of red blood cell-hemoglobin is an endogenous metabolic source of carbon monoxide. The rate of production of carbon monoxide can be measured in the patient's blood from an increase in carboxyhemoglobin. These data have been used to calculate the lifespan of

Table 2
FECAL UROBILINOGEN EXCRETION IN NORMAL VOLUNTEERS AND NONTRANSFUSED PATIENTS WITH TRAUMATIC INJURIES

		Fecal urobilinogen (mg/day)	=	Calculated hemoglobin destroyed[a] (g/day)	% of red cell mass
Normal volunteers	Mean	95.4		2.7	0.415
(n = 8)	S.D.	38.4		—	0.166
	S.E.	13.6		—	0.058
	Range	57—133		—	0.23—0.66
Traumatic injuries	Mean	75.0		2.1	0.492
(n = 12)	S.D.	46.4		—	0.287
	S.E.	12.4		—	0.077
	Range	20—208		—	0.14—1.10

[a] Each gram of hemoglobin destroyed = 35 mg of fecal urobilinogen.

Table 3
FECAL UROBILINOGEN EXCRETION IN NORMAL VOLUNTEERS AND NONTRANSFUSED PATIENTS WITH TRAUMATIC INJURIES WITH AND WITHOUT ANTIBIOTIC THERAPY

		Fecal urobilinogen (mg/day)	=	Calculated hemoglobin destroyed[a] (g/day)	% of red cell mass
Normal volunteers	Mean	95.4		2.7	0.415
(n = 8)	S.D.	38.4		—	0.166
	S.E.	13.6		—	0.058
	Range	57—133		—	0.23—0.66
Traumatic injuries	Mean	74.3		2.1	0.520
— no antibiotic	S.D.	28.5		—	0.268
treatment (n = 8)	S.E.	10.1		—	0.094
	Range	41—134		—	0.25—1.03
Traumatic injuries	Mean	50.3		1.4	0.338
— antibiotic	S.D.	21.2		—	0.136
treatment (n = 4)	S.E.	10.6		—	0.068
	Range	20—66		—	0.14—0.44

[a] Each gram of hemoglobin destroyed = 35 mg of fecal urobilinogen.

red blood cells, assuming that 15% of the carbon monoxide does not originate from destroyed red blood cells. Our carbon monoxide studies, which were done in collaboration with Dr. F. L. Rodkey of the Naval Medical Research Institute, Bethesda, Maryland, showed no increase in carbon monoxide production in our patients with traumatic injuries under basal conditions. A subsequent study of other patients before and after the transfusion of multiple units of compatible preserved red blood cells also gave no sign of an increase in carboxyhemoglobin related to the degradation of the nonviable red blood cells present in the transfused blood products.

The absence of any apparent increase in the normal breakdown products of hemo-

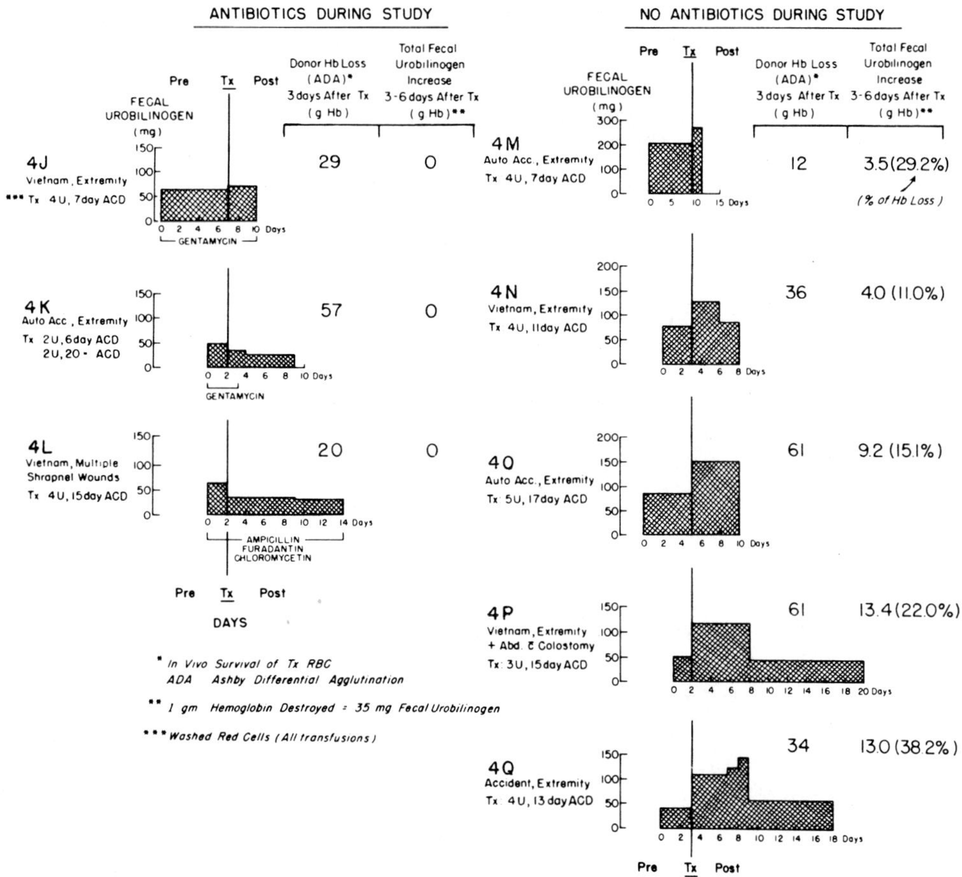

FIGURE 10. The fecal urobilinogen excretion prior to and following transfusion of compatible donor red blood cells is shown. Three patients were treated with systemic antibiotics during the study and five patients were not.

globin, i.e., fecal urobilinogen, suggested an alternative pathway of red blood cell-hemoglobin degradation in our patients, with production of porphyrins and iron. Our failure to detect an increase in carbon monoxide production may have been an indication of the integrity of the alpha-methene bridge, preventing release of carbon monoxide and unfolding of the protoporphyrin molecule to produce fecal urobilinogen breakdown products. On the other hand, it may have been that the method used for detection of carboxyhemoglobin was not adequate.

PORPHYRIN PATHWAY OF HEMOGLOBIN DEGRADATION

Published data have shown that some substances will degrade hemoglobin into porphyrin and iron without producing the bilirubin-urobilinogen complex (Veech et al., 1967; Rowlands et al., 1968). For example, hemoglobin may be degraded into porphyrin and iron when metabolites of catecholamines are present (Figure 11), and epinephrine in plasma can be degraded into adrenochrome-adrenolutin and melanin (Figure 12) (Hochstein and Cohen, 1963; Hegedus and Altschule, 1967, 1968, 1970a, 1970b; Janssen and Discher, 1967; Houlihan et al., 1968; van Woert, 1968; Altschule et al., 1969; Shafritz et al., 1969; Lalone and Houlihan, 1971; Misra and Fridovich, 1972; Valeri et al., 1972; Brunori et al., 1975; Altschule and Hegedus, 1976; Babior and Kipnes, 1976; Hegedus, 1977).

HEMOLYSIS PATHWAYS

A) ORDINARY

A) INTRAVASCULAR
HGB IN URINE

B) IN RE CELLS
HGB → HEME → BILIRUBIN + Fe
↘ GLOBIN

B) CATECHOLAMINE METABOLITES

HGB → HEME → PORPHYRIN + Fe
↘ GLOBIN

FIGURE 11. Schematic diagram showing the classic pathway of red blood cell destruction resulting in hemoglobinemia and hemoglobinuria, and red blood cell destruction within the reticuloendothelial tissues producing bilirubin-urobilinogen breakdown products. Red blood cell destruction may also produce porphyrins in the presence of catecholamine metabolites.

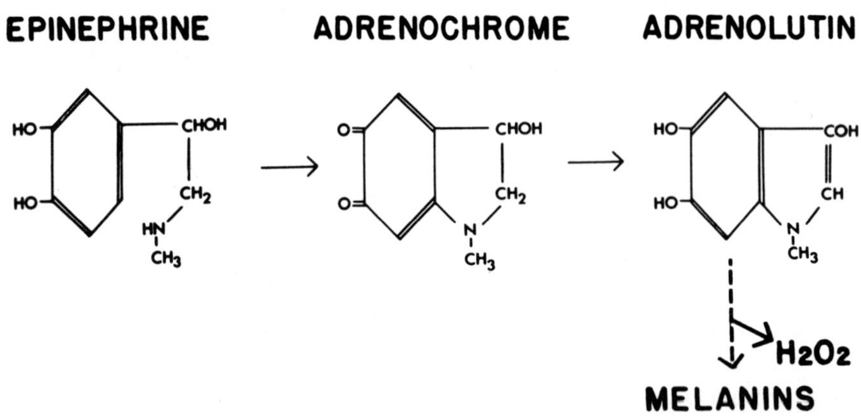

FIGURE 12. The degradation of epinephrine in plasma into adrenochrome, adrenolutin, and into melanins with the production of hydrogen peroxide is shown. (Reproduced with kind permission from PJD Publications Limited, Westbury, N.Y., and S. Karger AG, Basel. From Valeri, C. R., Altschule, M. D., and Pivacek, L. E., *Journal of Medicine,* 3: 20—24, 1972.)

The observation in our patients of destruction of both the patient's own red blood cells and the compatible donor red blood cells without detection of the usual breakdown product of fecal urobilinogen might have been due to a degradation of red blood cell-hemoglobin into porphyrins. Porphyrin materials are excreted in the urine and they also accumulate in granulation tissue (Figge et al., 1948; Kikkawa et al., 1955; Rasmussen-Taxdal et al., 1955; Cohen, 1963; Kopper, 1964; Stone et al., 1964; Williams and Bridges, 1964; O'Shaughnessy et al., 1966; Stone, 1966; Nemir et al., 1967;

Haining et al., 1969; Sauer and Funk, 1969; Pimstone et al., 1971; Gemsa et al., 1972). Data have been reported demonstrating that hemoglobin in the presence of adrenolutin, for example, can be degraded in vitro into porphyrins (Veech et al., 1967); other free radicles act similarly (Rowlands et al., 1968). Whether or not carbon monoxide is produced by degradation of hemoglobin through this alternate pathway is not known (Pimstone et al., 1971).

Our next undertaking was to search for degradation products of hemoglobin in the form of oxyporphyrin, dipyrroles, and monopyrroles in the urine, feces, and tissue, and in this endeavor we were fortunate to have the expertise of several other investigators. The dipyrroles were measured in the stool and urine samples of our patients by Dr. Martha Kreimer-Birnbaum and Dr. Robin M. Bannerman of the Health Sciences Center at the State University of New York, Buffalo General Hospital, Buffalo, New York. Six lyophilized urine samples were found to be negative for dipyrroles, and the fecal excretion of dipyrroles was not increased (Kreimer-Birnbaum et al., 1966). Attempts in our laboratory to measure monopyrroles in the urine were not successful.

Dr. Donald Borg and Dr. Donald vander Kolk of the Brookhaven National Laboratory, Upton, New York, used emission spectrophotometry to assay the lyophilized urines obtained from three of our patients with traumatic injuries and from three normal healthy individuals. The urines of the three patients that were excited at 465 mu revealed a yellow fluorescent material at 490 to 530 mu in amounts twice that found in the normal urines, but it was only at the excitation band at 465 mu that the urines of the patients differed from those of the normal persons. The yellow fluorescent material had its emission maximum at a wavelength consistent with that of oxyporphyrin.

To study further the possibility that the breakdown products of the red blood cell-hemoglobin might be degraded to porphyrin-type substances that fluoresce, the granulation tissues of the patients' wounds were observed under ultraviolet light. Granulation tissue, which is known to accumulate porphyrins, is rich in fluorescent material, much or all of it being porphyrin in nature. Fluorescent materials were searched for in the granulation tissue of the wounds of the extremities using an ultraviolet lamp at wavelengths of 2600 Å and 3500 Å. Studies were made before and after the transfusion of multiple units of compatible donor red blood cells. As discussed previously, nonviable compatible preserved donor red blood cells were destroyed with little production of fecal urobilinogen breakdown products of red blood cell-hemoglobin and with no increase in carbon monoxide production. Observation under an ultraviolet lamp with a wavelength of 3500 Å revealed little fluorescence in the wounds prior to the transfusion, but during the 72-hr posttransfusion period a golden yellow fluorescence appeared in granulation tissue at the wound margin. The golden yellow fluorescence first appeared within 2 to 4 hr after transfusion, persisted during the 24- to 72-hr posttransfusion period, and then disappeared into the bluish background. It seemed clear from all these studies that the breakdown of donor cells in our patients was accompanied not by the production of bile pigments but by the production of oxyporphyrin-like substances.

KNOWN FACTORS CONTRIBUTING TO HEMOLYSIS

Other tests also were employed to learn the mechanism of the reduced survival of red blood cells in our patients with traumatic injuries. Hemolysis as a result of Heinz body-type hemolytic anemia was ruled out because the response of the red blood cells to oxidative stress using acetylphenylhydrazine showed normal Heinz body response (Table 4). Likewise, no similarity to paroxysmal nocturnal hemoglobinuria was observed. The sugar water test was negative (Hartmann and Jenkins, 1966), and tests for

Table 4
SUSCEPTIBILITY OF THE RED BLOOD CELLS TO ACETYLPHENYLHYDRAZINE OXIDATIVE HEMOLYSIS

Heinz Bodies (normal 0—20%)	Miscellaneous diagnoses	Traumatic injuries with antibiotics	Traumatic injuries without antibiotics
N	15	21	25
Mean	19.2	11.9	10.7
S.D.	12.9	9.3	2.9
S.E.	3.2	2.0	0.6

hemosiderin gave negative results in the urine. Studies on lipid peroxidation of the red blood cells (Kaplan, 1967; Hyde and Rawson, 1969; Carolla et al., 1974; Henderson et al., 1978; Yoshioka et al., 1979) were not done, however.

The normal red blood cell morphology, negative Heinz body test, negative sugar water test, normal osmotic fragility — all indicated no intrinsic abnormality in the patient's own red blood cells. The data did suggest that one or more extracorpuscular factors might have been involved in the reduced survival of the patient's own red blood cells and of the compatible donor red blood cells in the circulation. The findings of shortened and biphasic survival of compatible donor red blood cells supported the idea of the presence of an extracorpuscular factor(s), a toxic substance, which might also have been responsible for the observed suppression of red blood cell production and ineffective erythropoiesis (Chapter 3).

There was no clear histologic evidence that bone marrow function was depressed in the syndrome discussed here (Chapter 3). However, in massive hemolysis (Kattlove et al., 1970) and in febrile states (Clark and Davidson, 1972) bone marrow macrophages have been found to contain a lipofuscin pigment. The pigment is believed to comprise remnants of ingested cells or of material derived from cell fragments. These granules are called hemosiderin because of their yellow color; however, they contain no iron and they fluoresce like lipofuscin. Lipofuscin is made up of oxidized unsaturated fatty acids, combined with protein and melanin. It would be interesting to know whether these granules accumulate in the bone marrow in patients with the hypovolemic anemia of trauma.

Red blood cell destruction has been studied in animals and men in hemorrhagic shock (Hardaway et al., 1964, 1979; Suzuki et al., 1964, 1965; Hardaway, 1978; Heideman et al., 1978); in burns (Troell et al., 1955; Loebl et al., 1973); and in traumatic shock (Bergentz and Danon, 1965; Dern, 1968; Taube et al., 1971). Results of these studies suggest the presence in blood of extracorpuscular substances that are released from injured tissue and produce hemolysis (McKay et al., 1969; Whitaker et al., 1969; Liu, 1971). Although these findings have not received much support, our results generally are in agreement with them.

SUSCEPTIBILITY OF THE RED BLOOD CELLS TO HEMOLYSIS CAUSED BY ADRENOCHROME

Because adrenochrome, an epinephrine metabolite, hemolyzes red blood cells in vitro, we decided to use it in an in vitro test to determine susceptibility of the red blood cells to hemolysis (Valeri et al., 1972). An additional factor in our decision to use this particular substance was the fact that adrenolutin, its isomer, breaks down hemoglobin in the production not of bilirubin but of protoporphyrin (Veech et al., 1967). Moreover, adrenochrome is stable but adrenolutin is not (Figure 12). Admittedly, this type of testing is not very sophisticated, but it was the only one available to us at the time. Blood for this test was collected in the acid-citrate-dextrose anticoagulant from 26 patients and 9 healthy volunteers. The blood of each was incubated in the absence and presence of adrenochrome under sterile conditions at 37°C for 48 hr.. The hemolysis of the red blood cells was quantitated by measuring the supernatant hemoglobin concentration using the benzidine reaction or the supernatant optical density at 400 mu.

Blood samples from 18 of 26 patients so studied exhibited increases in hemolysis similar to those in blood samples from healthy volunteers after incubation *with* adrenochrome (Group A, Figure 13), whereas samples from the other eight patients (Group B, Figure 13) showed greater increases in hemolysis than were seen in the normal controls. After incubation without adrenochrome, increases in hemolysis were not significantly different in the blood samples from the 26 patients and in the 9 normal volunteers.

Further studies were made of blood samples from 14 patients over a 4-month period of treatment with surgical debridement of wounds, antibiotic treatment, and transfusions of washed liquid-stored red blood cells and washed previously frozen red blood cells. During this 4-month period of follow-up, nine blood samples incubated *without* adrenochrome showed decreases in hemolysis toward normal from their initially increased values (Figure 14). One blood sample (Case G in Figure 14) that initially had shown minimal hemolysis subsequently showed significant hemolysis. Eight blood samples incubated *with* adrenochrome showed lessening degrees of hemolysis during this 4-month follow-up period (Figure 15).

Incubation with adrenochrome produced significantly increased hemolysis in the blood samples of about 30% of the patients with traumatic injuries. No significant increase in hemolysis was seen when blood samples from anemic patients with neoplastic disorders and infection were incubated with adrenochrome (Figure 16).

EVIDENCE OF A PLASMA FACTOR AFFECTING HEMOLYSIS

Further studies were made to determine the cause of the increased hemolysis in blood incubated with adrenochrome (4X, 4Y, and 4Z) (Figure 17). Studies were made of: (a) the red blood cells and plasma obtained from heparinized blood of the patient, (b) normal washed compatible donor red blood cells incubated with the patient's heparinized plasma, and (c) washed red blood cells of the patient incubated with normal compatible donor heparinized plasma. Each of the red blood cell-plasma mixtures was incubated with adrenochrome at 37°C for 48 hr (Figure 17), and the level of hemolysis in each mixture after incubation was measured. In Case 4X, the level of hemolysis was increased to the same degree whether the patient's plasma was combined with his own red blood cells or with normal compatible washed donor red blood cells. In Case 4Y, the mixture of normal compatible donor plasma with the patient's washed red blood cells resulted in the least hemolysis, while the greatest hemolysis was seen when the patient's plasma was combined with normal washed compatible donor red blood cells. Conversely, in Case 4Z, similar levels of hemolysis regardless of the combination of red blood cell-plasma mixture were observed (Figure 17). These data suggest the presence or lack of a substance in plasma of patients with traumatic injuries which causes increased hemolysis in the presence of adrenochrome.

In another study, serum samples from ten other seriously wounded patients in Danang, South Vietnam, were collected before operation and 3 hr and 24 hr after, and were shipped in the frozen state to our laboratory for evaluation (Figure 18). These patients had received initial resuscitation with colloid, crystalloid, and blood products to treat the hemorrhagic shock related to their trauma.

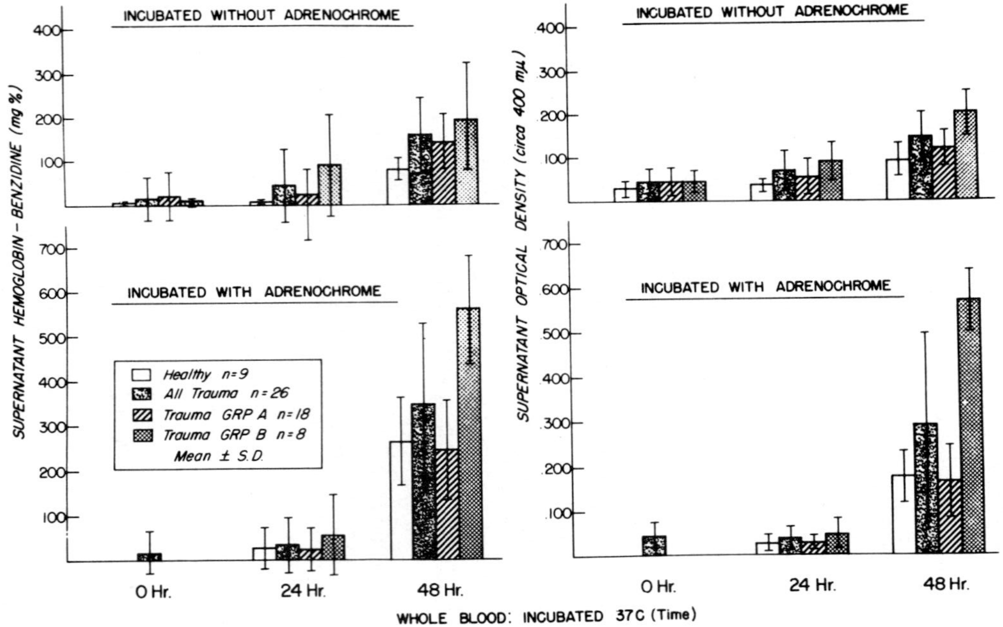

FIGURE 13. The hemolysis of red blood cells in whole blood anticoagulated with acid-citrate-dextrose during incubation under sterile conditions at 37°C for 48 hr in the absence and presence of adrenochrome. Blood was collected from healthy individuals and from patients with traumatic injuries before transfusion. Plasma hemoglobin was measured by the benzidine reaction method, and the hemolysis present in plasma was measured by the optical density recorded at 400 mu. Approximately 30% of the patients (Group B) exhibited increased susceptibility to adrenochrome hemolysis. (Reproduced with kind permission from PJD Publications Limited, Westbury, N.Y. and S. Karger AG, Basel. From Valeri, C. R., Altschule, M. D., and Pivacek, L. E., Journal of Medicine, 3: 20—24, 1972.)

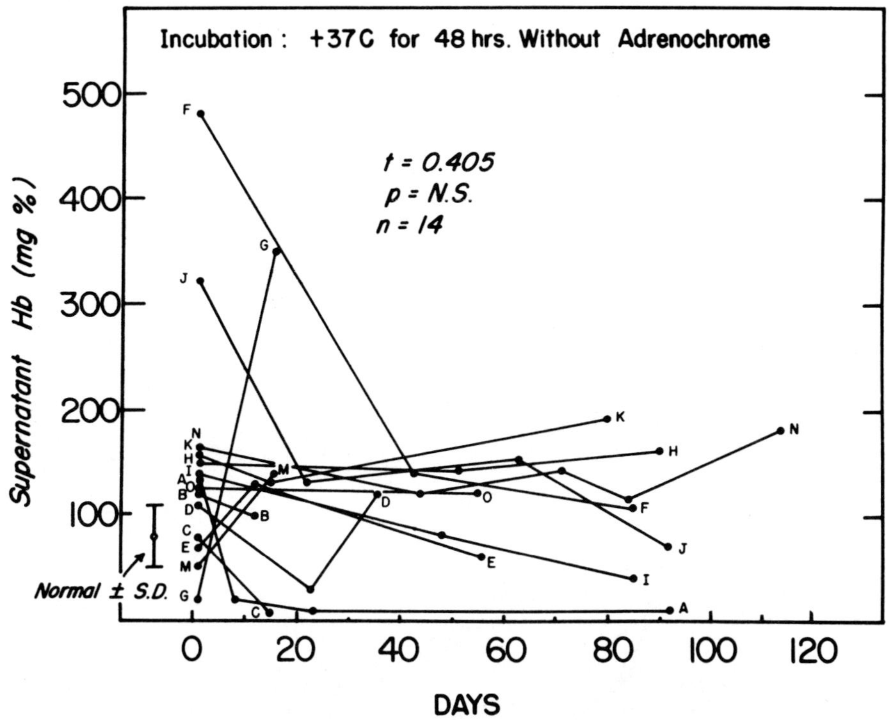

FIGURE 14. The hemolysis of the red blood cells in acid-citrate-dextrose-anticoagulated whole blood during incubation under sterile conditions at 37°C for 48 hr in the absence of adrenochrome is shown. The blood was collected from patients with traumatic injuries before and after red blood cell transfusions to restore the patient's red blood cell mass towards normal. The hemolysis was assessed from measurements of supernatant hemoglobin made by the benzidine reaction method.

At the time of our testing, the frozen serum was thawed, mixed with washed compatible donor red blood cells from healthy volunteers, and incubated under sterile conditions with adrenochrome at 37°C for 48 hr. Five preoperative samples incubated with adrenochrome exhibited increased hemolysis; five 3-hr postoperative samples showed reduced hemolysis; and four of five 24-hr postoperative samples showed increased hemolysis. In another five serum samples incubated with adrenochrome as described above, all five preoperative and 3-hr postoperative samples exhibited normal hemolysis, as did four of the five 24-hr postoperative samples (Figure 18). These data suggest the presence of (or lack of) a substance in the sera of five of the ten seriously wounded patients studied. We did not have detailed clinical data on these patients which might help us explain why half the patients had increased hemolysis or whether this increased hemolysis was related to, or a feature of, the *missing blood syndrome.*

SUMMARY OF BLOOD DESTRUCTION STUDIES

As indicated in the previous chapters, our patients with severe injuries had marked hypovolemia despite adequate treatment at the time of trauma (Chapter 2). These patients exhibited decreased red blood cell production, owing apparently to the effects of some toxic factor on the bone marrow (Chapter 3), as well as accelerated destruction of the patient's own red blood cells measured by a ^{59}Fe labeling technique. Survival

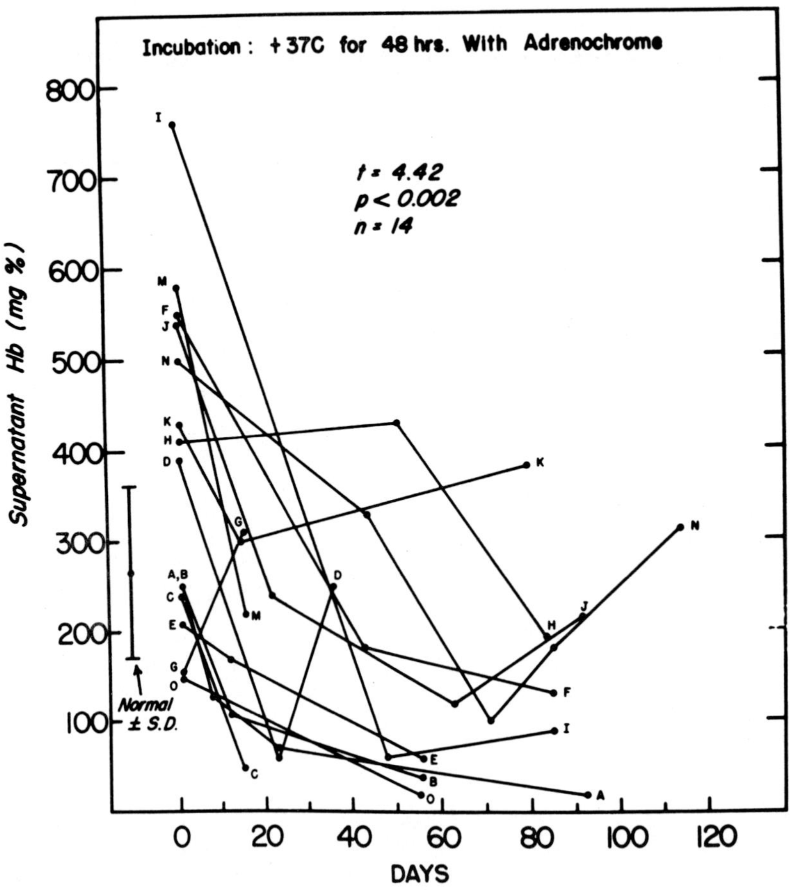

FIGURE 15. The hemolysis of red blood cells in acid-citrate-dextrose-anticoagulated whole blood during incubation under sterile conditions at 37°C for 48 hr in the presence of adrenochrome. The blood was collected from patients with traumatic injuries before and after red blood cell transfusions to restore the patient's red blood cell mass towards normal. The hemolysis was assessed from measurements of supernatant hemoglobin made by the benzidine reaction method.

measurements on the transfused compatible donor red blood cells showed normal, markedly reduced, moderately reduced, and biphasic survival curves. In the biphasic curves, the first portions showed accelerated red blood cell destruction and the second portion showed normal rates of destruction, suggesting that the transfusion of red blood cells either removed or neutralized whatever it was that was causing the accelerated red blood cell destruction.

Red blood cell destruction was evaluated from measurements of the breakdown products of red blood cell-hemoglobin. Degradation of hemoglobin usually is accompanied by the liberation of carbon monoxide when the alpha-methene bridge of the protoporphyrin molecule is open, after which protoporphyrin is degraded to bilirubin and urobilinogen in the gastrointestinal tract. Patients who did not receive blood transfusions showed no increase in carbon monoxide production. Moreover, there was no increase in carbon monoxide production associated with the destruction of the nonviable compatible red blood cells during the posttransfusion . Fecal urobilinogen excretion, a quantitative measurement of red blood cell destruction, was lower in the patients before transfusion than in the normal volunteers. Posttransfusion increases in

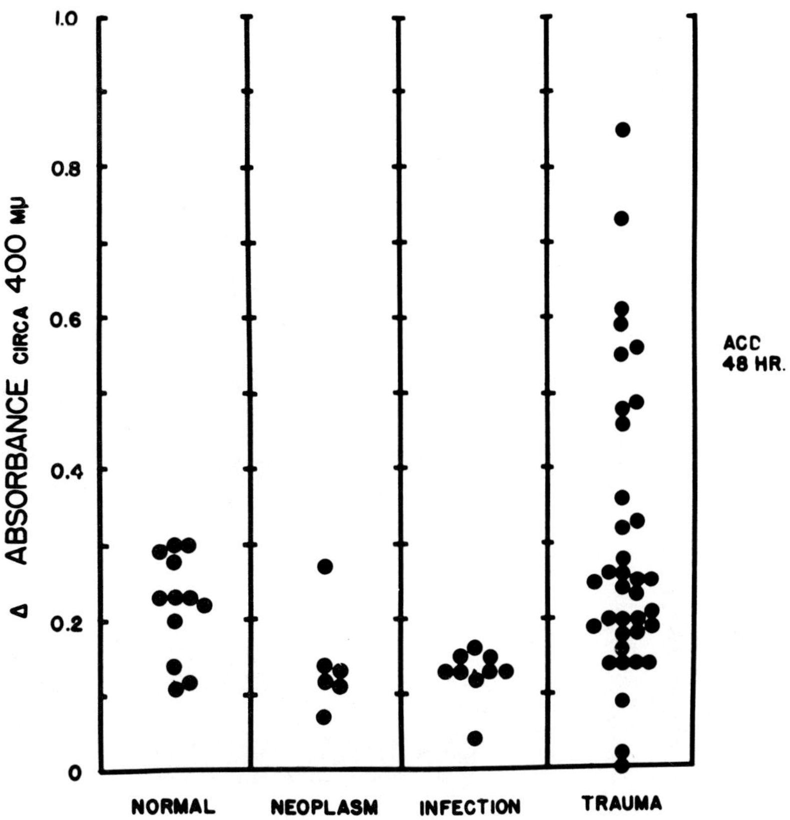

FIGURE 16. The hemolysis of red blood cells in acid-citrate-dextrose-anticoagulated whole blood during incubation under sterile conditions at 37°C for 48 hr in the presence of adrenochrome. Hemolysis was measured by the supernatant optical density at circa 400 mu. Blood samples were obtained from the normal volunteers and the patients with carcinoma, infection, and traumatic injuries before transfusion.

fecal urobilinogen seen in patients not receiving systemic antibiotics accounted for only 25% of the destroyed nonviable compatible red blood cells. The patients who were treated with systemic antibiotics showed no posttransfusion increase in fecal urobilinogen associated with the destruction of nonviable compatible donor red blood cells.

Studies also were made of the degradation of red blood cell-hemoglobin directly into porphyrins, dipyrroles, and monopyrroles. Dipyrroles could not be detected in the urine samples of our patients, and there was no increase in the excretion of dipyrroles in their stools either before or after transfusion. An increase in oxyporphyrin-like substances was observed in the urine of our patients, and their wounds contained a fluorescent material that appeared after the transfusion of red blood cells, indicating that as the nonviable red blood cells were destroyed a fluorescent material accumulated in the wounds. This finding in conjunction with the finding of an accumulation of only the ^{59}Fe in the wound dressings of patients after transfusion of ^{59}Fe-labeled and ^{51}Cr-labeled autologous red blood cells suggests that red blood cell destruction gave rise to the accumulation of iron and fluorescent porphyrin-like compounds. ^{59}Fe is known to label the heme portion and ^{51}Cr to label the globin portion of hemoglobin. The degradation of red blood cell-hemoglobin through the pathway producing iron and porphyrin compounds has been produced in vitro by Veech et al. (1967) by the incubation

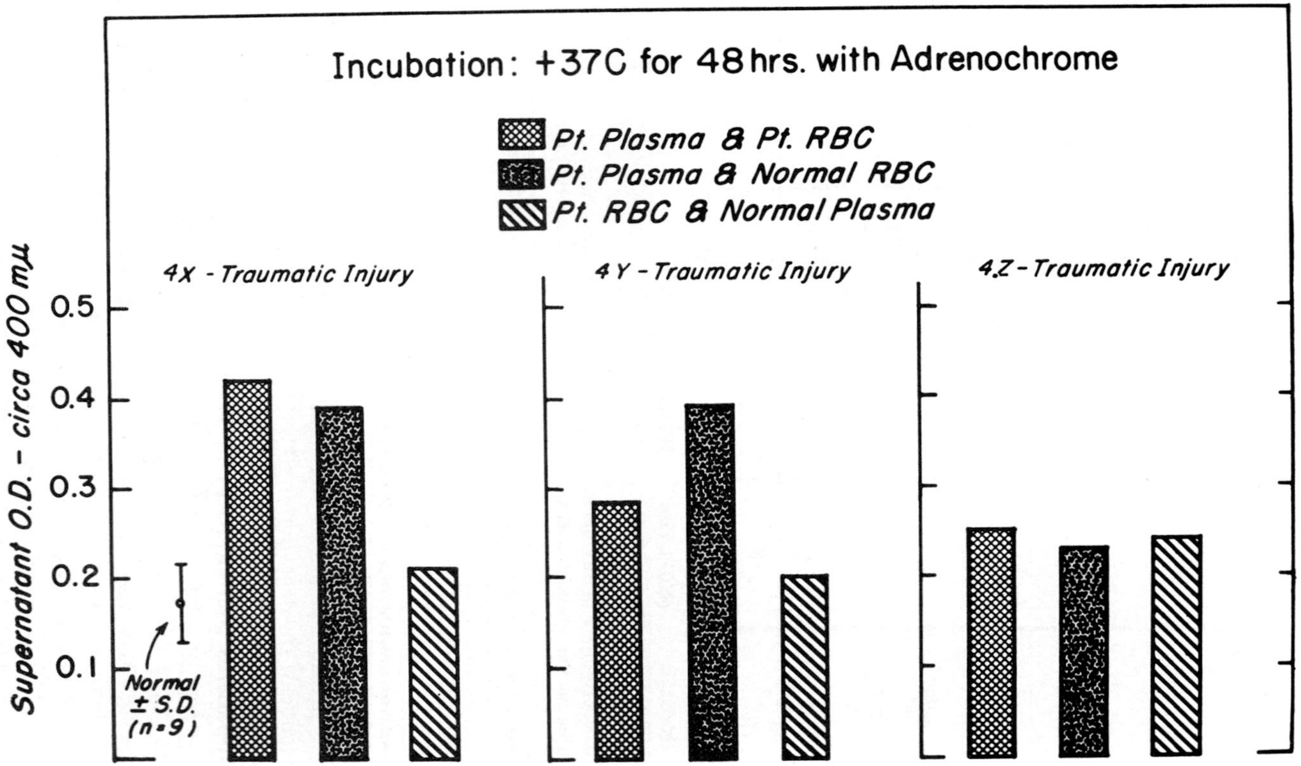

FIGURE 17. The hemolysis of the red blood cells in heparinized blood obtained from three male patients with traumatic injuries. Studies were made of (a) patient red blood cells in patient plasma, (b) normal washed compatible donor red blood cells in patient plasma, and (c) washed patient red blood cells in compatible normal donor plasma. The hemolysis measured by the supernatant optical density at circa 400 mu was measured after 48 hr of incubation at 37°C under sterile conditions in the presence of adrenochrome.

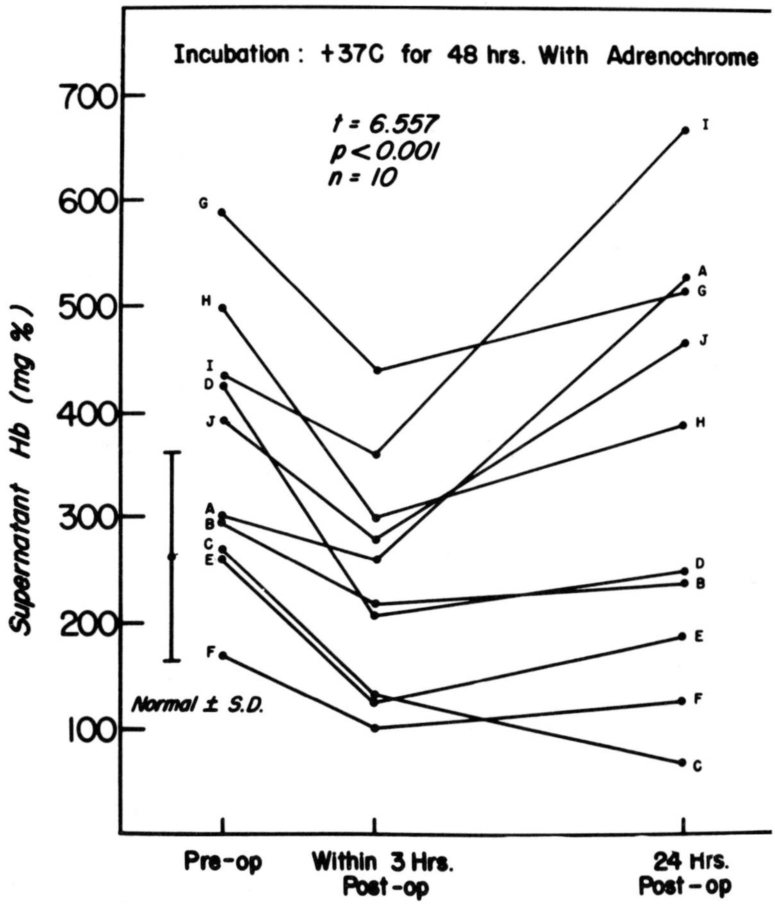

FIGURE 18. The hemolysis of normal washed compatible donor red blood cells incubated in compatible sera obtained from patients with traumatic injuries before operation, within 3 hr after operation, and 24 hr after operation. The normal washed donor red blood cells in compatible patient sera were incubated at 37°C under sterile conditions for 48 hr in the presence of adrenochrome. The hemolysis in the supernatant was measured by the benzidine reaction method.

of red blood cells with adrenolutin, a breakdown product of epinephrine, although other substances also may be involved.

The data presented in this chapter suggest that the plasma or serum of wounded men may contain one or more substances with hemolytic qualities. Whether these substances would also account for the bone marrow suppression described in Chapter 3 cannot be stated. The question that arises is whether our presumed toxic substance is the same as the toxic heme derivatives found in the blood in the acute phase of shock (Lillihei, 1958; Nemir et al., 1967; Friedman-Mor et al., 1978).

Observations made in our patients with traumatic injuries that were related to the missing blood syndrome include: (1) a significant loss of transfused red blood cells with only minimal increase in fecal urobilinogen excretion and no increase in carbon monoxide production; (2) the presence of fluorescent material and iron in wound dressings; (3) the presence of oxyporphyrin in the urine; and (4) the increased hemolysis that was observed when blood was treated with adrenochrome in vitro. It was our conclusion that as red blood cells are destroyed they yield red blood cell-hemoglobin breakdown products of iron and oxyporphyrin-like substances, and that unless these breakdown products are looked for specifically, hyperhemolysis may be overlooked.

Chapter 5

HEMODYNAMIC CHANGES — EFFECT OF BLOOD TRANSFUSION

Our patients came to the Chelsea Naval Hospital 2 weeks or more after having been treated for acute hypovolemia caused by their war wounds. Here they were found to have red blood cell and blood volume deficits of about 40% (Chapter 2). As discussed previously, although they were treated for their initial blood loss at the time they were wounded, their blood volume deficit soon recurred, this time because of hemolysis and depressed bone marrow function. It is important to compare the physiologic effects of these two consecutive states.

HEMODYNAMIC EFFECTS OF ACUTE SHOCK

The physiological changes that occur in the acute phase of hemorrhagic shock are well documented. They include decreases in red blood cell and plasma volumes (Suzuki et al., 1964, 1965; Simmons et al., 1969a); pulmonary dysfunction (Simmons et al., 1969c, 1969d; Smith et al., 1973; Holleman et al., 1978); cardiovascular dysfunction (Carey et al., 1965, 1967, 1969; Cohn and DelGuercio, 1966; Gudwin et al., 1968; Shoemaker, 1971; Byrnes et al., 1978); redistribution of blood flow (Cannon et al., 1917; Kety, 1950; Campbell et al., 1967; Forsyth et al., 1970; Couch et al., 1971; Rutherford and Trow, 1973; Selmyer et al., 1973; Slater et al., 1975; Laks et al., 1976; Badder et al., 1978; Berlin, 1979; Lovelace et al., 1979; Manny et al., 1979); acid-base disturbances (Cloutier et al., 1969); endocrine changes (Elmadjian, 1954; Elmadjian and Davis, 1955; Pace et al., 1956; Skillman et al., 1967; Carey et al., 1971; Noel et al., 1972; Watkins et al., 1974b; Gann and Pirkle, 1975); hypoperfusion of tissue (Seibert and Ebaugh, 1967; Aviado, 1968; Gilbert, 1968; Neill et al., 1969; Shoemaker and Reinhard, 1973; Eldridge, 1974; Eldridge et al., 1974; Sheps et al., 1979); metabolic changes (Imamura et al., 1975); alterations of the microcirculation (Braasch, 1971; Litwin and Relihan, 1973); venoconstriction (Alexander, 1955); disturbance of the reticuloendothelial system (Warner and Dobson, 1954); predisposition to sepsis and septic shock (Cavanagh and Rao, 1969; Rao and Cavanagh, 1971); coagulopathies (Hardaway, 1966, 1973; Salzman, 1968; Simmons et al., 1969b; Hirsch et al., 1971; Caprini et al., 1977; Effeney et al., 1978; Canoso et al., 1979); and acute renal insufficiency (Lauson et al., 1944; Bradley and Bradley, 1947; Frega et al., 1973; Selmyer et al., 1973; Siegel et al., 1973; Hermreck et al., 1977; Mitch and Walker, 1977).

Our patients had been adequately treated at the time of trauma, as judged by current standards, and had not suffered subsequent bleeding, so the syndrome we observed was an unusual one. The basic issue seemed to be the need for the body to adapt to a 30 to 40% decrease in the total circulating blood volume in order to provide adequate oxygen and nutritional substrates to the crucial tissues, and to remove the products of metabolism from these tissues.

ADAPTATION TO HYPOXIA

We concentrated our attention mainly on the delivery of oxygen since this need is the most demanding. The transport of oxygen from ambient air to the tissue involves ventilation, cardiac output and distribution to the various organs, the total number of red blood cells, and the function of the circulating red blood cells (Rahn, 1966; Finch and Lenfant, 1972) (Figure 1).

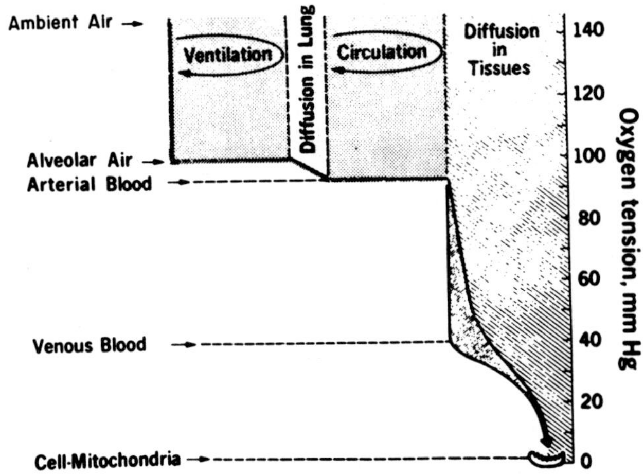

FIGURE 1. Diagram of factors involved in the transport of oxygen from ambient air to the tissue; ventilation, cardiac output, the number of red blood cells, and the red blood cell affinity for oxygen are involved.

The body adapts to tissue hypoxia produced by so-called anemic hypoxia, i.e., a reduction in the total number of red blood cells, and to the so-called hypoxic hypoxia, i.e., impairment of ventilatory and cardiac function, in various ways. These compensatory changes may include an increase in cardiac output, redistribution of blood volume and flow, an improvement in the function of circulating red blood cells, and an increase in red blood cell production (Table 1) (Finch and Lenfant, 1972). The regulation of blood flow and distribution to tissue provides substrates and oxygen for cellular metabolism according to the body's needs (Lamb et al., 1964; Miller et al., 1965; Chase et al., 1966; Saltin et al., 1968; Bohnn et al., 1970). The autoregulation of coronary and cerebral blood flow ensures proper maintenance of critical supplies of oxygen to the myocardium and the brain (Valeri, 1974, 1976). The blood flow to the vital organs, i.e., brain, heart, kidney, and adrenal glands, is maintained at the expense of nonvital organs such as the skin, muscles, gastrointestinal tract, and extremities (Fromm, 1973; Hechtman et al., 1979). Thus, our study involved not only the cardiac output but also its distribution to different parts of the body.

Before we discuss our findings and their significance, it is important that we analyze some of the factors that regulate cardiac output and the distribution of blood flow. Although fundamentally cardiac output is dependent on the venous return and normal function of the myocardium, it also is influenced by the red blood cell affinity for oxygen at different mixed venous pO_2 tensions (Plzak, 1973; Bowen and Fleming, 1974). At mixed venous pO_2 tensions of 35 mm Hg (low), 40 mm Hg (normal), or 45 mm Hg (increased), an increased oxygen affinity state is accompanied by increased cardiac output, and a decreased oxygen affinity state is associated with reduced cardiac output (Figure 2) (Plzak, 1973; Rice et al., 1975; Krall et al., 1978). The red blood cell affinity for oxygen conventionally is expressed by a number which, like all abstractions, is imaginary and exists only in the mind or on a graph. However, it is a useful convention for expressing in simple terms a complex relationship. This number is the P_{50}, the oxygen tension (mm Hg) at which 50% of the hemoglobin is saturated. The actual value of 50% saturation may never occur in a patient; nevertheless, the value is used as a convenient way to express the complicated relations that make up the oxygen affinity curve of blood.

Table 1
FACTORS COMPENSATING FOR TISSUE HYPOXIA RELATED TO ANEMIC HYPOXIA AND HYPOXIC HYPOXIA

1.	Cardiac output		
2.	Alteration of flow distribution		
	Vital organs		Nonvital organs
a.	Brain	a.	Skin
b.	Heart	b.	Muscle
c.	Kidney	c.	Extremities
d.	Adrenal		
3.	Shift of the oxyhemoglobin dissociation curve		
a.	Temperature		
b.	pH and pCO_2		
c.	Red cell 2,3 DPG, ATP, and P_i		
d.	HbCO and Meth HB		
4.	Increased erythropoiesis		

The factors that affect red blood cell affinity for oxygen are discussed elsewhere (Chapter 6). Here it is sufficient to point out that the state of affinity affects cardiac output, although the mechanism of this effect is totally unknown. Other factors also influence cardiac output. For example, acidosis increases total cardiac output (Andersen and Mouritzen, 1966), although the effects of acidosis and of carbon dioxide tension seem to be more marked with respect to local flow (Figure 3). Thus, a reduction in CO_2 tension reduces cerebral flow whereas an increase in CO_2 tension increases cerebral blood flow (Valeri, 1976). A reduction in blood pH increases coronary blood flow whereas an increase in blood pH reduces coronary blood flow (Valeri, 1976).

RED BLOOD CELL 2,3 DPG LEVELS

A basic compensatory mechanism that ensures optimum oxygen transport function in patients with a decrease in red blood cell volume is an increase in red blood cell 2,3 DPG (Figure 4). Although the red blood cell volume may be reduced so that the hemoglobin concentration falls from 15 g to 10 g, optimum tissue oxygen tension is maintained in the critical organs that require oxygen without an increase in cardiac output (Finch and Lenfant, 1972; Charache et al., 1978). With a 40% reduction in the red blood cell volume, a patient usually compensates for the reduced number of red blood cells by increasing the level of 2,3 DPG from 0.8 *M* DPG per *M* Hb to 1.6 *M* DPG per *M* Hb (Figure 4). This improves oxygen delivery to tissue, maintaining high tissue oxygen tensions (Valeri and Fortier, 1969a, 1969b). The increase in red blood cell 2,3 DPG concentration obviates the need for an increase in cardiac output.

The low blood volumes in our patients demanded that adequate blood flow in some areas of the body be achieved at the expense of other areas. In patients in whom total blood volume is reduced, the blood flow is maintained to the heart, brain, kidneys, and adrenal glands by redistribution of blood flow away from nonvital organs like the skin, muscle, extremities, and bone marrow. This redistribution of blood flow helps to maintain the critical oxygen tension of the brain, heart, kidneys, and adrenal glands and reduces the oxygen tension of other organs.

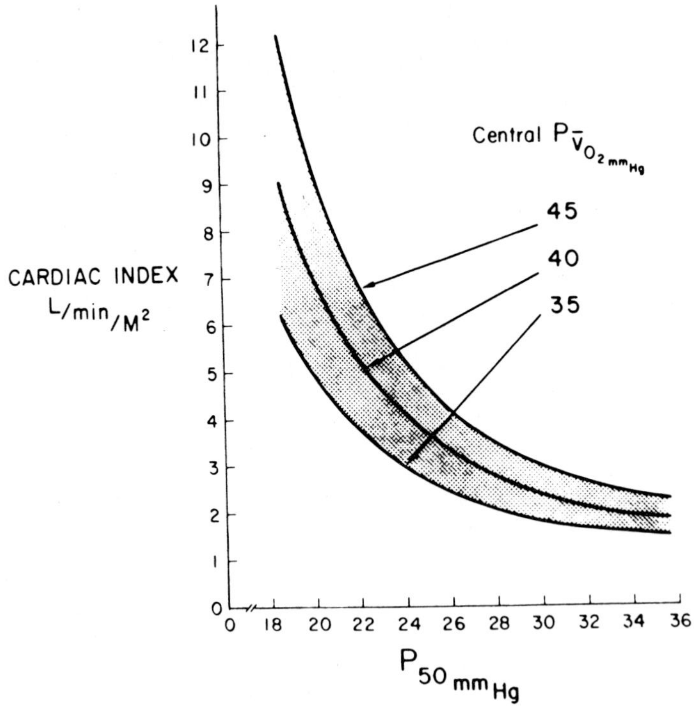

FIGURE 2. The relation between cardiac index and the P_{50} (mm Hg) at central venous pO_2 tensions of 35, 40, and 45 mm Hg. (From Plzak, L. F., Jr., in *Preservation of Red Blood Cells,* Chaplin, H., Jr., Jaffe, E. R., Lenfant, C., and Valeri, C. R., Eds., National Academy of Sciences, Washington, D.C., 1973, 35. With permission.)

Studies of blood flow and distribution were made in our patients from 1969 to 1971 using dye dilution cardiac output (Valeri and Collins, 1971). Renal blood flow was evaluated indirectly from renal function (see below). Distribution of blood flow also was appraised indirectly by measuring extracellular muscle pH with a pH electrode (Couch et al., 1971; Laks et al., 1976), although these data were not useful in assessing blood flow and blood volume in the extremities of our patients.

When we observed the hypovolemic anemia in our patients, we chose to restore the red blood cell volume deficit with washed liquid-stored red blood cells or washed previously frozen red blood cells, rather than attempt to treat the reduced plasma volume with crystalloid or colloid solutions. It has been suggested that rapid transfusion may precipitate cardiopulmonary insufficiency (Brannon et al., 1945; Sharpey-Schafer, 1945; Blumgart and Altschule, 1948; Schnabel et al., 1959; Frye and Braunwald, 1960; Duke et al., 1964; Duke and Abelmann, 1969; Gardner et al., 1975), but we believed this theory to be uncritically overemphasized (Altschule, 1954), and in any case it did not develop in our patients. Washed red blood cells were transfused to our patients to improve tissue perfusion, one effect of which was to increase oxygen available to tissue in order to accelerate healing of their indolent wounds (Freeman, 1943; Conolly et al., 1969; Hugo et al., 1969; Stephens and Hunt, 1971; Niinikoski et al., 1972).

OXYGEN TRANSPORT

When we transfused preserved red blood cells to restore the red blood cell volume

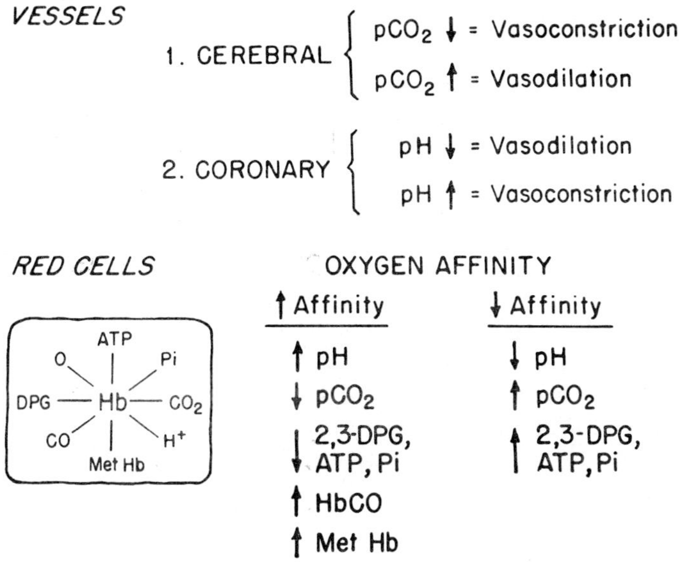

FIGURE 3. The effects of pH, pCO_2 and pO_2 on blood vessels and red blood cells. (From Valeri, C. R., in *Blood Banking and the Use of Frozen Blood Products,* CRC Press, Cleveland, Ohio, 1976. With permission.)

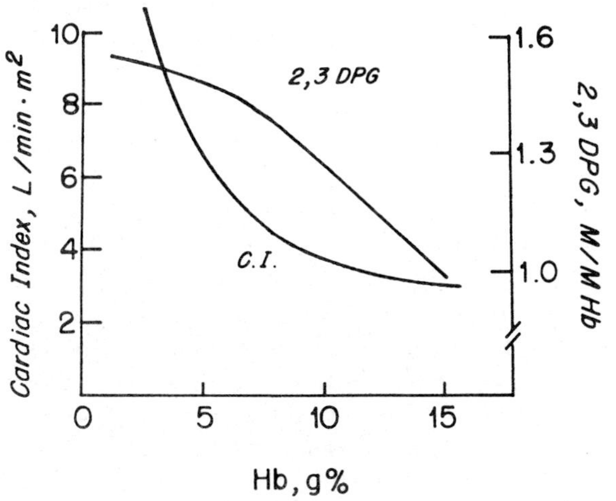

FIGURE 4. The relationships among cardiac index, hemoglobin concentration, and red blood cell 2,3 DPG level. (From Finch, C. A. and Lenfant, C., *New Engl. J. Med.,* 286, 407, 1972. With permission.)

deficits in our patients, we made every effort to ensure the quality and compatibility of these donor red blood cells and to guarantee a 24-hr posttransfusion survival value of greater than 70%. The donor red blood cells were stored in the acid-citrate-dextrose (ACD) anticoagulant at 4°C for up to 3 weeks after collection; this particular anticoagulant was being used during the period from 1968 to 1972 when our patients were being studied. Citrate-phosphate-dextrose (CPD) was not in use then. After 2 to 3 days of liquid storage in ACD, the preserved red blood cells had a decreased ability to deliver oxygen, a defect that we now realize is an important consideration when preserved blood is used for transfusions.

In 1954 Valtis and Kennedy reported deficient oxygen transport function in red blood cells after storage of the blood at 4°C in ACD for less than 1 week, a defect that was restored to normal usually within 24 hr after transfusion. In 1967 Benesch and Benesch, and Chanutin and Curnish identified red blood cell 2,3 DPG as the compound within the red blood cells that affected the oxygen affinity. Many investigators subsequently have studied the factors responsible for the in vitro and in vivo restoration of this respiratory defect in preserved cells (Beutler and Wood, 1969; Bunn et al., 1969; Valeri and Hirsch, 1969; Sugerman et al., 1970; Duhm et al., 1971; Oski et al., 1971b; Bowen and Fleming, 1974; Duhm, 1974; Rubinstein and Warrendorf, 1975; Bristow et al., 1977; Pollock et al., 1977). Although the relation between the 2,3 DPG level and the oxygen transport function of red blood cells has been established, official standards governing the transfusion of compatible preserved red blood cells contain no regulations for the functional state of the red blood cells. The emphasis is on the oxygen carrying capacity, i.e., the ability to survive in the circulation, and not on the oxygen delivery capability.

In a study of clinically stable anemic patients with chronic and subacute hypovolemia, we assessed the physiologic changes occurring after the transfusion of three to five units of preserved red blood cells. We found that the low 2,3 DPG concentrations were rapidly restored toward normal during the 24-hr posttransfusion period and then slowly to normal within one week (Figures 5A and 5B), and that the red blood cell adenosine triphosphate (ATP) level was completely restored usually within 3 hr after transfusion (Figure 6) (Fortier et al., 1969). These patients, who before treatment had respiratory alkalosis with slightly elevated arterial pH and reduced arterial pCO_2, were transfused with three to five units of red blood cells with low 2,3 DPG levels and increased affinity for oxygen. They had adequate dietary intakes of phosphorus from the gastrointestinal tract. Conditions in these subjects were optimal for synthesis in vivo of the red blood cell 2,3 DPG levels of the preserved units. Red blood cell 2,3 DPG may be synthesized at a retarded rate if the patient is acidotic or hypercarbic or has depleted levels of blood inorganic phosphate (Chapter 6) (Valeri, 1976).

The following important considerations should be known for proper interpretation of the results of our study (Fortier et al., 1969). Before the transfusion of the three to five units of compatible liquid-stored red blood cells with low 2,3 DPG levels and increased affinity for oxygen, the patients had been in stable condition for weeks after their traumatic injuries. Their measured hypovolemia was due to reductions in both red blood cell and plasma volumes averaging approximately 40%. Their oxygen consumption was measured directly from expired gases at intervals throughout the 24-hr posttransfusion period (Figure 7). Arterial and pulmonary artery blood samples were collected for measurement of oxygen content, percent saturation, in vivo and in vitro P_{50} values, red blood cell 2,3 DPG, ATP, and inorganic phosphate levels, and blood pH, pCO_2, and pO_2. Carboxyhemoglobin and methemoglobin concentrations also were measured. Cardiac output was calculated from the measured oxygen consumption and the arteriovenous oxygen content difference in the systemic circulation as well as directly by the dye method. It should be noted that when the dye method is used, measurements of cardiac output may not be accurate if there are changes in blood flow through the bronchial vessels (Valeri and Collins, 1971). Since this flow almost certainly increased during and after transfusion, we felt that the data obtained with the dye method were questionable and so are not reporting them. However, we did use these data in calculating pulmonary blood volume, for here any errors due to recirculation are compensated for in the mean transit time.

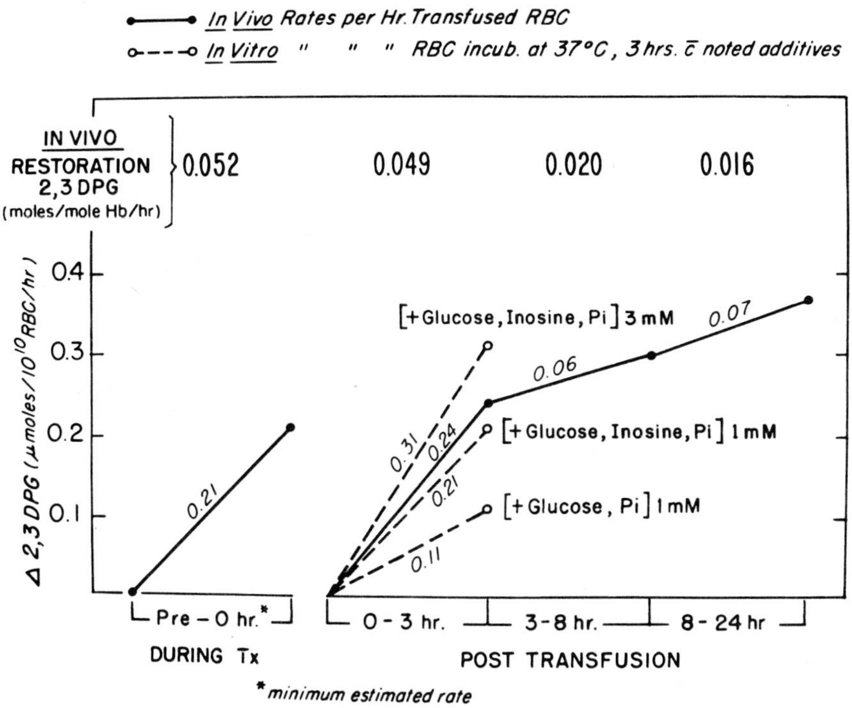

FIGURE 5A. The rates of restoration of red blood cell 2,3 DPG in vivo and in vitro. (From Fortier, N. L., Hirsch, N. M., and Valeri, C. R., *Forsvarsmedicin,* 5, 250, 1969. With permission.)

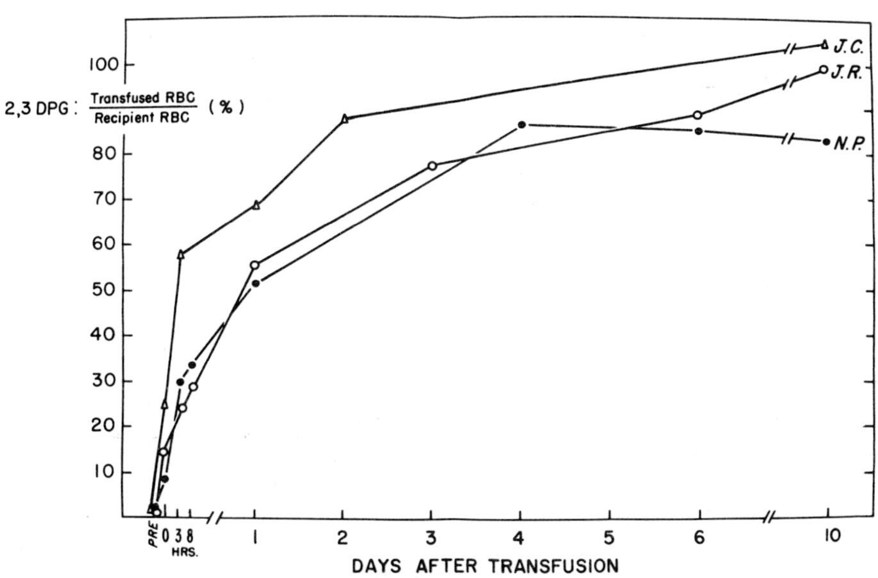

FIGURE 5B. The in vivo restoration of 2,3 DPG-depleted donor red blood cells is reported as a percentage of the recipient's level of 2,3 DPG for each of the patients studied. (From Fortier, N. L., Hirsch, N. M., and Valeri, C. R., *Forsvarsmedicin,* 5, 250, 1969. With permission.)

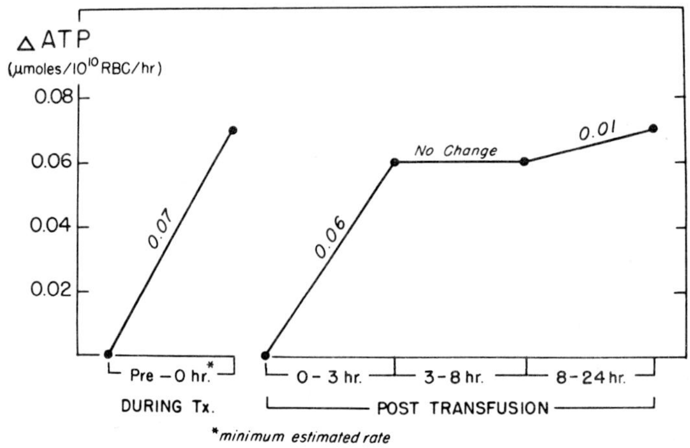

FIGURE 6. The rate of restoration of ATP in vivo. (From Fortier, N. L., Hirsch, N. M., and Valeri, C. R., *Forsvarsmedicin*, 5, 250, 1969. With permission.)

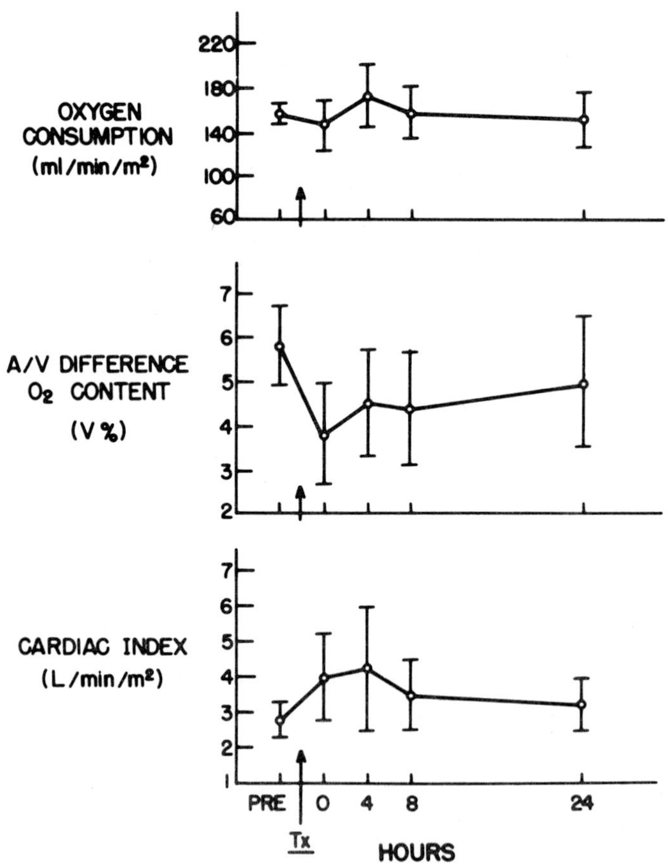

FIGURE 7. Oxygen consumption, arteriovenous difference in oxygen content, and cardiac output prior to and following transfusion of preserved red blood cells with low 2,3 DPG levels and with increased affinity for oxygen. (From Valeri, C. R., *Clin. Haematol.*, 3, 649, 1974. With permission.)

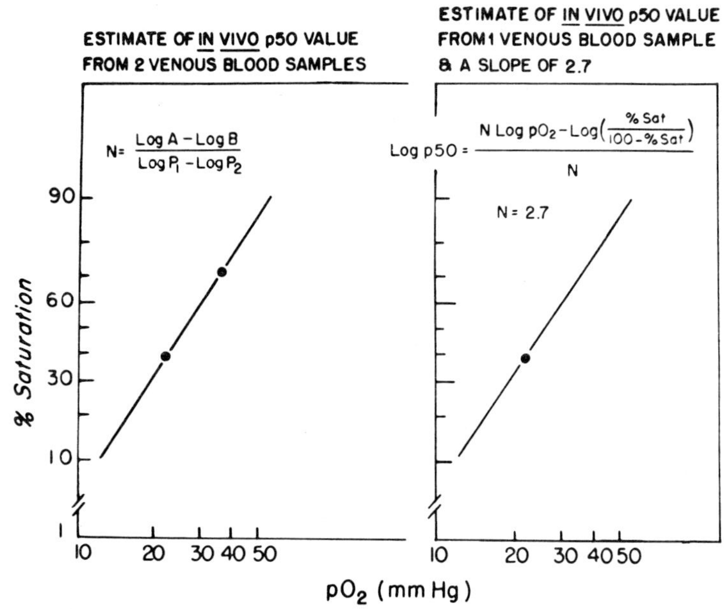

FIGURE 8. The estimate of the in vivo P_{50} value from two venous blood samples and from one venous blood sample and a slope of the oxyhemoglobin dissociation curve of 2.7. (From Valeri, C. R., in *Blood Banking and the Use of Frozen Blood Products,* CRC Press, Cleveland, Ohio, 1976, 145. With permission.)

It cannot be too strongly emphasized that because the blood used in these transfusions had a defective oxygen delivery capacity, the effects of transfusion must be examined in relation to two groups of factors. One group encompasses the effects of restoration of the blood volume. The other concerns the way in which the body handled the transfusion of red blood cells with low 2,3 DPG levels and increased affinity for oxygen.

In vitro p_{50} values were measured by the Bellingham-Huehns procedure (1969a, 1969b) using washed red blood cells at 37°C with a pH of 7.2 and a pCO_2 of 0 mm Hg, and by the Instrumentation Laboratory procedure using blood maintained at 37°C, pH 7.4, and a pCO_2 of 40 mm Hg (Valeri, 1976). The differences in the results obtained by these two techniques were due to the differences in pH and pCO_2 at which the measurements were made. In vivo P_{50} values were estimated. The two methods used gave comparable results. With one method the P_{50} is derived from two venous blood samples collected from different areas of the body, each with a percent saturation of between 30 and 70% (Figure 8). The other method permits estimation of the in vivo P_{50} value from a single anaerobically collected venous blood sample collected from the pulmonary artery, superior vena cava, or a peripheral vein and having an oxygen saturation between 40 and 60% and an assumed slope of 2.7 of the oxyhemoglobin dissociation curve (Figure 8).

There was a good correlation between the in vivo and in vitro P_{50} measurements in patients before and after transfusion. Examination of the patients 8 hr after they had been given red blood cells with low 2,3 DPG levels revealed a rise in the 2,3 DPG concentration and an increase in the P_{50} value, but the mixed venous blood oxygen tensions did not decrease during the posttransfusion period (Figure 9). Theoretically, the mixed venous oxygen tension should have decreased at the time the red blood cell

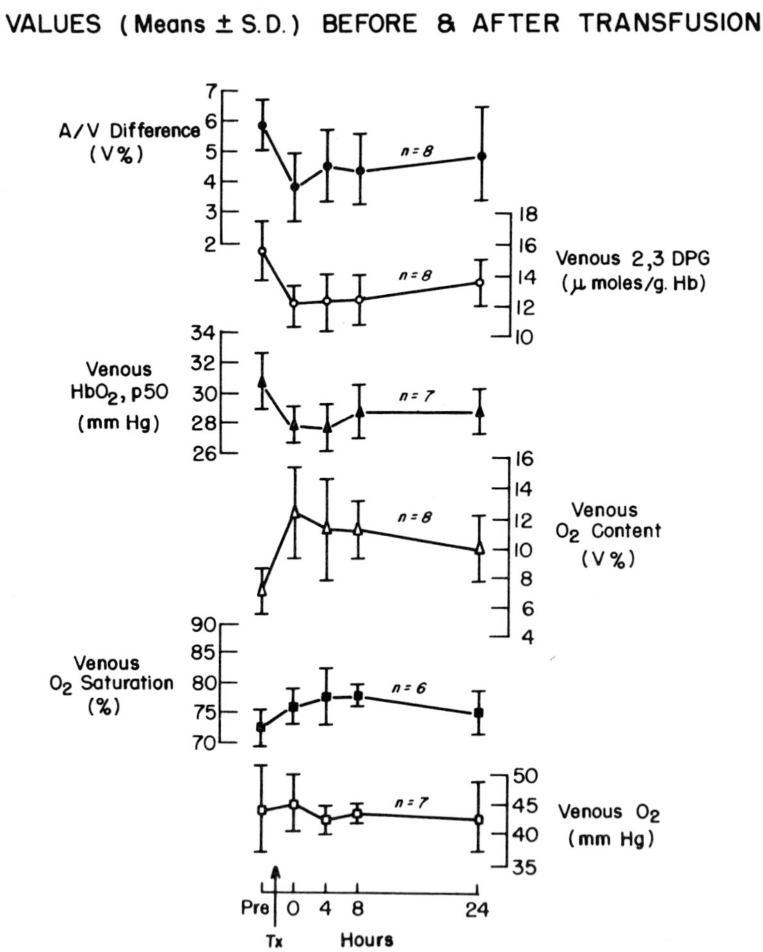

FIGURE 9. The effect of transfusion of three to five units of preserved red blood cells with low 2,3 DPG levels and with increased affinity for oxygen on arteriovenous difference in oxygen content, 2,3 DPG levels, in vitro P_{50} values measured by the Bellingham and Huehns procedure (1969b), and the blood oxygen content, percent saturation, and pO_2 tension in venous blood. These measurements were made before and for 24 hr after transfusion. (From Valeri, C. R. and Collins, F. B., *J. Appl. Physiol.*, 31, 823, 1971. With permission.)

oxygen affinity increased, but it actually rose slightly, indicating there was an increase in cardiac output (Figure 7).

The transfusion of red blood cells with low 2,3 DPG levels precipitated an immediate reduction in the arteriovenous blood oxygen difference, from 5.8 vol% to 3.8 vol% in the systemic circulation (Figures 7 and 9) (Valeri and Collins, 1971). Later, during the 24-hr posttransfusion period, the arteriovenous oxygen content difference rose gradually from 3.8 vol% to 4.5 vol%. During the 8 hr after transfusion the cardiac index as measured by the Fick method increased from 2.8 ℓ to 4.0 ℓ/m²/min (Figure 7), and then returned to a level of around 3.0, somewhat above the control level.

The observation that patients with anemic hypoxia due to red blood cell mass deficits and patients with hypoxic hypoxia due to cardiopulmonary insufficiency produce red blood cells with two times normal 2,3 DPG stimulated our interest in the possibility of biochemically modifying liquid red blood cells to increase their red blood cell 2,3 DPG and ATP levels to 1½ to 2 times normal prior to freeze-preservation with glycerol. In a baboon study, the transfusion of red blood cells with increased 2,3 DPG levels and improved oxygen delivery capacity reduced cardiac output, whereas transfusion of red blood cells with low 2,3 DPG levels and decreased oxygen delivery capacity increased cardiac output (Rice et al., 1975; Valeri et al., 1975).

Once we were convinced of the importance of the red blood cell 2,3 DPG level in maintaining the oxygen transport function in our patients, we utilized a process of biochemical modification to restore or increase the 2,3 DPG levels of preserved red blood cells. In two patients (5A and 5B) who received biochemically modified red blood cells with 2,3 DPG levels increased to twice normal, the 2,3 DPG levels and P_{50} values were markedly increased during the 48 hr after transfusion, and four days after transfusion these values were normal (Figures 10 and 11) (Valeri, 1974, 1976). In these two patients elevations in the blood carboxyhemoglobin level were observed before and after transfusion, related to their smoking habits (Figures 10 and 11) (Ayres et al., 1965; Clark et al., 1978).

DISTRIBUTION OF BLOOD

Since our patients were hypovolemic with reductions in both red blood cell mass and plasma volume, the distribution of these volumes before and after transfusion was an important aspect of their clinical evaluation. Before the deficit in the total number of circulating red blood cells was restored by transfusion, the central red blood cell volume remained normal at the expense of the peripheral red blood cell volume. It is not surprising, therefore, that wound healing in the extremities was poor. In a group of patients who were transfused with three to five units of preserved red blood cells with low 2,3 DPG levels and with increased affinity for oxygen, measurements were made before and after transfusion of the total red blood cell volume, the central red blood cell volume (i.e., red blood cells in the heart and lungs) and the peripheral red blood cell volume (Valeri and Collins, 1971). The red blood cell volume was measured before transfusion using ^{51}Cr-labeled autologous red blood cells; after transfusion it was estimated from the pretransfusion measurement and the estimated increase in red blood cell volume produced by the donor red blood cells in the circulation calculated from the volume and survival percentage of the transfused donor red blood cells. The automated differential agglutination procedure was used to measure the donor red blood cell survival. The central blood volume was calculated from the cardiac output measured by the indocyanine green dye dilution method and the mean transit time (Hamilton et al., 1932, 1948; Carleton et al., 1959; Levinson et al., 1959; Thompson et al., 1964; Cohn and DelGuercio, 1966, 1967; Siegel et al., 1968). The red blood cell volume in the heart and lungs was calculated using the mean hematocrit of the blood obtained from the brachial artery and the pulmonary artery. The peripheral red blood cell volume was calculated from the total red blood cell volume minus the central red blood cell volume (Figures 12 and 13).

The central red blood cell volume was significantly increased 4 hr after the transfusion of the three to five units of preserved red blood cells with low 2,3 DPG levels, but when measured 8 hr after transfusion had returned to the pretransfusion value (Figures 12 and 13). Prior to transfusion, our patients with a 30 to 40% reduction in total blood volume showed a redistribution of blood volume that maintained the central blood volume but reduced the peripheral blood volume, although the peripheral red blood cell volume was restored to or toward normal after transfusion (Figures 12 and 13). These findings suggest that when the peripheral red blood cell volume is re-

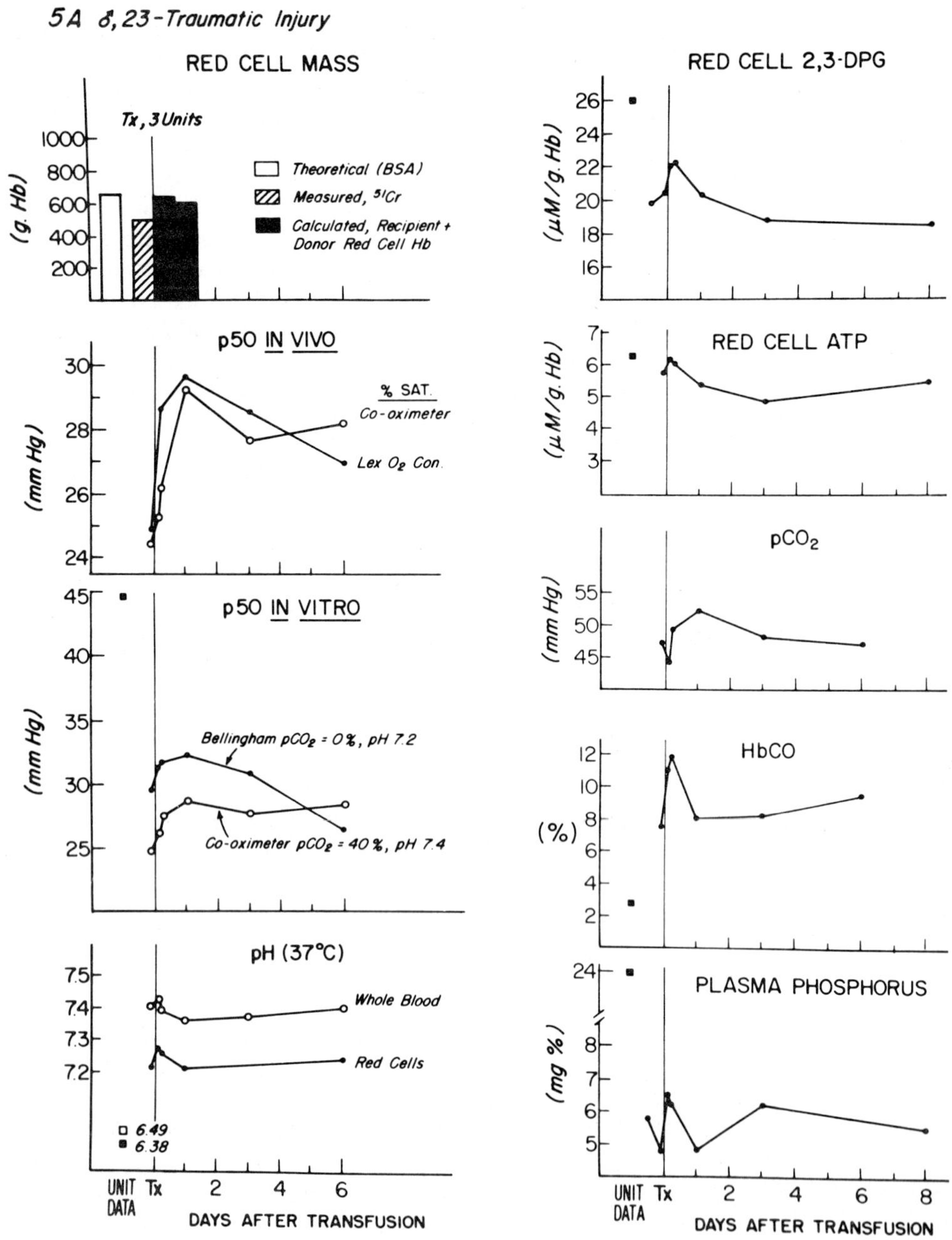

FIGURE 10. Measurements of red blood cell mass, in vivo P_{50}, in vitro P_{50}, blood and red blood cell pH, red blood cell 2,3 DPG and ATP, blood pCO_2, carboxyhemoglobin, and plasma phosphorus in Patient 5A, a 23-year-old male with traumatic injuries, after transfusion of three units of rejuvenated washed previously frozen red blood cells. The red blood cells were stored in ACD for two days, rejuvenated with PIGPA solution B to increase their 2,3 DPG levels to two times normal, frozen with 40% W/V glycerol and stored at −80°C, washed in the IBM® Blood Processor with 2.2 ℓ of sodium chloride solutions and stored at 4°C for 24 hr in sodium chloride-glucose-phosphate solution prior to transfusion. At the time of transfusion the red blood cells were concentrated by centrifugation to remove the supernatant solution and the red blood cell concentrates with a hematocrit value of 80 vol% were administered. (From Valeri, C. R., *Clin. Haematol.*, 3, 649, 1974. With permission.)

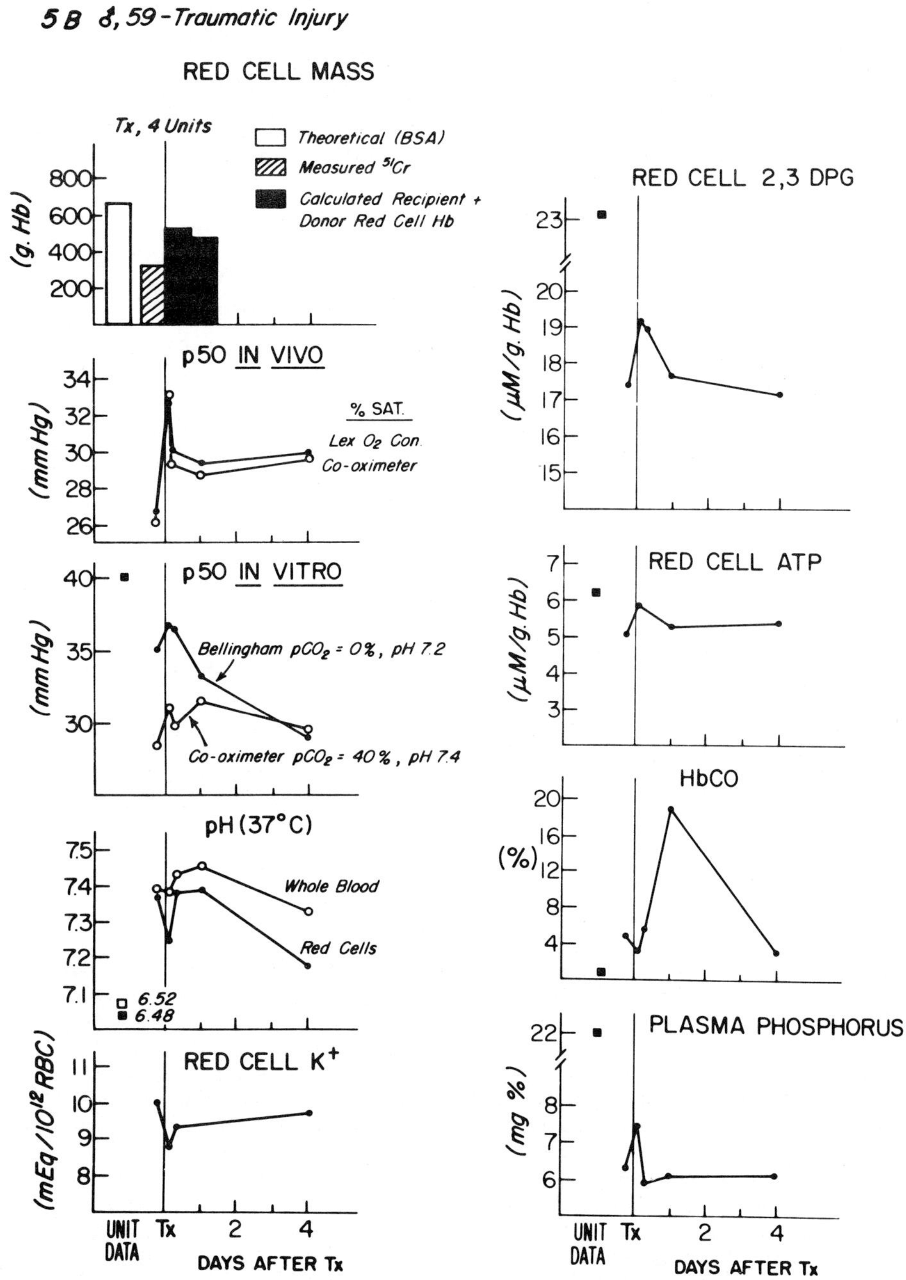

FIGURE 11. Measurements of red blood cell mass, in vivo P_{50}, in vitro P_{50}, blood and red blood cell pH, red blood cell potassium ion, 2,3 DPG and ATP, carboxyhemoglobin, and plasma phosphorus in Patient 5B, a 59-year-old male with traumatic injuries after the transfusion of four units of rejuvenated washed previously frozen red blood cells. The red blood cells were stored in ACD, rejuvenated with PIGPA Solution B to increase their 2,3 DPG levels to two times normal, frozen with 40% W/V glycerol and stored at −80°C, and stored at 4°C for 24 hr in sodium chloride-glucose-phosphate solution prior to transfusion. At the time of transfusion, the red blood cells were concentrated by centrifugation to remove the supernatant solution, and red blood cell concentrates with hematocrit values of 80 vol% were administered.

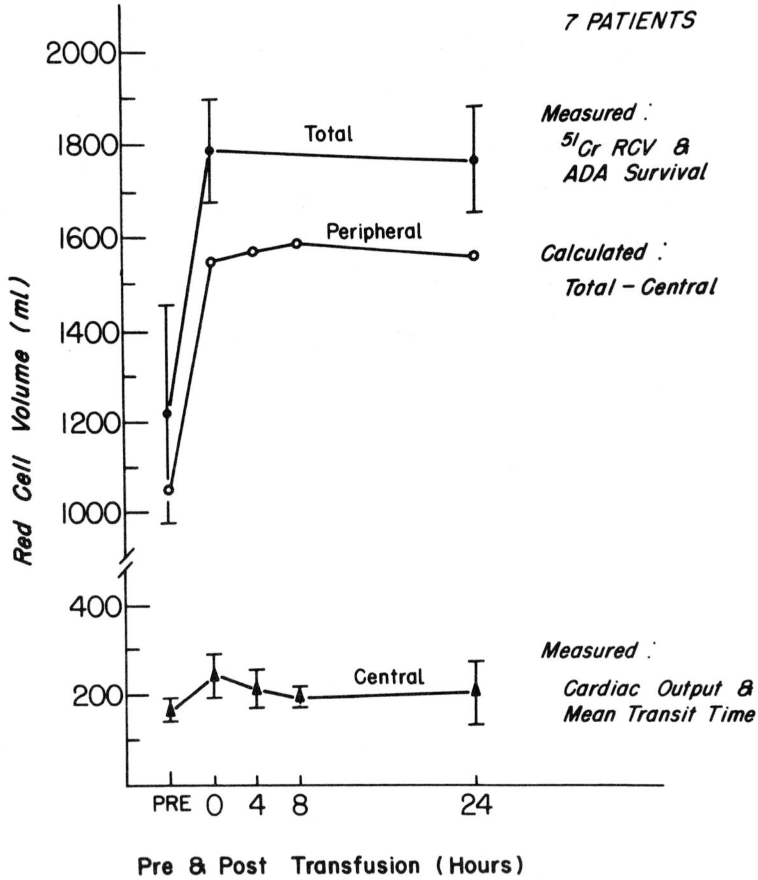

FIGURE 12. The total, central, and peripheral red blood cell volumes measured prior to and following transfusion of three to five units of preserved red blood cells with low 2,3 DPG and with increased affinity for oxygen in seven patients. The central red blood cell volume was measured from the cardiac output, the pulmonary circulation mean transit time, and the hematocrit of the blood circulating through the lungs. Before transfusion, the red blood cell volume was measured using ^{51}Cr-labeled autologous red blood cells, and after transfusion it was estimated from the red blood cell volume measured before transfusion and the increase in red blood cell volume due to the circulating donor red blood cells calculated from the volume and survival percentage of the transfused donor red blood cells. The automated differential agglutination procedure was used to measure the donor red blood cell survival. The peripheral red blood cell volume was calculated from the total red blood cell volume minus the central red blood cell volume.

duced, there may be a liberation of toxic substances from hypoperfused tissue which may trigger a reduction in blood volume, as found in our patients before transfusion. The restoration of the peripheral red blood cell volume and the peripheral blood flow after transfusion is accompanied by improved delivery of substrates and oxygen to tissues, and possibly by a reduction in the toxic substances produced by the hypoperfused tissues.

RENAL BLOOD FLOW

One might expect that our patients with moderate to severe subacute and chronic

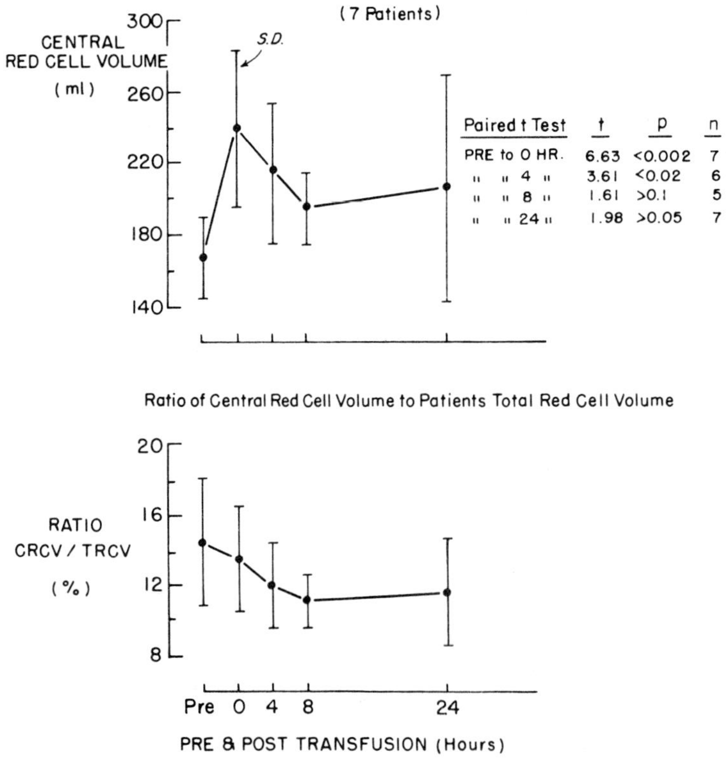

FIGURE 13. The central red blood cell volume and ratio of the central red blood cell volume to the total red blood cell volume measured prior to and following the transfusion of three to five units of preserved red blood cells with low 2,3 DPG levels and increased affinity for oxygen in seven patients with traumatic injuries.

trauma before transfusion would have had reduced renal blood flow, and that as a consequence renal function would be so compromised as to produce prerenal azotemia. Instead, we found that the renal function as measured by urine output and calcium, phosphate, creatinine, and uric acid clearance and excretion, as well as sodium and potassium excretion, were similar to the values observed in normal healthy persons studied at the same time (Figures 14, 15, and 16). There was no correlation between the red blood cell volume deficit and serum creatinine or serum uric acid levels in patients with extremity injuries (Figure 17).

Renal function, as studied by noninvasive methods, was clearly normal in our patients. In a sense, the renal function was under some stress, for patients with muscle injury are known to exhibit a considerable increase in the delivery of uric acid to the kidney (Knochel et al., 1974). Yet, our patients exhibited no such increase, and clearly showed no limitation in ability to excrete increased loads of that substance. The finding of normal renal function in these patients was not expected. They had all been in shock or close to it at the time of the original trauma and before resuscitation, and at that time presumably had exhibited the changes in renal status, including a fall in renal blood flow, that occur in shock. As a matter of fact, renal blood flow may be significantly decreased for some time after hemorrhage even while the cardiac output is still normal (Forsyth et al., 1970). Accordingly, we commence our discussion of the reported effects of hemorrhage and shock on renal blood flow.

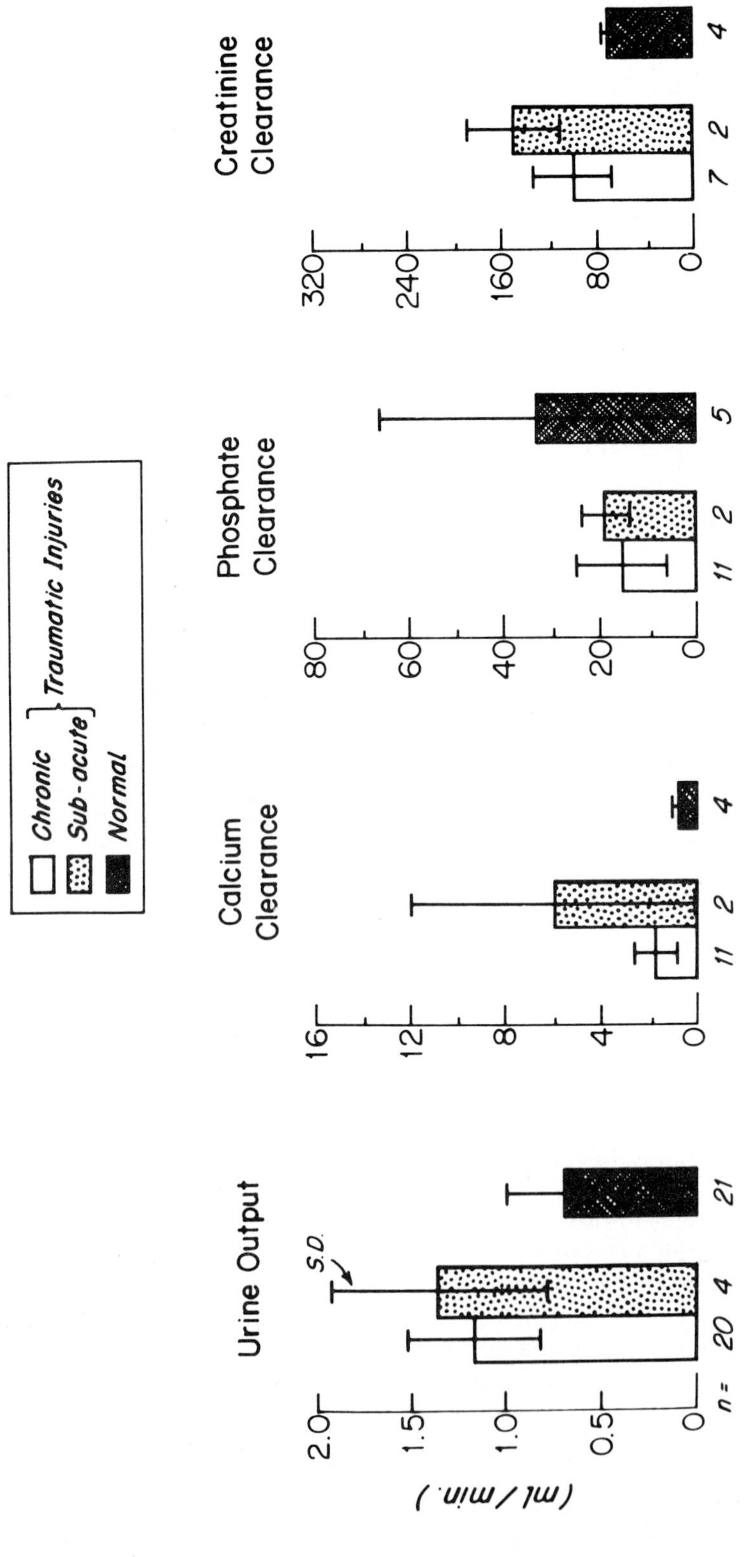

FIGURE 14. Renal function in normal volunteers and in patients with chronic and subacute traumatic injuries. Urine output and calcium, phosphate, and creatinine clearance are reported.

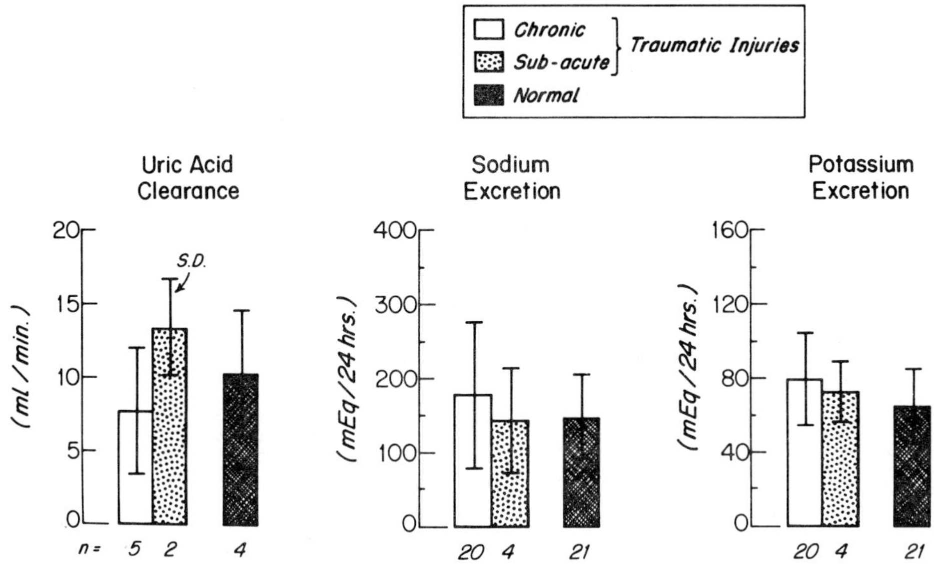

FIGURE 15. Renal function in normal volunteers and in patients with chronic and subacute traumatic injuries. Uric acid clearance and sodium and potassium excretion are reported.

Impaired renal function, manifested by oliguria, is a well-known phenomenon in trauma and shock (Lauson et al., 1944). The report of Manny et al., (1979) appears discrepant in its description of a small rise in renal blood flow in bled dogs instead of a fall as reported by others. However, this discrepancy is more presumed than real, for close study of the experimental protocol used by these investigators shows that the animals, which weighed between 20 and 25 kg, received Ringer's lactate solution in amounts of around 4 mℓ/min before, during, and after bleeding. Rather than regard the study of Manny et al., (1979) as a study on the effects of hemorrhage, it is better considered a study of preventive and restorative resuscitation from the effects of hemorrhage. The renal failure always found in shock is important in itself, but it must also be discussed in relation to the hyperphosphatemia seen in our patients (Chapter 6).

The renal failure that occurs in hemorrhage is due to marked renal ischemia caused by intense afferent arteriolar constriction (Lauson et al., 1944; Forsyth et al., 1970; Frega et al., 1973; Rutherford and Trow, 1973; Siegel et al., 1973; Badder et al., 1978). However, the renal lesion is not always reversed by attempts to counteract the ischemia with transfusions (Lauson et al., 1944; Rutherford and Trow, 1973) or with infusions of Ringer's lactate solution with or without albumin (Siegel et al., 1973). This seems to be owing to persistent changes in the filtering membranes (Hermreck et al., 1977). Many experiments designed to elucidate the phenomenon have been made in dogs, but since the renal physiology is different in that species, the findings cannot be applied to man (Hermreck et al., 1977). When persistent renal damage in man occurs in hemorrhage, it is not due to excessive secretion of renin or angiotensin. One study showed increased concentrations of both in the serum in patients with so-called "shock kidney"; the patients exhibited oliguria, rising serum creatinine levels, and low urine osmolality values. In patients in whom hypotension was purposely induced to promote hemostasis during their operations there was no evidence of renal insufficiency although their serums had greatly increased amounts of renin and angiotensin (Mitch and Walker, 1977). It is evident that neither of these substances causes "shock kidney".

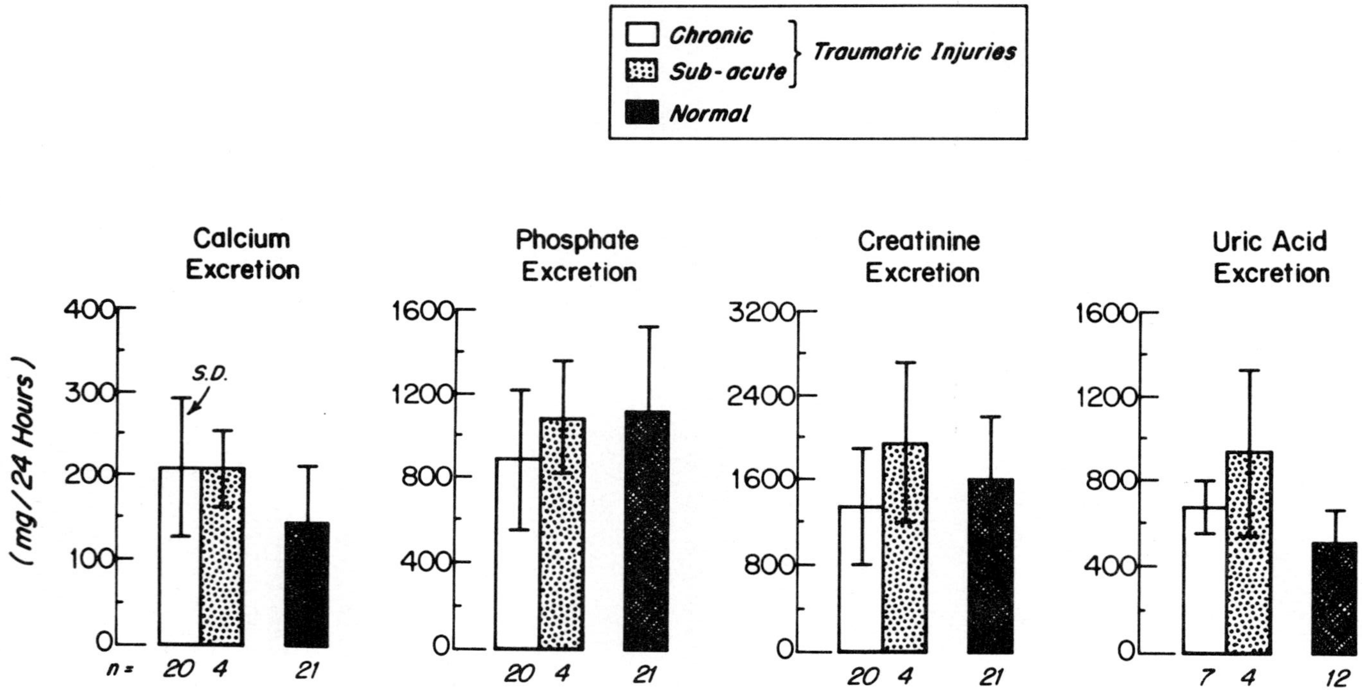

FIGURE 16. Renal function in normal volunteers and in patients with chronic and subacute traumatic injuries. Calcium, phosphate, creatinine, and uric acid excretion are reported.

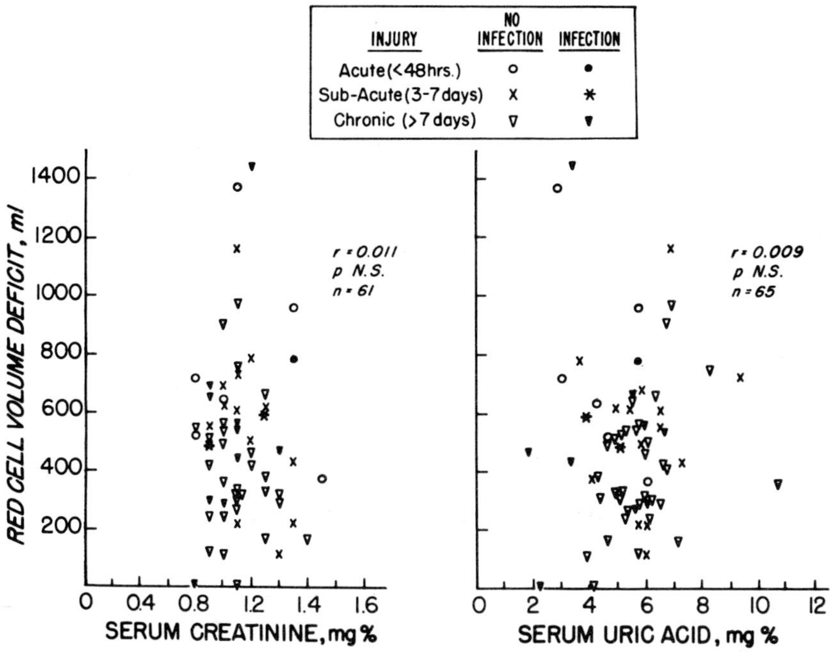

FIGURE 17. The relations between red blood cell volume deficit and serum creatinine and uric acid levels in 18- to 26-year-old male patients with traumatic injuries.

The cause of "shock kidney" has never been established. We were particularly puzzled by its absence in our patients, despite the fact that their blood volumes were lowered, in some cases by almost 50%. Other findings in patients with ordinary chronic anemias contrast with the findings of normal renal dynamics in our patients. In the former group, the glomerular filtration rate was somewhat lower than normal and the renal blood flow was markedly reduced (Bradley and Bradley, 1947). Although restoration of renal blood flow to normal is not immediate in patients in hemorrhage and shock despite what appears to be successful cardiovascular resuscitation (Rutherford and Trow, 1973), the renal blood flow is usually found to be normal some weeks later (Lauson et al., 1944). However, there are indications that even during the acute phase of shock, the changes in blood chemistry that occur with renal insufficiency are far greater than can be accounted for by decreased renal circulation (Sevitt, 1966). Urinary creatinine excretion may decrease for as long as 2 weeks following injury (Schiller et al., 1979). What has been overlooked is the fact that one response to severe acute stress is a marked breakdown of body protein as part of increased gluconeogenesis. This causes the delivery of massively increased amounts of urea to the kidney so that the blood urea increases to a degree that cannot be accounted for solely on the basis of decreased renal blood flow (Altschule and Rosenfeld, 1947).

In addition to oliguric renal failure consequent to the reduced renal blood flow of hemorrhagic shock, nonoliguric failure may also occur. This is most likely to develop during surgical procedures after resuscitation and is not necessarily associated with clinical manifestations of shock (Shin et al., 1979). The nonoliguric type of renal failure seems to occur in a small number of trauma patients in whom the oliguric type had been prevented by emphasis on restoring the blood volume to normal (Shin et al., 1979). It probably is due to persistent renal tubular damage following restoration of the renal blood flow to or toward normal.

RENAL VASOCONSTRICTION

A persistent severe renal vasoconstriction has been seen in patients in hemorrhage or shock owing to selective vasoconstriction, involving skin and muscle among other parts (Forsyth et al., 1970). Some patients have a normal renal circulation within weeks (Lauson et al., 1944), whereas some who appear otherwise to be making a good recovery exhibit a permanent and sometimes serious impairment of renal function. Our patients had all been resuscitated successfully but had been left with poorly healing wounds of the extremities. They had normal renal circulations but they still had marked vasoconstriction involving the extremities. In other words, the selective vasoconstriction of hemorrhage and shock in these patients (as well as some other conditions, as discussed in Chapter 7) had been replaced by a different pattern of selective vasoconstriction by the time we saw them. Whatever it is that causes the renal vasoconstriction and its associated glomerular damage in shock (we do not know which is primary) disappears or is counteracted in the many patients who survive with aggressive treatment. The disappearance of the renal vasoconstriction of shock saves the patients' lives, but the persistence of the extremity vasoconstriction prevents wound healing.

In summary, the hemodynamic studies showed that our patients with subacute and chronic hypovolemia due to reductions in plasma and red blood cell volumes had normal cardiac output, blood pressure, and heart rate. The major alteration in hemodynamics was a redistribution of blood volume and blood flow to the vital organs, i.e., heart, brain, kidneys, and adrenal glands. The skin, the muscles of the extremities, and perhaps bone marrow were deprived of blood volume and blood flow. Restoration of the red blood cell volume deficit by transfusion increased the peripheral but not the central red blood cell volume.

Clinical observation showed that the repeated transfusions administered to correct our patients' persistent hypovolemia were attended by clinical improvement. The initial process in this improvement was an increase in blood volume and flow in the extremities. When this process becomes sustained rather than temporary after a transfusion, clinical improvement goes forward rapidly. Does the increase in blood volume and the increase in bone marrow perfusion allow the depressed bone marrow to function normally? Does the increase in perfusion of the wounded extremities stop the production in them of toxic substances that, among other things, depress the bone marrow? We have no definitive answer to these questions on the basis of our present knowledge. However, our findings have suggested the presence in our patients of a circulatory toxin unrelated to infection. Does this necessarily originate in the wounded parts? We do know that the restoration of the blood volume and flow in the extremities was followed by wound healing and improvement in mental status and appetite, as well as by a lessening of antibiotic and narcotic requirements. The transfusions were effective in restoring the total blood volume and red blood cell volume in the extremities, and this improvement in peripheral tissue perfusion seemed to initiate clinical improvement, despite the fact that the oxygen delivery capacity of the transfused blood was defective for 4 to 8 hr after transfusion. The obvious question is whether more rapid improvement might have occurred if the transfused blood had normal or improved oxygen delivery function.

Chapter 6

METABOLIC CHANGES — EFFECTS OF BLOOD TRANSFUSION

The clinical syndrome discussed in the present monograph posed a number of important questions for us. (1) What was the underlying pathophysiology of this syndrome in our patients? The fundamental disorder proved to be a markedly reduced blood volume (Chapter 2). (2) What were the causes of the basic pathophysiological disorder? Depressed bone marrow function and shortened erythrocyte lifespan were involved (Chapters 3 and 4). (3) What were the compensatory mechanisms that permitted survival but did not permit normal function in the patients? Part of the answer to this was presented in Chapter 5, which described redistribution of available blood to central areas of the body and away from the periphery which in our patients, unfortunately, included the wounded parts. Here we will describe another change that compensated for the reduced blood volume, i.e., a modification in the metabolic status of the red blood cells, which was touched upon earlier (Chapters 2 and 3) and is being discussed thoroughly here.

These changes in the red blood cell metabolic status are affected to a great extent by biochemical phenomena in the muscles and bones which were also studied. The first matter under discussion here is the improvement in oxygen delivery function that compensated to a degree for the reduced red blood cell mass in our wounded patients. A change within the red blood cells, an increase in the organic phosphate compound, 2,3 DPG, produces an improvement in oxygen delivery to the tissues at high tissue oxygen tensions (Guest and Rapoport, 1941; Rodman et al., 1960; Chance et al., 1962; Hilpert et al., 1963; Keitt, 1966; Chanutin and Curnish, 1967; Benesch and Benesch, 1967, 1969; Astrup et al., 1968; Bauer et al., 1968; Eaton and Brewer, 1968; Edwards et al., 1961, 1968, 1971; Lenfant et al., 1968; Brody and Coburn, 1969; Oski, 1969, 1973; Oski et al., 1969, 1971a; Valeri and Fortier, 1969a, 1969b, 1970; Bauer, 1970; Battaglia et al., 1970; Miller et al., 1970a; Salhany et al., 1970; Schaefer et al., 1970; Bellingham et al., 1971; Biron et al., 1972; Edwards and Canon, 1972; Finch and Lenfant, 1972; Sugerman et al., 1972; Valeri and Kopriva, 1972; Wranne et al., 1972; Bryan-Brown et al., 1973; Bellingham and Grimes, 1973; Rosenthal et al., 1973; Sheldon, 1973a, 1973b; Canizaro et al., 1974; Thomas et al., 1974; Valeri, 1974; Watkins et al., 1974a; Meldon and Garby, 1975; Cymerman et al., 1976; Greenburg et al., 1976, 1977; Harken and Woods, 1976; Bakker et al., 1976a, 1976b, 1977; Arturson, 1977; Harken, 1977; Hlastala et al., 1977; Sheldon and Fuchs, 1977; Schrumpf et al., 1977; Bard et al., 1978; Broadie and Herman, 1978; Shaklai et al., 1978; Woodson et al., 1978; Jeul, 1979; Malmberg et al., 1979; Samaja and Winslow, 1979; Sheps et al., 1979; Smith et al., 1979; Tapper et al., 1979).

The red blood cell 2,3 DPG level can be used to distinguish a compensatory from an adaptive anemia. In compensatory anemia, a reduction in the total number of red blood cells is accompanied by a simultaneous increase in the red blood cell 2,3 DPG concentration. In adaptive anemia, on the other hand, the red blood cell 2,3 DPG level is normal despite a reduction in the total number of red blood cells (Torrance et al., 1970; Rodriguez and Shahidi, 1971; Fondu and Mandelbaum, 1975; Fondu et al., 1978). An increase in the red blood cell 2,3 DPG level means that increased red blood cell function is necessary to meet requirements for oxygen. Thus, when early in the study we observed elevated red blood cell 2,3 DPG levels in our patients, we concluded that what we were seeing was not an adaptive anemia but rather a compensatory response to a significant reduction in the total number of red blood cells, i.e., the improvement of oxygen delivery to tissue (Valeri and Fortier, 1969a, 1969b; Biron et al., 1972). A correlation was seen between red blood cell affinity for oxygen and the peripheral hemoglobin and hematocrit values: a reduction in the total number of red blood cells was accompanied by improved oxygen transport function of the red blood cells. The red blood cell affinity for oxygen was influenced by the red blood cell 2,3 DPG and ATP levels (Table 1).

REGULATION OF ERYTHROCYTE 2,3 DPG LEVEL

It is important to recognize the factors that affect the 2,3 DPG level of red blood cells. The acid-base status of the blood and the plasma inorganic phosphate level both play a role in the regulation of 2,3 DPG. Alkalosis, hypocarbia, and hyperphosphatemia increase the red blood cell 2,3 DPG concentration, whereas acidosis, hypercarbia and hypophosphatemia decrease it (Hilpert et al., 1963; George et al., 1964; Lichtman et al., 1969a, 1969b; Lichtman and Miller, 1970; Sheldon, 1973a, 1973b; Territo and Tanaka, 1974; Valeri, 1974; Miller et al., 1976; Sheldon and Fuchs, 1977; Knochel et al., 1978; Lentz et al., 1978; Shields, 1978). The alkalosis stimulates red blood cell glycolysis, and in the presence of inorganic phosphate, red blood cell 2,3 DPG is produced. Growth hormone and the hormonal changes associated with pregnancy also stimulate red blood cell 2,3 DPG synthesis (Rorth and Bille-Brahe, 1972). There are also some data to suggest that pyruvate may stimulate 2,3 DPG synthesis in vivo (Rorth et al., 1972). Red blood cell 2,3 DPG has been synthesized in vitro with substrates and cofactors such as inosine, pyruvate, inorganic phosphate, methylene blue, ascorbate, dihydroxyacetone, PGE_2, thyroid, and methyl prednisolone (Table 2).

The body's oxygen requirements, determined by the metabolic rate of the tissue, generally affect the total number of red blood cells and their oxygen affinity. Patients with panhypopituitarism and hypothyroidism have reduced oxygen requirements, and patients with hyperthyroidism have increased oxygen requirements (Evans et al., 1958; Meineke and Crafts, 1959). However, there have been conflicting reports on the effect of thyroid hormones on red blood cell affinity for oxygen and red blood cell 2,3 DPG (Miller et al., 1970b,c; Snyder and Reddy, 1970a,b; Zaroulis et al., 1978). Studies of the effects of mineralcorticoids and corticosteroids on red blood cell 2,3 DPG also have borne variable results (Bauer and Rathschlag-Schaefer, 1968; McConn and Del Guercio, 1971; Böning et al., 1976). Red blood cell affinity is affected by the hemoglobin type, e.g., fetal hemoglobin (F) has greater affinity for oxygen than adult hemoglobin. The red blood cell affinity for oxygen affects the red blood cell mass in patients with hemoglobinopathy (Bellingham and Huehns, 1969a,b; Valeri, 1979) (Figure 1). Hemoglobinopathies in which the affinity for oxygen is increased are associated with an increased red blood cell mass, whereas those in which oxygen affinity is decreased are associated with a decreased red blood cell mass (Valeri, 1974, 1976, 1979; Charache et al., 1978) (Figure 1).

Of course 2,3 DPG alone does not control the oxygen affinity state of red blood cells. The pH effects and the nature of the hemoglobin also play a role. In vivo conditions of metabolic acidosis, respiratory acidosis and hyperthermia decreased red blood cell affinity for oxygen, whereas those of metabolic alkalosis, respiratory alkalosis, and hypothermia increase red blood cell affinity for oxygen. Red blood cell affinity for oxygen is reduced under circumstances in which red blood cell 2,3 DPG, ATP, inorganic phosphate, and MCHC are increased (Figure 2). Red blood cell affinity for oxygen is increased by reductions in red blood cell 2,3 DPG, ATP, inorganic phosphate, and MCHC, and by increases in carboxyhemoglobin and methemoglobin. Red blood cells with increased affinity for oxygen usually cause increased erythropoietin

Table 1
RELATIONS BETWEEN THE OXYHEMOGLOBIN DISSOCIATION CURVE (P_{50}, mm Hg) AND 11 VARIABLES

	r	p	n
Red cell ATP (μmol/g Hb)	0.399	>0.05	20
Red cell 2,3 DPG (μmol/g Hb)	0.683	<0.002	20
Red cell ATP + 2,3 DPG (μmol/g Hb)	0.655	<0.002	20
Plasma inorganic phosphorus (μmol/mℓ plasma)	0.279	>0.2	20
Plasma pyruvate (μmol/mℓ plasma)	0.338	>0.1	20
Venous blood pH	−0.047	>0.8	20
Venous blood lactate (μmol/mℓ WB)	0.224	>0.2	20
Red cell creatine (μmol/g Hb)	0.600	<0.01	20
Red cell ADP (μmol/g Hb)	0.074	>0.5	20
Peripheral venous hematocrit (V%)	−0.671	<0.002	20
Peripheral venous hemoglobin (g%)	−0.707	<0.002	20

Table 2
IN VITRO AND IN VIVO FACTORS INVOLVED IN THE INCREASE IN THE 2,3 DPG LEVEL IN HUMAN RED CELLS

In vivo	In vitro
↓pCO_2	↑Blood pH; ↑RBC pH
↑Blood pH	Inosine
↑RBC pH	Pyruvate
↓Mean RBC HbO_2	Inorganic phosphorus
Inorganic phosphorus	Methylene blue
Growth hormone	Ascorbate
Pregnancy	Dihydroxyacetone
Pyruvate?	PGE_2
	Thyroid
	Methyl prednisolone

From Valeri, C. R., *Clin. Haematol.*, 3, 649, 1974. With permission.

production, whereas red blood cells with decreased affinity for oxygen usually suppress erythropoietin production (Rörth, 1974; Miller, 1975).

PHOSPHATE METABOLISM

The observation of elevated 2,3 DPG levels in the red blood cells of our patients with traumatic injuries directed our attention to their phosphate metabolism, because the serum inorganic phosphate level controls the levels of certain organic phosphate compounds in circulating erythrocytes (George et al., 1964; Lichtman et al., 1969a, 1969b; Lichtman and Miller, 1970; Sheldon, 1973a, 1973b; Territo and Tanaka, 1974). The changes in concentrations of two of the organic phosphates of the erythrocyte, ATP and 2,3 DPG, are similar in direction though not necessarily synchronous in time (Miller et al., 1976). A change in serum inorganic phosphate concentration is not the

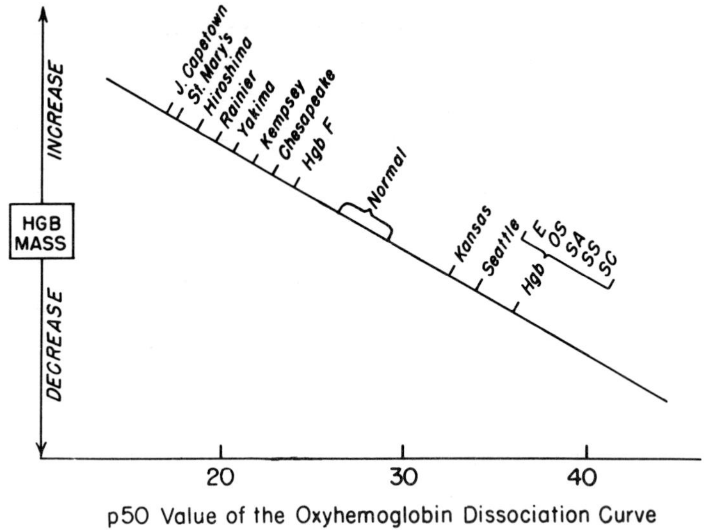

FIGURE 1. The relation between red blood cell-hemoglobin mass and the P_{50} value of the oxyhemoglobin dissociation curve. (From Valeri, C. R., *Best & Taylor's Physiological Basis of Medical Practice,* 10th ed., Brobeck, J. R., Ed., © Williams & Wilkins, Baltimore, 1979, chap. 4. With permission.)

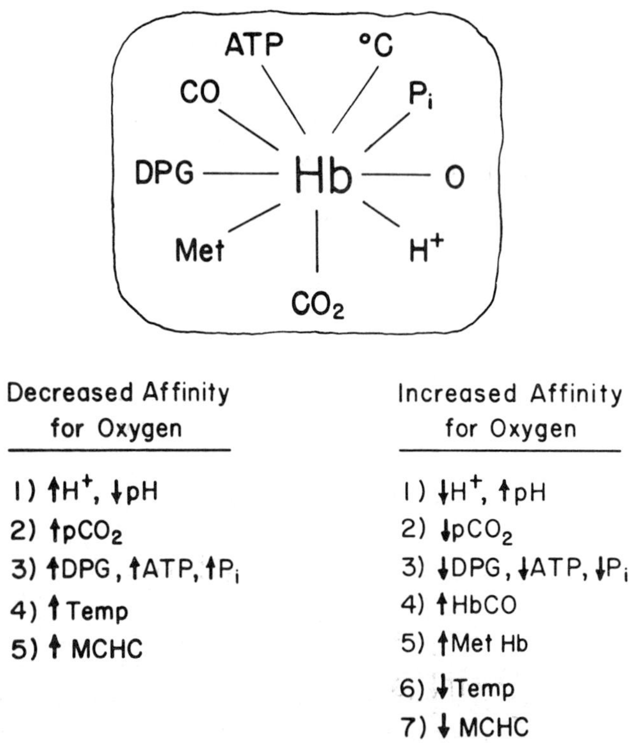

FIGURE 2. The factors influencing red blood cell affinity for oxygen — effect of pH, pCO_2, 2,3 DPG, temperature, inorganic phosphorus, methemoglobin, carboxyhemoglobin, and mean corpuscular hemoglobin concentration (MCHC). (From Valeri, C. R., *Clin. Haematol.*, 3, 649, 1974. With permission.)

only cause of a change in the red blood cell 2,3 DPG level. There is evidence that other factors also operate. Phosphate is present in muscle in large amounts, and damage to skeletal muscle may produce changes in blood inorganic phosphate level (Matsumoto et al., 1969; Knochel et al., 1974). Acute damage to other tissues such as occurs in intestinal infarction (Jamieson et al., 1979) and in chemical burns of skin and muscle (Bowen et al., 1971) may have the same effects. Very severe hypophosphatemia may occur in hyperalimentation, nutritional replenishment following starvation, treatment of diabetic lacticacidosis, alcohol withdrawal, congestive cardiomyopathy, antacid abuse especially when combined with dialysis or a phosphorus-poor diet, and prolonged respiratory alkalosis (O'Connor et al., 1977; Darsee and Nutter, 1978; Fuller et al., 1978; Lentz et al., 1978). Stress alone may be a cause of hypophosphatemia (Kaplan et al., 1969; Altschule, 1970). None of these types of hypophosphatemia occurred in our patients. Moreover, since the mechanisms of this phenomenon are not known, nothing would be gained from our further analysis of them here. High serum inorganic phosphate levels found in a few of our patients were considered to be secondary to hypocalcemia seen in desperately ill patients during and for a short time after resuscitation with citrate-containing blood products (Sibbald et al., 1977), but our patients were beyond this stage in their treatment.

CATABOLIC STATE AFTER TRAUMA

Our interest was directed toward the findings of Cuthbertson (1929, 1930, 1931, 1932), subsequently corroborated by many other workers, who called attention to marked changes in phosphate metabolism occurring in trauma involving limbs. Shortly after the trauma there is a massive outpouring of phosphate in the urine, together with nitrogen and sulfate, and although it diminishes considerably after a few days, it persists in some degree for many weeks. The chemical pattern, according to Cuthbertson, indicates widespread changes in skeletal muscle occurring both in the injured and the uninjured limbs. Increased outputs of phosphate, sulfate, and nitrogen together indicate a catabolic state, although the mechanism of this catabolic state is not known. It is true that a negative nitrogen balance occurs in markedly increased adrenal corticoid secretion, but this clearly cannot be a factor for very long in trauma. Moreover, adrenal steroid lowers serum inorganic phosphate concentrations (Henneman et al., 1955a, 1955b) whereas trauma raises it. One factor that seems to be involved in the phenomenon is immobility, but this accounts for only a small part of the losses (Cuthbertson, 1929).

Cuthbertson (1930), who reviewed the early publications in this field and described the common finding of elevated serum inorganic phosphate levels in trauma, demonstrated that this phenomenon was not immediate in onset. The delayed onset raises some doubt as to its relationship to the negative phosphate balance of trauma since it develops as the intensity of the body's loss of phosphate begins to subside. Reiss et al. (1970) found that the ability of the normal kidney to excrete phosphate is limited, leading one to expect a rise in serum inorganic phosphate level soon after a loss of phosphate from the tissues into the extracellular fluid. Hence, there must be some other explanation. It is interesting that the rise in serum phosphate described by Reiss et al. (1970) was followed immediately by a slight fall in calcium level and then by an increase in the amount of parathormone in the blood. This increase in blood parathormone level, a type of secondary hyperparathyroidism, has been invoked to explain the late hypercalcemia of immobilization (Lerman et al., 1977; Pezeshki and Brooker, 1977); a rise in the blood parathormone level may cause hypercalcemia but this is not commonly the case. Interpretation of the changes in the calcium level is made difficult by the fact that changes in serum calcium levels may be due solely to changes in protein intake in trauma patients (Schenk and Moylan, 1979).

Still another explanation of the disturbances in inorganic phosphate and calcium metabolism in patients with muscle injury was offered by Knochel et al. (1974). The rise in serum inorganic phosphate level associated with acute muscle injury occurring during strenuous exertion in hot climates was explained as being reciprocal to the observed fall in serum calcium level, the latter being ascribed to trapping of the calcium in necrotic muscle. It is worthy of note that the small number of our patients with high serum phosphate levels also exhibited low calcium concentrations. Further complicating the issue is a study by Sibbald et al. (1977) showing normal serum inorganic phosphate levels with hypocalcemia in patients with trauma.

We were aware that the changes in serum calcium and phosphorus were not well defined and, at any rate, most of our patients were well beyond the acute stages of their trauma and had normal serum calcium and phosphorus levels and only slightly elevated serum alkaline phosphatase activity (Table 3). The mean blood levels of calcium and phosphorus were normal, although elevated and decreased levels were seen in a few patients. Serum inorganic phosphate is known to influence synthesis of red blood cell 2,3 DPG in patients with red blood cell mass deficits. In most of our patients we saw no correlation between the red blood cell volume deficit and the levels of serum inorganic phosphate and calcium (Figure 3). Neither was any correlation seen between these levels and the number of extremities injured or the presence or absence of infection (Figure 4).

Observations of normal serum inorganic phosphate levels in most of our patients, and even low levels in a few, would appear to be inappropriate in view of commonly reported findings of elevated red blood cell 2,3 DPG levels. This is not actually as discrepant as it seems at first glance since serum values are not necessarily an indication of the phosphorus levels inside the erythrocytes (George et al., 1964). Our observations on serum inorganic phosphate levels (and of serum calcium levels) gave us no insight into the mechanism of the increased levels of red blood cell organic phosphate compounds exhibited by our patients and, in fact, offered nothing to elucidate the known ambiguities of inorganic phosphate metabolism in patients with trauma to the extremities.

CREATINE METABOLISM

Studies of creatine metabolism were made in our patients for several reasons, one being that red blood cell creatine levels are thought by some to be an indication of the age of the erythrocyte, as discussed below. In addition, marked disturbances of creatine metabolism are seen in several disorders of skeletal muscles. Creatinuria apparently is due to leakage of creatine from injured muscles, and our patients who had suffered serious injury to skeletal muscle at the time of wounding had persistent muscle damage at the time of our studies. Creatinuria also may occur as a result of the widespread breakdown of muscle protein during the catabolic reaction to severe stress (Altschule and Rosenfeld, 1947), although most of our patients were probably well beyond that phase of their injury. Nevertheless, a few of them still did have a slightly negative nitrogen balance when studied. In addition, creatinuria apparently occurs owing to muscle hypoxia (Altschule, 1954) as a consequence to a low cardiac output in chronic cardiac decompensation, and when treatment improves this condition the creatinuria disappears. The creatinuria in our hypovolemic wounded patients disappeared following restoration of the red blood cell deficits with transfusion and hence was probably hypoxic in origin.

Table 3
SERUM CALCIUM AND PHOSPHATE LEVELS, ALKALINE PHOSPHATASE LEVEL, AND URIC ACID LEVEL IN PATIENTS WITH TRAUMATIC INJURIES WITH AND WITHOUT ANTIBIOTICS, PATIENTS WITH CARCINOMA, PATIENTS WITH CARDIOPULMONARY DISEASE, AND PATIENTS WITH MISCELLANEOUS DIAGNOSES

Group	Calcium (9—11 mg%)	Phosphate (3—5 mg%)	Alkaline phosphatase (12—40 I.U.)	Uric acid (2—7 mg%)
I				
n	42	41	39	11
Mean	9.6	4.5	47.7	5.3
S.D.	0.8	1.7	16.2	1.8
S.E.	0.1	0.3	2.6	0.6
II				
n	99	100	89	19
Mean	9.5	4.4	43.5	5.5
S.D.	1.2	0.9	16.2	1.6
S.E.	0.1	0.1	1.7	0.4
III				
n	9	8	4	19
Mean	10.2	3.9	51.0	5.9
S.D.	1.1	1.2	28.3	2.2
S.E.	0.2	0.4	14.1	0.5
IV				
n	12	19	6	19
Mean	9.7	3.4	41.7	5.7
S.D.	1.2	1.2	26.3	1.8
S.E.	0.4	0.3	10.7	0.4
V				
n	10	10	9	23
Mean	9.7	4.3	43.1	4.6
S.D.	0.9	2.2	20.2	2.5
S.E.	0.2	0.5	4.7	0.5

Note: Group I — traumatic injuries without antibiotics. Group II — traumatic injuries with antibiotics. Group III — patients with carcinoma. Group IV — patients with cardiopulmonary disease. Group V — miscellaneous diagnoses.

The finding of creatinuria in our wounded patients prompted us to study the plasma and red blood cell creatine levels in many of them (Figure 5) (Biron et al., 1972). The value of plasma creatine in normal healthy volunteers was 0.02 ± 0.01 μmol/mℓ plasma, whereas in our patients with traumatic injuries, as well as those with uremia, cardiopulmonary insufficiency, and infection, the plasma creatine levels ranged from 0.034 to 0.23 μmol/mℓ plasma (Table 4). The patients with cardiopulmonary insuffi-

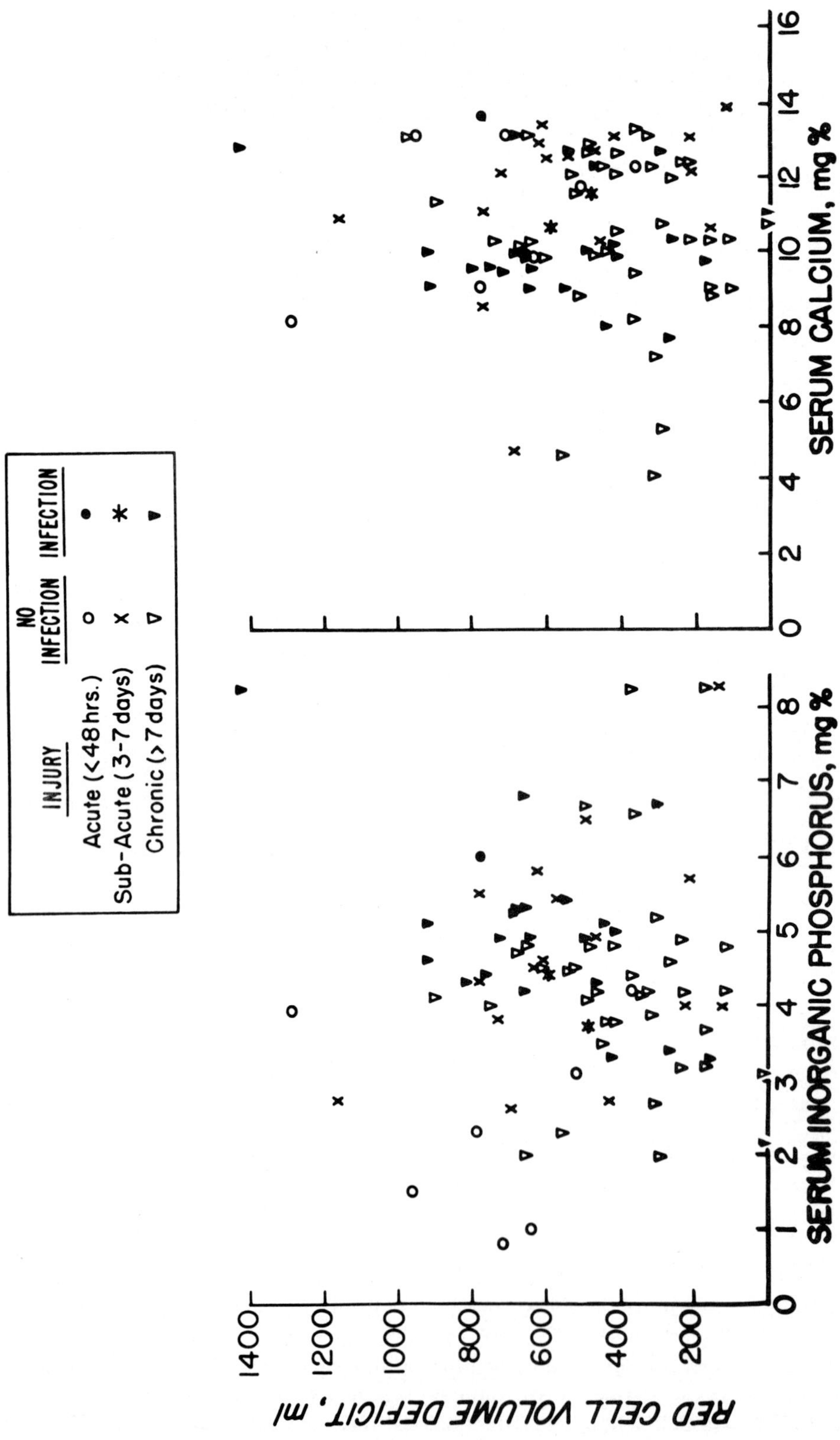

FIGURE 3. The relations between red blood cell volume deficit and the serum inorganic phosphorus level and serum calcium level.

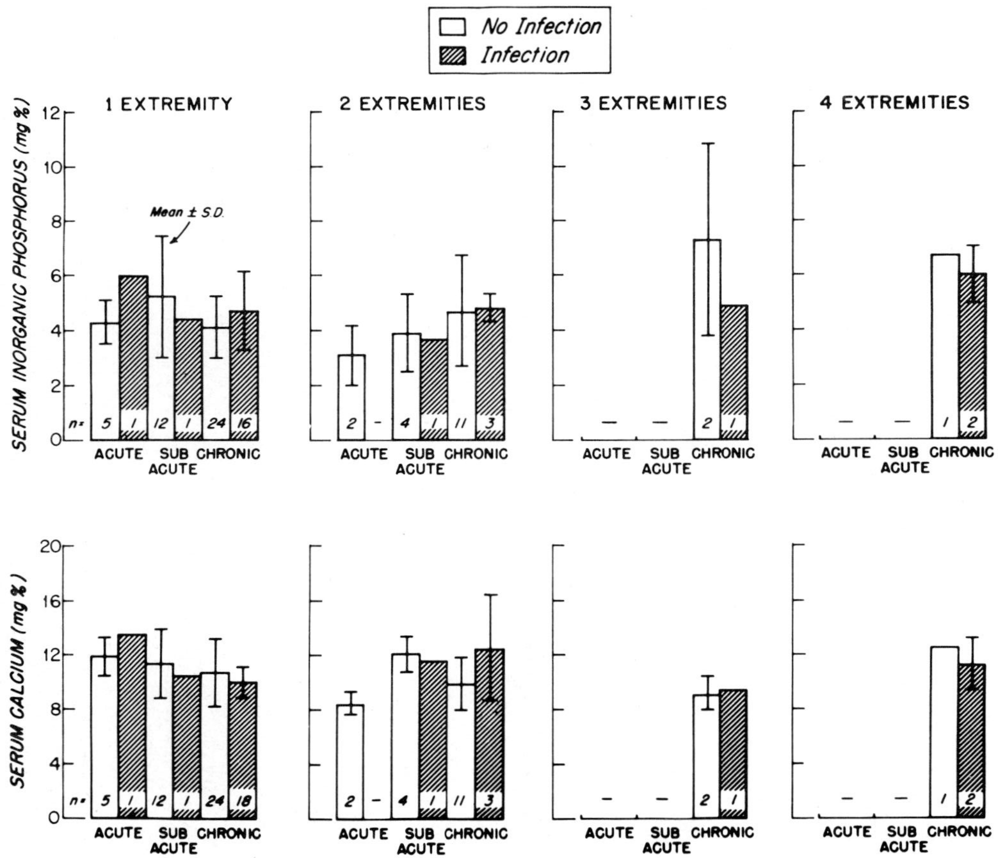

FIGURE 4. The levels of serum inorganic phosphorus and calcium in patients with acute, subacute, and chronic traumatic injuries involving one, two, three, or four extremities with or without infection.

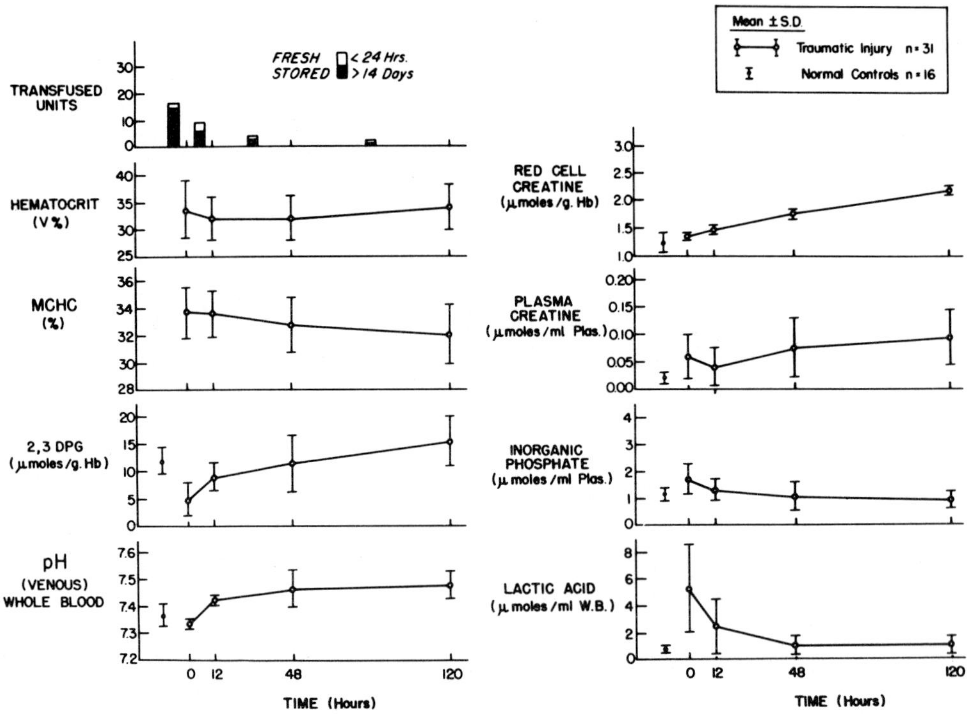

FIGURE 5. The effect of massive transfusion of red blood cells to 31 patients with traumatic injuries in hemorrhagic shock. Some of the red blood cell units were stored at 4°C for greater than two weeks and some were fresh units, i.e., stored at 4°C for less than 24 hr. Hematocrit, MCHC, red blood cell 2,3 DPG and creatine levels, plasma creatine level, plasma inorganic phosphorus level, blood lactic acid, and pH of venous blood were measured for a period of 120 hr after transfusion. (From Kopriva, C. J., Ratliff, J. L., Fletcher, J. R., Fortier, N. L., and Valeri, C. R., *Ann. Surg.*, 176, 585, 1972. With permission.)

Table 4
PLASMA CREATINE AND OTHER HEMATOLOGIC MEASUREMENTS IN FOUR GROUPS OF PATIENTS

	Hct (V%)	Hb (g%)	MCHC (%)	RBC creatine μmol/g Hb (1.2 ± 0.6)	Blood creatine μmol/mℓ WB (0.18 ± 0.09)	Plasma creatine μmol/mℓ Pl (0.02 ± 0.01)	Plasma creatine (%)	Inorganic phosphate (mg%) (3.5 ± 1)	RBC 2,3 DPG μmol/g Hb (12 ± 1.2)	Blood lactic acid μmol/mℓ WB (1.0 ± 0.3)
Cardiopulmonary insufficiency										
n	9	9	9	9	9	9	9	9	9	9
Mean	45.4	14.2	31.6	3.09	0.443	0.052	4.60	3.44	16.74	1.32
± SD	7.1	2.5	0.9	2.65	0.370	0.085	3.31	2.08	2.77	0.65
Uremia										
n	9	9	9	9	9	9	9	9	9	9
Mean	27.2	9.2	34.1	4.77	0.434	0.034	6.54	7.12	18.40	1.79
± SD	7.6	2.4	1.7	2.58	0.188	0.014	4.40	2.08	5.12	0.54
Traumatic injuries with sepsis										
n	4	4	4	4	4	4	4	4	4	4
Mean	32.5	11.0	33.9	2.35	0.248	0.231	34.10	3.81	15.63	1.36
± SD	2.0	0.4	1.1	0.79	0.079	0.293	16.00	1.73	2.80	0.69
Traumatic injuries without sepsis										
n	82	82	82	82	82	82	82	82	82	82
Mean	42.7	13.9	32.7	2.11	0.308	0.035	6.26	3.93	13.90	1.49
± SD	4.0	1.5	1.3	0.68	0.171	0.023	3.63	1.64	1.97	0.53

ciency had normal hemoglobin and hematocrit values when their levels of plasma creatine were increased (Tables 4, 5A, and 5B), and this may be explained by the release of creatine from hypoxic muscle into the plasma. However, in our patients with traumatic injuries, plasma creatine levels differed markedly between those with sepsis and those without (Figure 6). Patients with traumatic injuries with sepsis had significantly higher plasma creatine levels than those without sepsis (Figure 6), a finding for which we can offer no explanation. Patients with uremia also had increased creatine levels, and perhaps this is one of the complicated biochemical abnormalities of that condition. The patients with increased plasma creatine levels also had slightly elevated blood lactic acid levels (Table 4).

Our studies on red blood cell creatine levels produced some surprises. For one thing, significantly elevated red blood cell creatine levels often were accompanied by only minimal increases in plasma levels. The red blood cell level of creatine was similar in the patients with traumatic injuries whether or not sepsis was present (Figure 6). Interpretation of the elevated red blood cell creatine levels in our patients is difficult. The role of red blood cell creatine has not been clearly established, although it is thought to reflect the mean red blood cell age (Griffiths and Fitzpatrick, 1967; Griffiths, 1968a, 1968b; Griffiths and Lothian, 1969; Opalinski and Beutler, 1971; Fehr and Knob, 1979).

We have data supportive of the findings of Griffiths and Fitzpatrick (1967) and Opalinski and Beutler (1971) who found increased red blood cell creatine levels associated with reticulocytosis and reduced mean red blood cell age in hemolytic anemia, and reduced red blood cell creatine levels associated with reduced reticulocyte production and increased mean red blood cell age in aplastic anemia (Figure 7 and Tables 5A and 5B). However, this has no bearing on our patients with trauma. Red blood cell hexokinase and glutamicoxaloacetic transaminase activities, both of which are elevated in young erythrocytes (as is 2,3 DPG also), were found to be abnormally high, as was the reticulocyte count, in our patients with elevated red blood cell creatine levels associated with hemolytic anemia and with cardiopulmonary insufficiency (Karmen et al., 1955; Edwards et al., 1961; Brewer and Powell, 1963; O'Connell et al., 1965; Brok et al., 1966; Edwards and Rigas, 1967; Valentine et al., 1967; Malone et al., 1968; Sabine and Kwok, 1968; Hillman and Finch, 1969; Keitt, 1969; Blum, 1970; Anderson et al., 1971; Edwards et al., 1971; Larkin et al., 1973). The significant increase in the red blood cell creatine level despite the slight reduction in the mean red blood cell age (45 days) in our wounded patients suggests that the creatine level was not related solely to the red blood cell age (Tables 5A and 5C and Figures 7, 8, and 9). Patients with traumatic injuries exhibited increases in red blood cell hexokinase, GOT, creatine, and 2,3 DPG levels, but had normal levels of reticulocytes (Tables 5A, 5B, and 5C). Posttransfusion measurements of mean red blood cell age in five patients with traumatic injuries revealed no correlation between the mean red blood cell age and red blood cell creatine (Figure 8). In these studies the mean red blood cell age was calculated from the serial measurements of red blood cell volume using ^{51}Cr-labeled autologous red blood cells before and after transfusion of identifiable compatible cells. It is evident that there must be one or more factors that affect red blood cell creatine in addition to red blood cell age.

We were surprised to find a correlation between the red blood cell creatine level and the 2,3 DPG level in our patients with traumatic injuries, and this prompted us to further analyze our data with regard to a possible correlation between the red blood cell creatine concentration and the red blood cell deficit (Figures 8 and 9). Red blood cell creatine levels were increased in our patients with red blood cell mass deficits independent of the mean red blood cell age (Figure 8). We do not know what causes

Table 5A

THE HEMATOLOGIC MEASUREMENTS IN SIX GROUPS OF PATIENTS AND IN A GROUP OF NORMAL VOLUNTEERS

		Normal volunteers (n = 31)	Traumatic injuries (n = 15)	Cardiopulmonary disorders (n = 4)	Carcinoma (n = 10)	Hemolytic anemia (n = 4)	Aplastic anemia (n = 2)	Uremia (n = 4)
Hematocrit (Vol %)	Mean	45.1	39.6	41.7	39.5	24.4	18.0	23.6
	SD	2.8	5.8	6.8	7.1	10.0	2.5	9.0
	SE	0.5	1.5	3.4	2.3	5.8	1.8	6.4
RBC 2,3 DPG (μmol/g Hb)	Mean	11.7	15.0	14.7	15.3	20.0	13.0	15.3
	SD	0.5	0.9	1.3	1.9	2.9	0.8	1.7
	SE	0.1	0.2	0.7	0.6	1.4	0.6	0.9
RBC Creatine (μmol/g Hb)	Mean	1.09	2.53	2.43	2.56	5.70	0.59	2.59
	SD	0.28	0.52	0.68	1.39	1.70	0.32	0.63
	SE	0.05	0.15	0.34	0.44	0.80	0.23	0.31
RBC Hexokinase (μmol/min/g Hb)	Mean	0.86	1.04	1.67	1.19	2.87	0.80	1.45
	SD	0.15	0.17	0.35	0.26	1.40	0.06	0.61
	SE	0.02	0.04	0.17	0.08	0.70	0.04	0.31
RBC GOT (μmol/min/g Hb)	Mean	2.64	3.50	4.32	3.10	3.65	1.25	4.39
	SD	0.54	1.10	2.32	0.78	1.50	0.38	1.77
	SE	0.09	0.30	1.16	0.24	0.70	0.27	0.89
Reticulocyte count (%)	Mean	0.94	1.00	2.02	0.69	12.8	0.25	1.67
	SD	0.62	0.52	0.52	0.38	14.8	0.07	1.87
	SE	0.11	0.14	0.26	0.12	7.4	0.05	0.93

Table 5B
T-TEST COMPARING THE VALUES FOR A GROUP OF NORMAL VOLUNTEERS WITH THOSE FOR EACH OF SIX GROUPS OF PATIENTS

		Traumatic injuries	Cardiopulmonary disorders	Carcinoma	Hemolytic anemia	Aplastic anemia	Uremia
Degrees of freedom		44	33	39	33	31	33
Hematocrit (vol%)	t	4.25	1.78	3.52	8.83	12.94	9.76
	p	<0.002	NS	<0.002	<0.002	<0.002	<0.002
RBC 2,3 DPB	t	−15.63	−8.43	−9.219	−13.95	−3.32	−8.77
(μmol/g Hb)	p	<0.002	<0.002	<0.002	<0.002	<0.01	<0.002
RBC Creatine	t	−11.92	−7.02	−5.42	−13.33	2.35	−7.61
(μmol/g Hb)	p	<0.002	<0.002	<0.002	<0.002	<0.05	<0.002
RBC Hexokinase	t	−3.57	−8.07	−4.87	−7.44	0.55	−4.33
(μmol/min/g Hb)	p	<0.002	<0.002	<0.002	<0.002	NS	<0.002
RBC GOT	t	−3.48	−2.12	−2.03	−2.57	3.47	−4.08
(μmol/min/g Hb)	p	<0.002	<0.05	<0.05	<0.02	<0.002	<0.002
Reticulocyte count	t	−0.32	−3.24	1.18	−4.30	1.53	−1.55
(%)	p	NS	<0.01	NS	<0.002	NS	NS

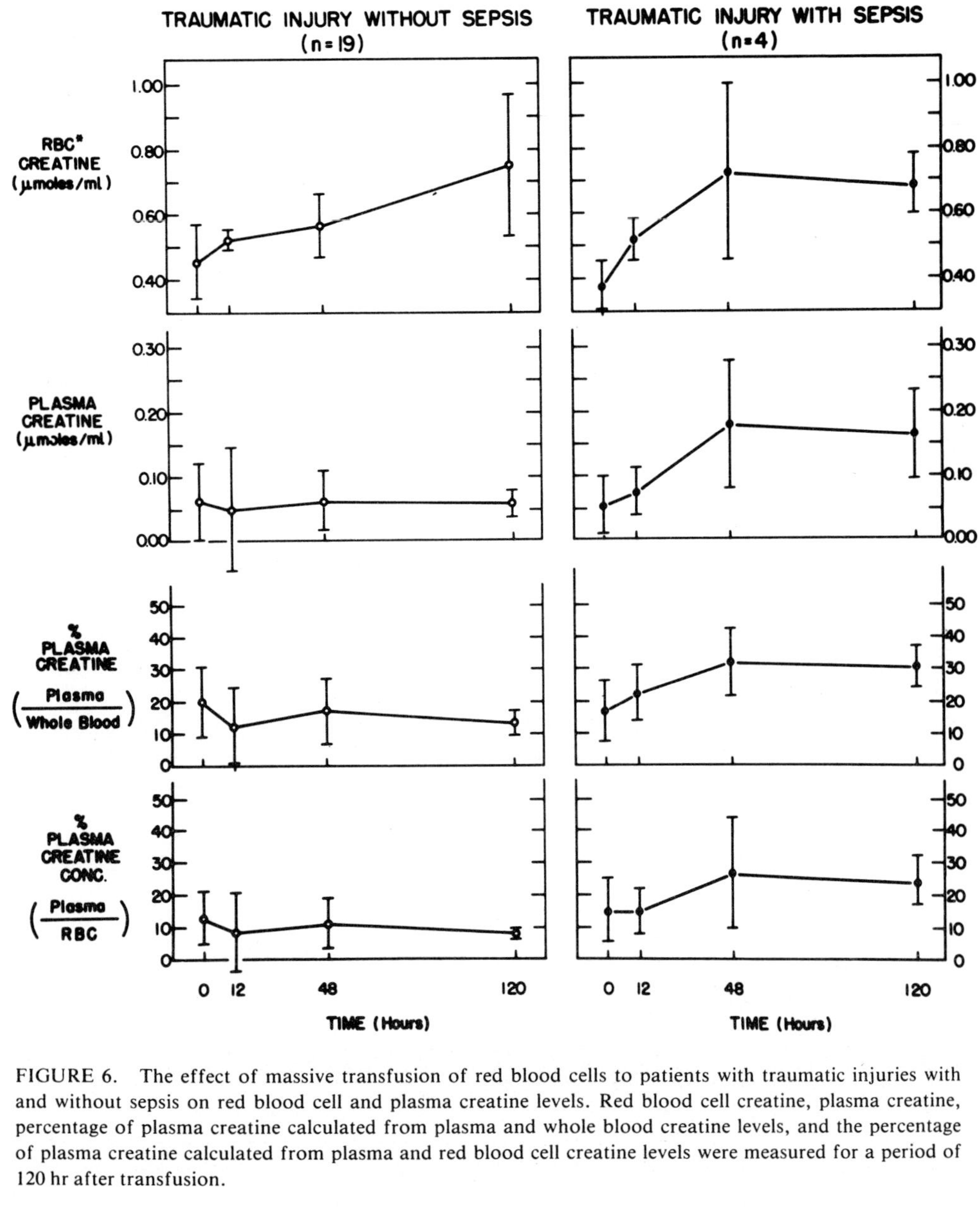

FIGURE 6. The effect of massive transfusion of red blood cells to patients with traumatic injuries with and without sepsis on red blood cell and plasma creatine levels. Red blood cell creatine, plasma creatine, percentage of plasma creatine calculated from plasma and whole blood creatine levels, and the percentage of plasma creatine calculated from plasma and red blood cell creatine levels were measured for a period of 120 hr after transfusion.

creatine to accumulate in red blood cells in vivo nor do we understand its role in the metabolism and function of the red blood cells (Valeri and Fortier, 1969b).

Although a significant correlation between red blood cell creatine and red blood cell 2,3 DPG levels in patients with anemic and hypoxic hypoxia was evident (Figure 10), it was also clear that unlike 2,3 DPG, creatine has no effect on the red blood cell affinity for oxygen (Paniker and Beutler, 1970; Valeri and Fortier, 1970). Rather it appears that these two measurements may act to monitor the magnitude of the red blood cell mass deficit (Valeri and Fortier, 1969b), and serve much better than peripheral hemoglobin and hematocrit values which are often normal or nearly so because of the simultaneous decreases in red blood cell and plasma volumes (Chapter 2). Thus, measurements of red blood cell 2,3 DPG and creatine concentrations could be instituted as part of regular clinical studies of patients following trauma in hospitals where measurements are not commonly made of red blood cell mass.

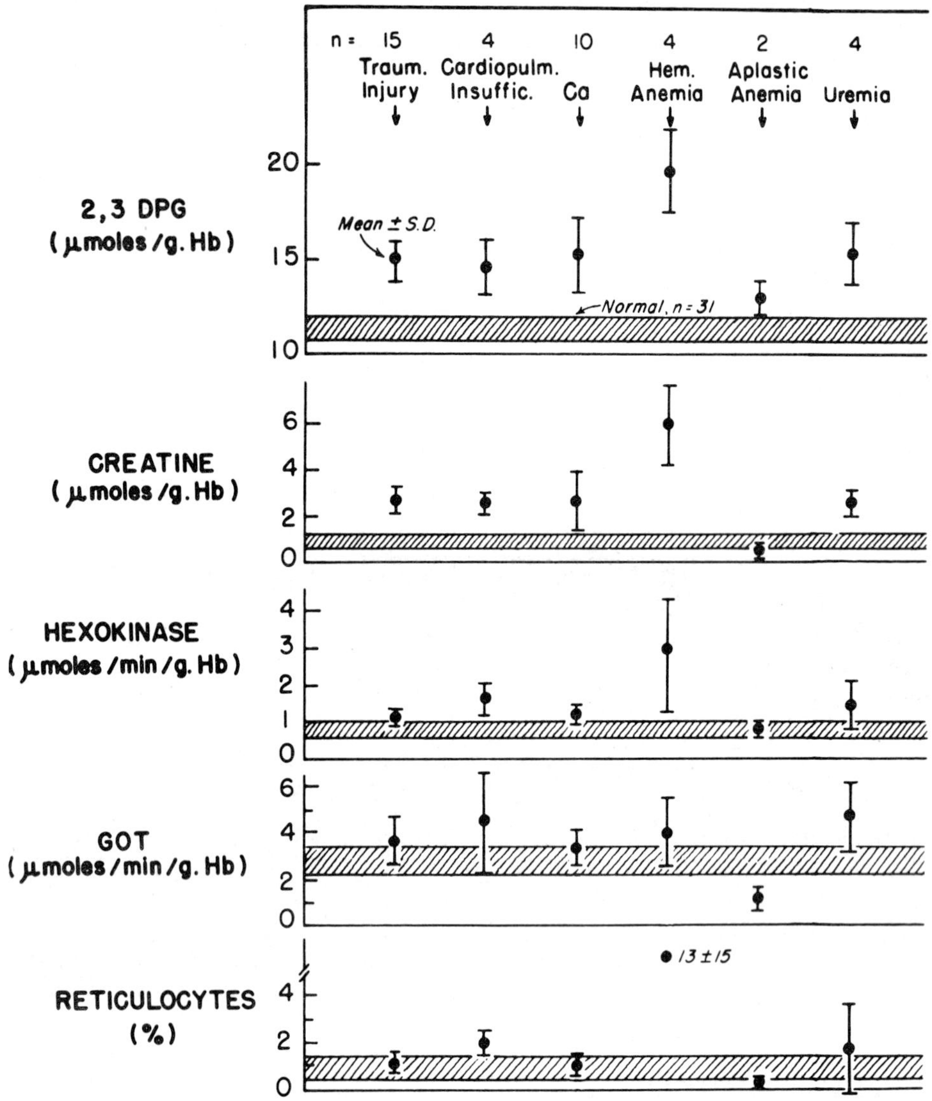

FIGURE 7. Red blood cell 2,3 DPG, creatine, hexokinase, and GOT levels and reticulocyte counts in patients with traumatic injuries, cardiopulmonary insufficiency, carcinoma, hemolytic anemia, aplastic anemia, and uremia.

Red blood cell 2,3 DPG and creatine levels and red blood cell mass and the reticulocyte count were measured before and after transfusion. In addition, red blood cell ATP concentration, in vitro P_{50} value, and venous blood pH were measured in some of the patients.

We must emphasize again, at the risk of redundancy, that the therapeutic transfusions administered to our patients and the measurements made to evaluate the effectiveness of the transfusions were part of a strict regimen of treatment for these men with traumatic injuries. Another point that must be made is that the blood transfused was not a source of creatine, since the plasma level of creatine increased only slightly during storage of the blood at 4°C for 21 days (Figure 11). Creatine levels in plasma do increase after storage of blood at 4°C for 30 to 40 days. Nevertheless, the amount

Table 5C

T-TEST BETWEEN THE VALUES OF EACH OF THREE GROUPS OF PATIENTS AND A GROUP OF NORMAL VOLUNTEERS COMPARED TO A GROUP OF PATIENTS WITH TRAUMATIC INJURIES

		Normal volunteers	Cardiopulmonary disorders	Carcinoma	Uremia
Degrees of freedom:		44	17	23	17
Hematocrit (vol %)	t	−4.25	−0.58	0.036	4.07
	p	<0.002	NS	NS	<0.002
RBC 2,3 DPG	t	15.63	0.51	0.51	0.45
(μmol/g Hb)	p	<0.002	NS	NS	NS
RBC Creatine	t	11.92	0.3	0.07	−0.18
(μmol/g Hb)	p	<0.002	NS	NS	NS
RBC Hexokinase	t	3.57	−4.82	−1.69	−2.17
(μmol/min/g Hb)	p	<0.002	<0.002	NS	<0.05
RBC GOT	t	3.48	−0.96	0.96	−1.18
(μmol/min/g Hb)	p	<0.002	NS	NS	NS
Reticulocyte count	t	0.32	−3.29	1.56	−1.16
(%)	p	NS	<0.01	NS	NS

of plasma creatine in the blood used in transfusions to our patients clearly could not explain the plasma creatine levels observed following massive transfusion (Figure 5).

BLOOD CREATINE STUDIES IN PATIENTS

We present here an analysis of data derived from studies of seven patients hospitalized for up to 2 years on the Orthopedic Service at Chelsea Naval Hospital. This prolonged period of observation permitted us to ascertain with confidence the normal body weights of our patients after their wounds had healed and their condition had improved. At the beginning of the study, one patient (Figure 12) had a normal red blood cell mass, and the other six patients (Figures 13 to 18) had reduced red blood cell masses. The patients with reduced red blood cell mass were usually transfused with whole blood during an operation. They were also given washed liquid-stored red blood cells and washed previously frozen red blood cells before and after the operation in order to restore the red blood cell mass deficits measured with the use of their own ^{51}Cr-labeled red blood cells. Reductions in red blood cell mass were accompanied by increased levels of red blood cell 2,3 DPG and creatine, and normal or low reticulocyte counts.

Patient 6A, a 20-year-old man (Figure 12), who had a normal red blood cell mass prior to operation, received four units of whole blood during his operation. Three days after this he was seen to be pale, weak, and drowsy, with tachycardia but no hypotension. His red blood cell mass had decreased by 65% and his hemoglobin and hematocrit values were also decreased. The loss of the patient's own and the compatible donor red blood cells transfused during the operation could not be explained solely by the bleeding that occurred during or after the operation, and this unexplained loss suggested the missing blood syndrome. A transfusion of five units of washed liquid-stored red blood cells corrected his reduced red blood cell mass. After 2 years of convalesc-

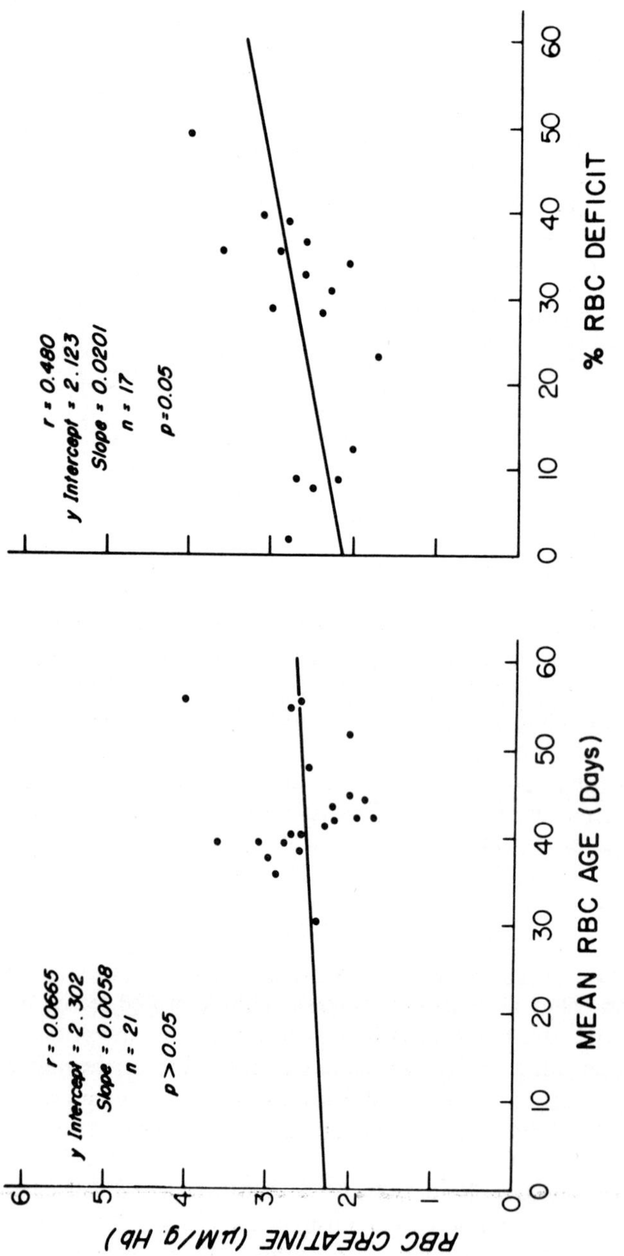

FIGURE 8. The relation of red blood cell creatine to the mean red blood cell age and the percent red blood cell deficit in five patients with traumatic injuries.

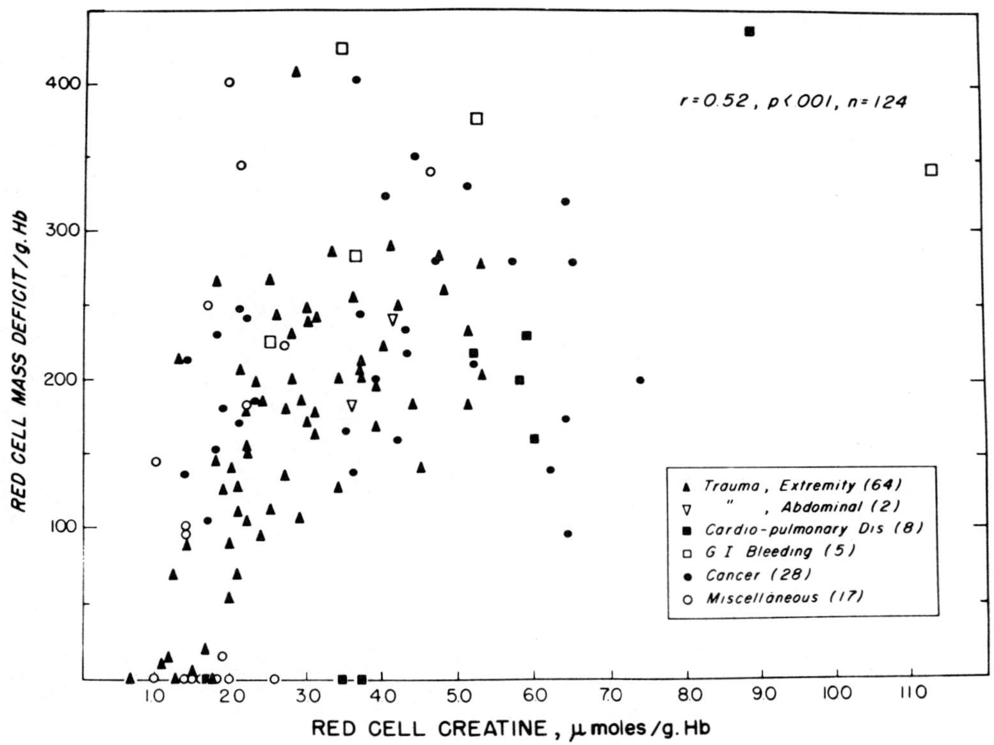

FIGURE 9. The relation between red blood cell creatine and the red blood cell mass deficit in patients with traumatic injuries, cardiopulmonary insufficiency, gastrointestinal bleeding, carcinoma, and miscellaneous diagnoses. (Reprinted by permission from Valeri, C. R. and Fortier, N. L., *New Engl. J. Med.*, 281, 1452, 1969.)

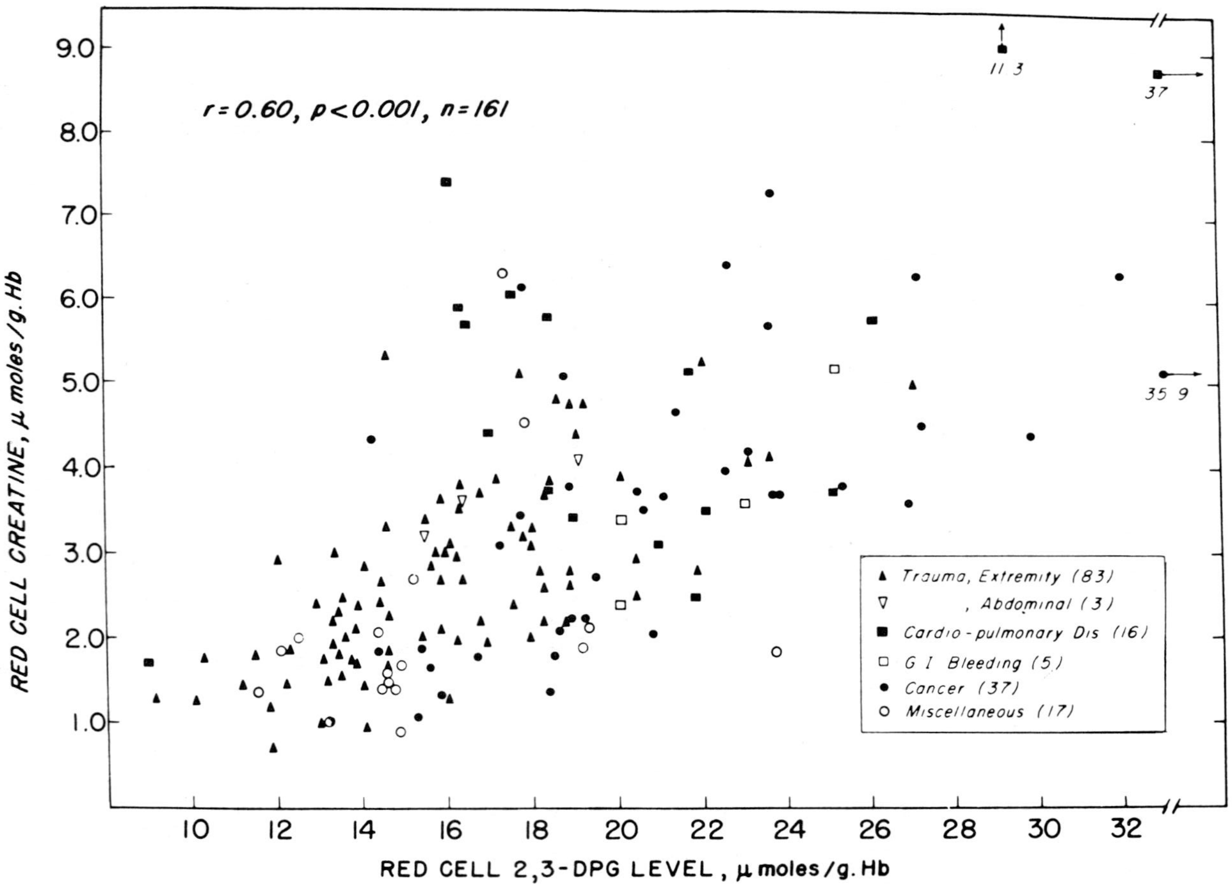

FIGURE 10. The relation between red blood cell 2,3 DPG and creatine levels in patients with traumatic injuries, cardiopulmonary diseases, gastrointestinal bleeding, carcinoma, and miscellaneous diagnoses. (Reprinted by permission from Valeri, C. R. and Fortier, N. L., *New Engl. J. Med.*, 281, 1452, 1969.)

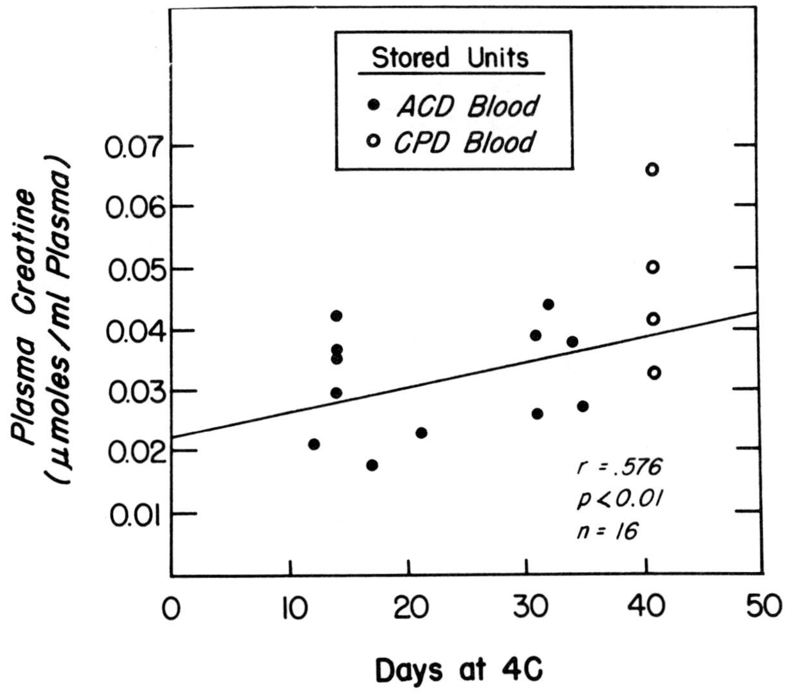

FIGURE 11. The plasma creatine level in acid-citrate-dextrose and citrate-phosphate-dextrose blood stored in the liquid state at 4°C for 42 days.

ence, this patient's red blood cell mass was found to be normal as estimated from his body surface area.

In the six patients described in Figures 13 to 18, red blood cell mass deficits of more than 40% were accompanied by reduced hemoglobin and hematocrit values, whereas deficits of less than 40% were accompanied by only slightly reduced hemoglobin and hematocrit values. Increased red blood cell 2,3 DPG and creatine levels were related to the red blood cell mass deficits, and when the transfusion increased the red blood cell mass, the red blood cell 2,3 DPG and creatine levels decreased. With restoration of the red blood cell mass to normal, red blood cell 2,3 DPG and creatine also returned to normal levels. In each of these patients (Figures 13 to 18) the red blood cell mass approached the theoretical volume when the patient's state of health returned to normal; this happened within 3 months to 2 years of convalescence (Figures 12 to 18). Most of the patients required repeated transfusions to restore the red blood cell mass to normal.

Another group of acutely wounded patients were observed to be anemic even after the massive transfusion of acid-citrate-dextrose (ACD) anticoagulated liquid-stored blood; red cell creatine and 2,3 DPG data indicated that the blood loss was not being adequately replaced and the red blood cell volume was decreased. Red cell 2,3 DPG and creatine levels increased over the 120-hr posttransfusion period and plasma creatine levels changed only slightly (Figure 5) (Kopriva et al., 1972). Each patient initially was given 15 units of 14-day-old blood, then five units that had been stored for less than 24 hr, and then five units stored at 4°C for longer than 14 days.

In another group of 15 anemic patients, the transfusion of three to five units of washed liquid-stored or washed previously frozen red blood cells reduced the red blood cell mass deficit, from 227 g to 81 g in 11 patients, whereas in the other four patients

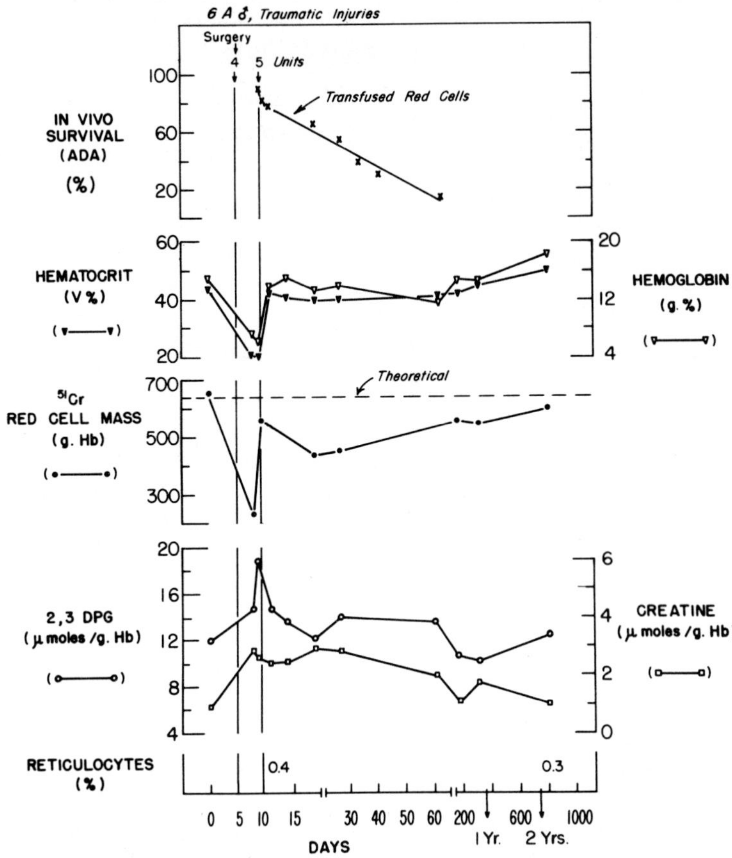

FIGURE 12. Hematocrit and hemoglobin concentrations, red blood cell mass, red blood cell 2,3 DPG and creatine levels, and reticulocyte counts in Patient 6A, a 20-year-old male with traumatic injuries who was treated and evaluated over a 2-year period. The red blood cell survival of five units of liquid-stored washed red blood cells was measured by the automated differential agglutination procedure. (From Biron, P. E., Howard, J., Altschule, M. D., and Valeri, C. R., *J. Bone Jt. Surg.*, 54(A), 1001, 1972. With permission.)

the red cell mass deficit actually increased during the 10-day posttransfusion period, from 170 to 253 g. In the eleven patients whose red blood cell mass deficit was reduced, the measured red cell creatine levels after transfusion were consistently lower than the calculated levels; in the four patients in whom the red blood cell mass deficit was increased after transfusion, the measured red cell creatine levels were consistently higher than the calculated levels (Table 6). The calculated level was arrived at by measuring the patient's red cell creatine prior to transfusion, the donor's red cell creatine, and the percentages of recipient and donor red blood cells after transfusion (Table 6). The percentage of identifiable donor red blood cells was measured by the automated differential agglutination procedure. Our data do not support the hypothesis of Fehr and Knob (1979) who suggest that a prolonged reduction in red cell creatine following transfusion is an indication of donor red blood cell compatibility and that a rapid increase indicates incompatibility. In all 15 of our patients the percentage of donor red blood cells was similar, indicating compatibility, despite the observed differences in red cell creatine levels (Table 6).

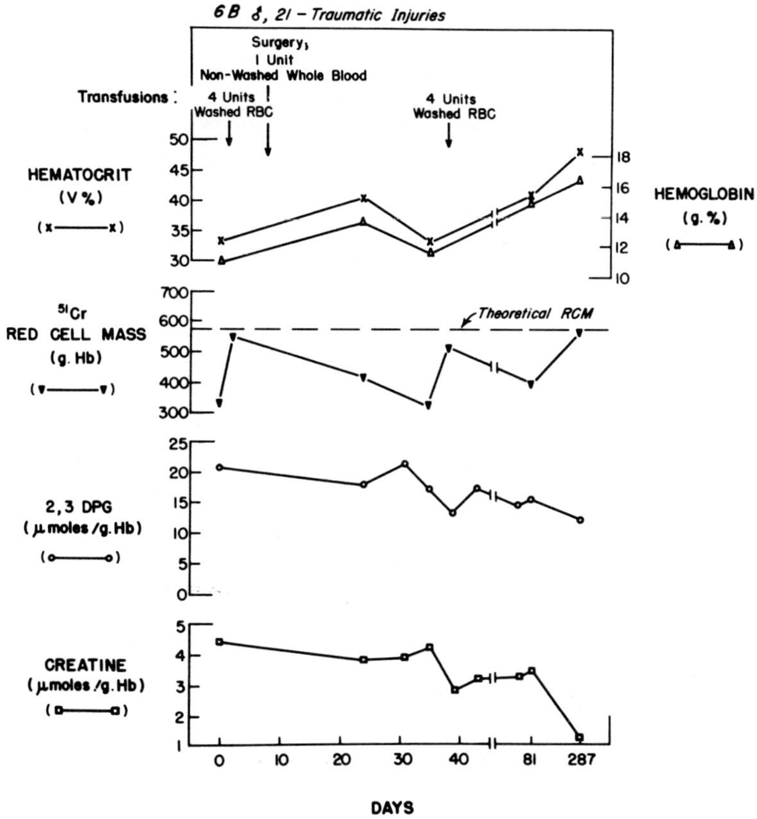

FIGURE 13. Hematocrit and hemoglobin concentrations, red blood cell mass, and red blood cell 2,3 DPG and creatine levels in Patient 6B, a 21-year-old male with traumatic injuries who was treated and evaluated for a 10-month period.

Our data collected before and after transfusion suggest that when the red blood cell mass deficit is not restored following transfusion, creatine enters the circulating red blood cells (Valeri and Fortier, 1969a, 1969b; Biron et al., 1972), and failure to restore the red blood cell mass will result in continued elevation or a further increase in red cell creatine. Our theory is that ischemic muscle releases creatine and this accumulates in the circulating red blood cells (Fitch and Rahmanian, 1969; Kreisberg et al., 1970). The entry of creatine into red blood cells has yet to be shown in vitro (Griffiths and Fitzpatrick, 1967; Griffiths and Lothian, 1969; Valeri and Fortier, 1970; Opalinski and Beutler, 1971) but our in vivo data showing a change in red blood cell creatine following transfusion (Table 6) suggest that in anemic hypoxia the red blood cells accumulate creatine presumably liberated from hypoxic muscle. When the red blood cell mass is restored to normal, the circulation to muscle is restored (Chapter 5). Elimination of the hypoperfusion and hypoxia of muscle results in cessation of the leak of creatine from muscle to plasma and red blood cells.

GENERAL COMMENTS

In summary, this chapter describes observations on the general metabolic effects of trauma that may induce biochemical changes which will affect the metabolism of red

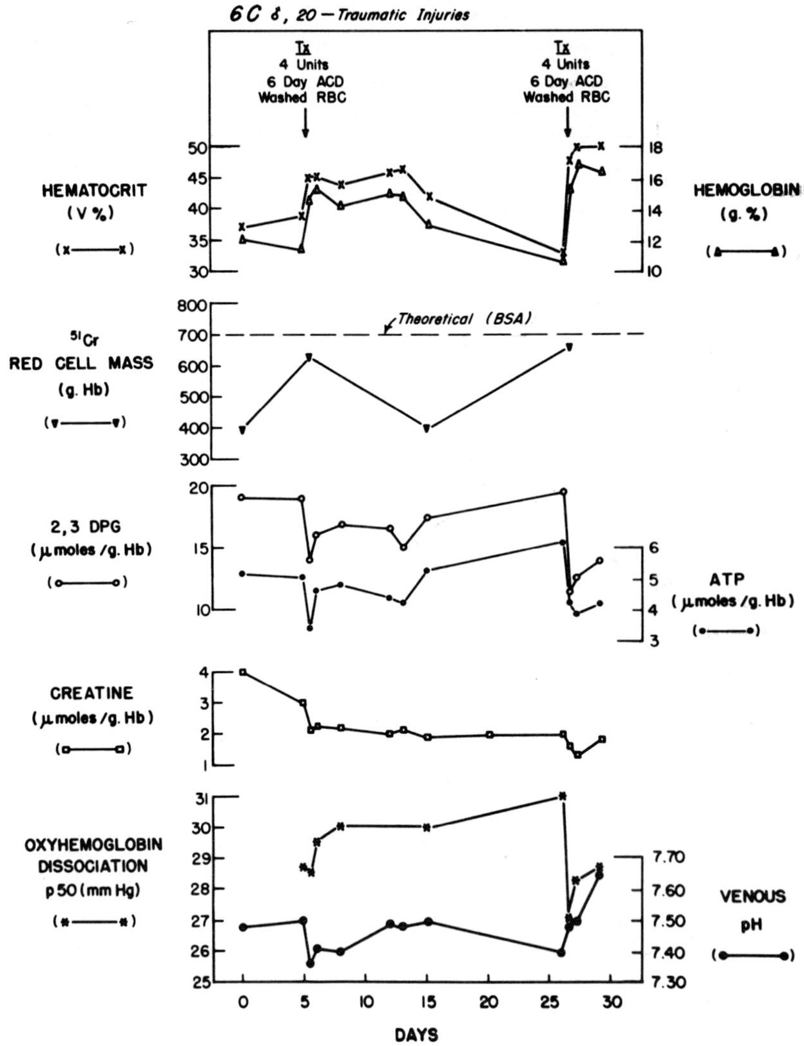

FIGURE 14. Hematocrit and hemoglobin concentrations, red blood cell mass, red blood cell 2,3 DPG, ATP, creatine, and P_{50} values, and the venous blood pH in Patient 6C, a 20-year-old male with traumatic injuries who was treated and evaluated for a 1-month period.

blood cells. The well-known role of inorganic phosphate in 2,3 DPG formation was studied. We also studied the creatine metabolism associated with trauma and observed changes in the erythrocyte creatine level not previously described and still not understood by us. Whatever the mechanisms may have been for these increases in red blood cell 2,3 DPG and creatine levels, these measurements served as accurate indications of red blood cell mass deficits in our patients.

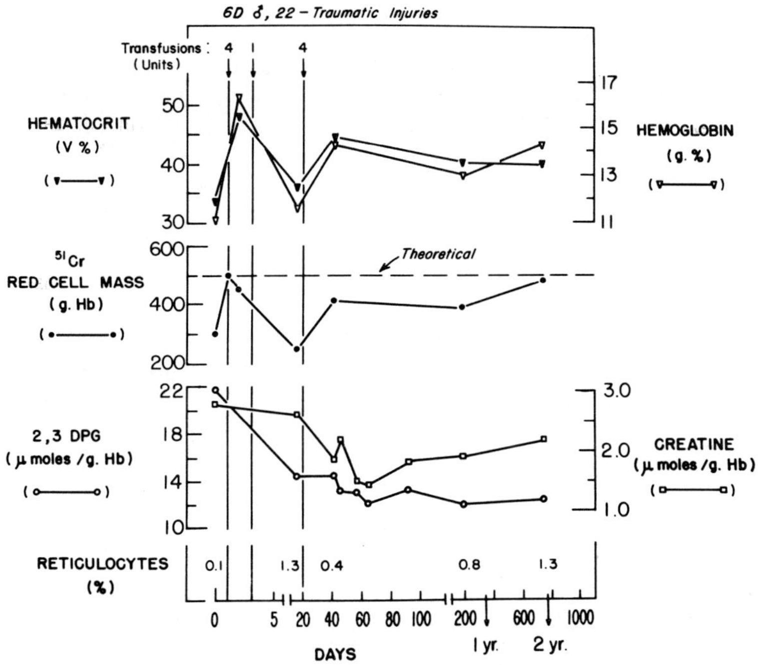

FIGURE 15. Hematocrit and hemoglobin concentrations, red blood cell mass, red blood cell 2,3 DPG and creatine levels, and reticulocyte count in Patient 6D, a 22-year-old male with traumatic injuries who was treated and evaluated over a 2-year period.

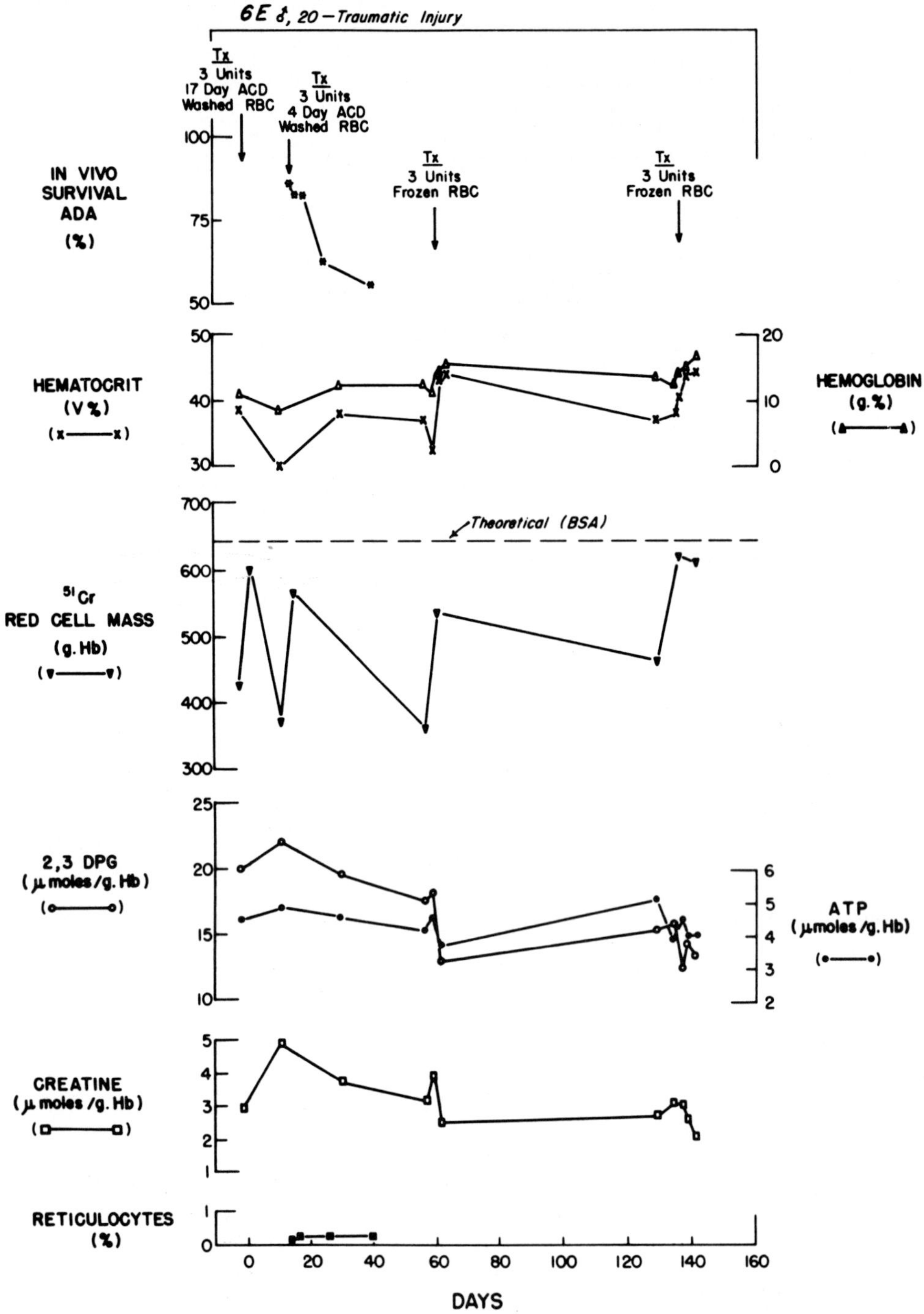

FIGURE 16. Hematocrit and hemoglobin concentrations, red blood cell mass, red blood cell 2,3 DPG, ATP, and creatine levels, and reticulocyte count in Patient 6E, a 20-year-old male with traumatic injuries who was treated and evaluated for a 5-month period. After one of the four red blood cell transfusions given this patient, the survival of the donor red blood cells was measured using the automated differential agglutination procedure. (From Biron, P. E., Howard, J., Altschule, M. D., and Valeri, C. R., *J. Bone Jt. Surg.*, 54(A), 1001, 1972. With permission.)

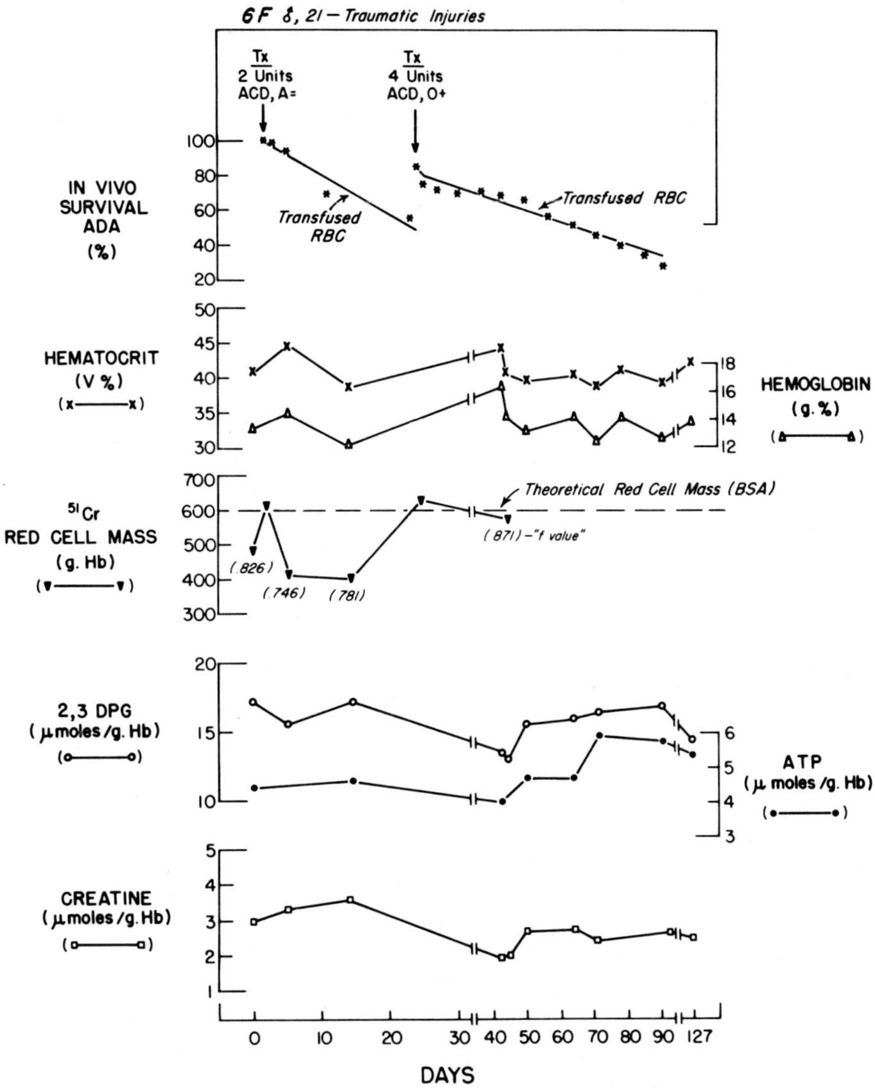

FIGURE 17. Hematocrit and hemoglobin concentrations, red blood cell mass, red blood cell 2,3 DPG, ATP, and creatine levels in Patient 6F, a 21-year-old male with traumatic injuries who was treated and evaluated over a 4-month period. After the two red blood cell transfusions given this patient, the survival of the donor red blood cells was measured using the automated differential agglutination procedure.

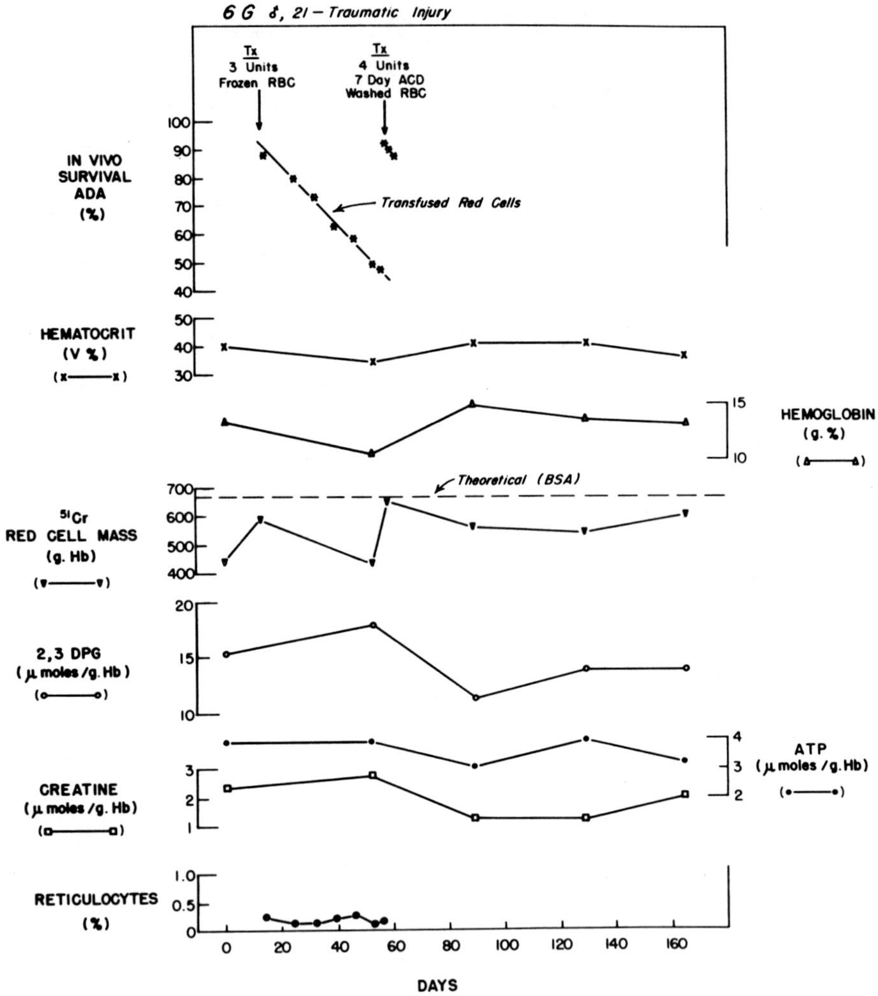

FIGURE 18. Hematocrit and hemoglobin concentrations, red blood cell mass, red blood cell 2,3 DPG, ATP, and creatine levels, and the reticulocyte count in Patient 6G, a 21-year-old male with traumatic injuries who was treated and evaluated over a 5½-month period. After the two red blood cell transfusions given this patient, the survival of the donor red blood cells was measured using the automated differential agglutination procedure. (From Biron, P. E., Howard, J., Altschule, M. D., and Valeri, C. R., *J. Bone Jt. Surg.*, 54(A), 1001, 1972. With permission.)

Table 6
THE EFFECTS OF TRANSFUSING ON PATIENTS WITH TRAUMATIC INJURIES ON RED BLOOD CELL CREATINE[a]

Patient	RBC mass deficit Pre Tx (g Hb)	Measured RBC creatine Pre Tx (μmol/g Hb)	Days Post Tx	RBC mass deficit Post Tx (g Hb)	Measured RBC creatine Post Tx (μmol/g Hb)	% Donor cells	Calculated RBC creatine Post Tx (μmol/g Hb)
Group A — Red Cell Mass Deficit Restored Towards Normal Following Transfusion							
1	259	3.0	10	73	2.6	22	2.9
2	193	2.8	3	21	1.5	21	2.4
3	175	4.9	10	119	3.3	20	4.1
4	193	2.0	10	18	1.3	30	1.7
5	221	4.3	6	0	2.6	22	3.6
6	218	3.6	2	45	2.2	34	2.8
7	150	2.7	5	144	2.1	14	2.5
8	303	4.1	10	161	2.7	28	3.3
9	194	2.8	5	45	2.4	21	2.4
10	230	4.1	6	176	3.3	27	3.3
11	355	2.3	5	87	1.4	44	1.8
Mean	227	3.3	7	81	2.3	26	2.8
SD	59	0.3	3	61	0.7	8	0.7

Table 6 (continued)
THE EFFECTS OF TRANSFUSING PATIENTS WITH TRAUMATIC INJURIES ON RED BLOOD CELL CREATINE[a]

Patient	RBC mass deficit Pre Tx (g Hb)	Measured RBC creatine Pre Tx (μmol/g Hb)	Days Post Tx	RBC mass deficit Post Tx (g Hb)	Measured RBC creatine Post Tx (μmol/g Hb)	% Donor cells	Calculated RBC creatine Post Tx (μmol/g Hb)
Group B — Red Cell Mass Deficit Increased Following Transfusion							
1	244	3.6	3	345	3.5	27	2.9
2	123	2.9	3	178	3.3	20	2.5
3	123	3.0	4	207	3.4	15	2.8
4	188	2.4	10	284	2.9	20	2.2
Mean	170	3.0	5	253	3.3	21	2.6
SD	58	0.5	3	76	0.3	5	0.3

[a] Red blood cell creatine was calculated from the patient's red cell creatine prior to transfusion, the red cell creatine in the donor red cells, and the percentages of the patient's own red cells and of the donor red cells in the circulation at the time of the repeat red cell mass measurement made within 10 days after transfusion. The percentage donor red cells was determined by the automated differential agglutination procedure and the red cell mass determined by ^{51}CR-labeled autologous red cells. The red cell mass deficit was calculated from the theoretical red cell mass and the ^{51}CR measured red cell mass. The measured creatine was compared to the calculated values.

Chapter 7

REGULATION OF THE CIRCULATION

A circulatory adjustment evidently occurred in our patients with traumatic injuries, and there are two aspects of this adjustment which must be considered. First, there are the factors that determine the blood volume, and second the factors responsible for the circulatory adjustments when blood volume is chronically decreased. Regarding the first, there was evidence that the factor principally responsible for the decreased blood volumes in our patients was a depression of erythropoiesis. In some cases, particularly after transfusion, abnormal hemolysis was an additional factor. Findings reported earlier (Chapters 2 and 3) ruled out the commonly recognized nutritional disorders that might have contributed to the syndrome. A disturbance in the regulation of the red blood cell mass was evident in our patients, although it was not completely explainable. A disturbance in the regulation of the plasma volume was equally difficult to understand.

LITERATURE REVIEW OF BLOOD VOLUME REGULATION

It is evident that to understand the regulation of the blood volume as a whole requires an understanding of the regulation of the plasma volume, which despite prolonged and extensive efforts, remains somewhat of a mystery. Studies that investigate only one or a few factors at a time prove little since the limited answers, when they do surface, are built into the method of investigation used. Thus, the disturbed plasma volume regulation in our patients was a puzzle to us. The fact that knowledge of the relevant physiological mechanisms is both incomplete and unreliable became apparent to us when we decided to review all the available physiological data in an attempt to gain some understanding of the mechanisms responsible for the decreases in blood and plasma volumes. The poverty of data in the literature is exemplified by the fact that the words "blood volume" are to be found only occasionally in *Annual Reviews of Physiology.* The most recent review of cardiovascular regulation (Oberg, 1976) does not mention it at all. However, four major monographs on the regulation of extracellular fluid volume have appeared since 1970 (Gauer et al., 1970; Guyton et al., 1972; Shore and Claybaugh, 1972; Andersson, 1977). In the main, they discuss the way in which the salt and water content of the body is regulated, relying on hormonal and neurogenic phenomena in their explanations. The blood volume as such is discussed in only one of them, the one by Gauer et al. (1970), and only in a superficial account a few hundred words in length:

DEFINITION OF BLOOD VOLUME CONTROL*

The control of plasma volume or blood volume centers about the need for a mechanism for the reciprocal adjustment of two variables, the blood volume and the size of the total vascular bed. The size of the vascular bed or its potential capacity is given by: the dimensions attained by the structural elements of the capacitance vessels and their elastic properties; and the tone of the vascular smooth muscles.

As Guyton points out, the various aspects of the long-term adaptation of the size of the vascular tree to the needs of the body are scarcely recognized as basic physiological problems. Yet Sjostrand has shown that blood volume is a function of body type, body size, age, climate, and, of particular importance, physical activity. From the viewpoint of blood volume control, we believe that the increased blood volume in response to greater metabolic demands is a two-step operation in which the dimensions of the heart and vascular bed

* From Gauer, O. H., Henry, J. P., and Behn, C., *Ann. Rev. Physiol.*, 32, 547, 1970. With permission.

are first increased, while the ensuing demand for a greater filling volume is satisfied in a second step. Observations of newborn infants held in an incubator speak in favor of this concept: Upon exposure to high oxygen tension the vessels already present in the immature retinal tissues shrink within hours, and if the high oxygen tension is maintained, they will fail to grow in sufficient number and size. The secondary pathological changes lead to the blindness of retrolental fibroplasia.

But metabolic demand is not the only factor inducing increased size of a vascular bed. When a high regional blood flow is enforced without an increase in oxygen consumption, as, for instance, in long-standing arteriovenous fistulas, anastomoses open up and the dimensions of the afferent and efferent vessels may increase grotesquely. A pertinent and very interesting observation is the development of wide anastomoses in the coronary circulation of dogs which have been treated with high doses of a coronary dilator drug for several weeks. So effective is the collateralization, that they may not show coronary infarction following ligation of a major vessel as do control. The mechanism by which these changes in the dimensions of the vascular bed are controlled is obscure.

A clear-cut example involving an adjustment of volume secondary to a change in vascular capacity is the observation that patients with gross varicose veins and, therefore, an oversized capacity of the vascular beds of the dependent legs exhibit an abnormally large blood volume. The increased blood volume often found in patients with idiopathic postural hypotension may be explained on a similar basis.

Recently Gauer (1974) put forward a hypothesis, unfortunately based on faulty data obtained with inaccurate methods, that several different processes, such as prolonged recumbency, total body immersion in water, and residence in a space vehicle, may activate a reaction, called the Gauer-Henry reaction, in which the heart acts as a sensor for a variety of reflex arcs that affect extracellular fluid volume. However, attempts by physiologists to study the Gauer phenomenon have produced discordant results, and the whole matter is in an unsettled and controversial state (Reinhardt et al., 1977). The complex interrelations among the various physiological mechanisms that come into play in total body immersion in water have been discussed by Farhi and Linnarsson (1977) who point out that many of the factors counteract one another, and hence no fixed pattern of response can occur. In fact, in the experiments of these authors, total body immersion in water did not displace all the peripheral blood into the thorax as Gauer's hypothesis required. Moreover, to apply the Gauer hypothesis to our patients would require that blood displaced from the periphery must lodge in the thoracic viscera, and we certainly did not see this. Another reported finding that we made note of but deemed irrelevant with regard to our patients was the small but significant decrease in red blood cell mass, with no significant change in plasma volume, occurring in the head-down position (Nixon et al., 1979). Whatever the applicability of the Gauer-Henry reaction might be in some instances of total body immersion in water or to residence in a spacecraft, or perhaps to the head-down position, it had no bearing on the conditions in our patients.

An even briefer and less informative discussion of the subject appears in Albert's monograph (1971) which bears the name *Blood Volume and Extracellular Fluid Volume;* however inadequate it may be in physiologic conceptualization, it nevertheless contains valuable clinical material. This scholarly physician probably was as disappointed as we over the paucity of physiologic work on the regulation of the blood volume.

Studies of clinical conditions in which changes in blood volume occur have revealed a controlling factor: namely, the size of the vascular bed. Thus the circulating blood volume normally varies with the size of the person, although increases can be found in patients with advanced mitral and tricuspid disease in which each auricle may contain 1 to 2 ℓ (instead of the normal 50 mℓ) (Altschule, 1954). The development of arteriovenous aneurysms is accompanied by increases in blood volume that correspond, as far as we can ascertain, to the volume of the markedly dilated veins that drain the aneurysm. Similarly, patients with cirrhosis of the liver, who have enormously dilated portal venous systems, also develop large blood volumes. Even in disorders of thyroid function, where the changes in blood volume have been ascribed to the changes in metabolic rate acting in some undefined way, the low blood volume of myxedema may actually reflect a marked cutaneous vasoconstriction, and the increased blood volume of Graves' disease may reflect a very marked cutaneous vasodilation (Albert, 1971). Likewise, the decrease in circulating blood volume found in patients with pheochromocytomas may be the result of the generalized arterial and venous constriction caused by the circulating catecholamines.

It would be wrong to conclude that the size of the circulatory bed alone determines the blood volume, for the volume is increased in chronic congestive heart failure and in polycythemia, the former representing edema of the blood. There must be other phenomena involved, for the large increases in circulating blood volume with normal hematocrit values found in chronic congestive heart failure seem to be the cause rather than the effect of an increase in the volume of the vascular bed. Moreover, there is an increase in plasma volume, without an increase in red blood cell mass in patients with splenomegaly (Bowdler, 1970; Donaldson et al., 1970; Hess et al., 1976). The explanation offered for this anomaly is an unexplained activation of the renin-angiotensin-aldosterone system, today's standard explanation for retention of salt and water. In monoclonal gammopathy, plasma viscosity increases owing to the formation of globulins of high molecular weight; the plasma volume subsequently increases until the plasma viscosity approaches or actually becomes normal (Alexanian, 1977). This suggests that *plasma* viscosity affects blood volume through some unknown mechanism. In contrast, the greatly increased *blood* viscosity of polycythemia vera does not lead to an increase in *plasma* volume. Intriguing as these possiblities may be, it is unlikely that they had any bearing on the status of our patients.

Although it can reasonably be concluded that the functional size of the circulatory bed is a primary determining factor in the circulating blood volume, the mechanism of this effect is totally unknown. A normal vascular bed volume seems to ensure a normal blood volume. The precision of this regulation is seen in chronic iron deficiency anemia, where the fall in total circulating red blood cell mass is accompanied by a rise in plasma volume, so that the total blood volume remains normal. Since in our patients the failure of the plasma volume to increase, as it does in iron deficiency or other anemias (Cropp, 1969), was due to a decrease in the size of the cardiovascular bed, it was necessary for us to analyze the circulatory adjustments and the patterns of vascular constriction.

REGIONAL BLOOD FLOW

One characteristic pattern found in all the patients we studied was a decrease in flow limited largely or entirely to the extremities. Despite hypoxia, as evidenced by the compensatory rise in red blood cell 2,3 DPG level, there was no overall increase in cardiac output such as occurs in hypoxia due to high altitude, chronic anemia, or chronic pulmonary disease. In these three hypoxic states, the total circulating blood volume is at least normal. Increases in cardiac output do not occur in all types of hypoxia; there is no increase in cardiac output in the acute hypovolemic hypoxia of shock states such as hemorrhage, burns, trauma, and acute pulmonary edema. There was no increase in cardiac output in our patients in the chronic hypovolemic state. The hypoxia was compensated for to a large degree by changes in red blood cell 2,3 DPG, and to a lesser degree by selective vasoconstriction. It is interesting to note that mature fetal lambs, whose vasomotor system is extremely sensitive to hypoxia, show decreases in renal and femoral blood flow despite increases elsewhere (Campbell et al., 1967).

Regarding the redistribution of regional blood flow to compensate for some of the effects of hypovolemic hypoxia, our patients showed some similarities in patterns with those seen in the acute hypovolemic states of hemorrhage, traumatic, and burn shock. In both acute and chronic hypovolemic states the blood flow to the extremities is greatly reduced, owing to differential vasoconstriction. However, in another respect, the acute and chronic states are totally different. In the acute hypovolemia of hemorrhage or trauma, severe renal vasoconstriction regularly occurs, often to the point of producing fatal renal insufficiency. It is interesting to note that in chronic cardiac decompensation, in which circulating blood volume is normal or increased, a similar though lesser degree of renal vasoconstriction occurs (Altschule, 1954). Even in severe chronic anemia, a condition in which the cardiac output increases, there may be some degree of renal vasoconstriction (Bradley and Bradley, 1947). Therefore, it is clear that renal vasoconstriction may be caused by factors other than hypovolemia, one such factor being hypoxia per se. Nevertheless, our patients showed no evidence of renal vasoconstriction despite their low blood volumes and the hypoxia manifested by the elevated erythrocyte 2,3 DPG levels.

The matter of differential vasoconstriction in hemorrhage and shock has been the subject of a great deal of discussion in physiology literature (Chien, 1967) with reference to the roles of autonomic function, local neurogenic vasomotor reactions, vasoactive hormones, and tissue products. However, as yet no formulation has evolved to explain the phenomena encountered in pathologic states in man or animals. Consequently, the physician's only recourse is to seek clues offered by other syndromes in which major redistribution of blood is characteristic. Such an analysis would require an understanding of how a decrease in blood volume leads to redistribution of blood. The theory of Gauer et al. (1970) that a fall in blood volume is a consequence solely of redistribution has no support in observation.

Observations made after acute hemorrhage showed the response to a low blood volume to be a redistribution of blood induced by acral and renal vasoconstriction. The flow to these areas is reduced. Specific studies of regional flow in hemorrhage have shown no effect on pulmonary flow in man (Hanson et al., 1973), or on cerebral blood flow except terminally (Kovach and Sandor, 1976). Renal blood flow is markedly reduced in shock in man (Chapter 1). Extensive studies in rabbits (Neutze et al., 1968) and dogs (Kaihara et al., 1969) show marked decreases in renal blood flow and increases in the percentage of cardiac output directed to other parts. There are, however, other syndromes with various etiologies in which redistribution of blood volume occurs. By far the most common factor in man leading to redistribution of the circulating blood is strong emotion or intense mental concentration (Altschule, 1953). Both these factors (which in fact may be only one) are always accompanied by acral *vasoconstriction* involving both veins and arteries. *Vasodilation* over the head, neck, and upper trunk occurs simultaneously. In certain circumstances strong emotion or intense mental concentration may cause facial pallor, but it is more common to see flushing of the face, stuffiness of the nose, and dilation of the visible head and neck veins. The ingenious observations of Mosso (1880) illustrate this redistribution. He balanced subjects lying on a plank on a knife edge. Mental effort caused a cephelad shift of weight indicating increased blood flow to the head end as shown by the tilt that developed. These vasomotor phenomena disappear during sleep. There is nothing to indicate that the blood that leaves the acral area accumulates in the lungs or that the physiological response to emotion is accompanied by a fall in blood volume (Altschule, 1953).

Another syndrome characterized by redistribution of blood is the chill phase of the febrile reaction (Altschule and Freedberg, 1945). In this syndrome intense cutaneous vasoconstriction is accompanied by shunting of blood to the gut, with no evidence of accumulation of the displaced blood in the lungs (Altschule and Freedberg, 1945). In febrile reactions the total circulating blood volume is not decreased.

There has been much discussion recently on the changes in blood flow caused by positive-pressure breathing. The findings and conclusions offered in the literature are inconsistent, which is not at all unusual in view of the marked variations in method and approach used and in the clinical circumstances under which these have been applied. Positive-pressure respiration usually causes a decrease in the venous return of blood to the heart, with a resultant fall in cardiac output. The observed decrease in renal blood flow is variously described as proportional to, more than, or less than, the fall in cardiac output. Interesting as these discussions may be, they had no bearing on the hypovolemic syndrome we studied.

SELECTIVE VASOCONSTRICTION

The occurrence of selective visceral vasoconstriction is not necessarily a manifestation of pathological processes. This kind of reaction, seen in seals during dives, may last as long as an hour (Kjekshus and Blix, 1977). In these circumstances blood flow to the muscles and the kidneys decreases markedly, whereas flow to the central nervous system is maintained (Scholander, 1962; Elsner et al., 1964, 1966). Circulatory phenomena of this type in seals (as well as in dogs) are determined in large measure by the action of the intrahepatic venous sphincters, but there is also extensive and marked selective peripheral arteriolar constriction. The mechanisms that activate these selective changes are not known, although there is a striking similarity between the vasomotor patterns in acute hypovolemic shock and in diving animals, suggesting a common neurogenic mechanism even if of different etiology. This unitary, albeit complicated, mechanism could not have been involved in our patients however, since the renal vasoconstriction was not present, although the diminution of blood flow to the extremities was clearly evident.

It is quite unlikely that there is any similarity between the pattern of redistribution of blood flow seen in our patients and that seen as responses to a variety of physiological states, including the state of shock. In all these disorders the selective vasoconstriction that occurs involves mainly the kidneys and extremities. In our patients the blood flow only to the extremities was decreased. This unusual type of selective constriction of blood vessels cannot be explained on the basis of accepted physiologic phenomena, but the following data should be considered. In the first place, when a leg is traumatized its circulation increases while that of the opposite leg decreases (Grega et al., 1971), undoubtedly because of the action of some neurogenic mechanism. We have no information on the duration of the increased circulation in the wounded leg, but it is known that it lasts for more than a few days or at least until the acute inflammation due to tissue damage in the wounded leg subsides. Regarding the opposite leg, we know only that its flow is decreased. At any rate, our patients presumably were beyond the stage of acute inflammation, although they clearly exhibited chronic inflammatory changes. One other mechanism to be considered in our patients is the possibility that the number of functioning capillaries in the extremities was reduced. We know that the number of capillaries increases in the muscles of persons who exercise regularly (Edström, 1968; Gollnick et al., 1972, 1974; Dubowitz et al., 1973; Andersen, 1975), and it is reasonable to assume that in a state of almost complete muscular inactivity the muscle capillary blood flow decreases.

SKELETAL MUSCLE FUNCTION

Skeletal muscle contains two types of fibers called in shorthand terms *fast twitch* (FT) and *slow twitch* (ST), although in the cat different muscles are made up almost entirely of one or the other (Folkow and Halicka, 1968). A large number of experiments in animals have shown that prolonged immobilization results in marked atrophy of muscles made up mainly of so-called ST fibers, the capillary-rich muscles (Booth and Seider, 1979), but no comparable data are available from human studies. In man most muscles contain both ST and FT fibers (Johnson et al., 1973; Andersen, 1975). The ST type sometimes called red because of the higher myoglobin content, has a high oxidative, low glycolytic metabolism, and a relatively high capillary surface area and blood flow. The FT type is sometimes called white because of its lower myoglobin content, although of course it is not devoid of it. It has a lower oxidative and higher glycolytic mechanism, and a relatively lower capillary surface area and blood flow (Edström and Nyström, 1969; Gollnick et al., 1972, 1974).

With regard to our patients, the question arises as to whether the proportion of ST muscle fibers (having a higher capillary flow) decreases, while the FT fibers (having lower capillary blood flow) increases, at least proportionately. If this were to occur, the capillary blood flow would fall to a level that might be adequate for low oxidative fibers at rest, but not adequate for the high metabolic requirements of healing tissues. Engle (1970) believes that the wasting associated with disease states causes selective atrophy of the FT fibers. There is evidence of selective atrophy of skeletal muscles in trauma patients (Gordon and Reinstein, 1979), but this did not help us to find which fiber types were involved in our patients. A finding of selective atrophy of high-blood-flow skeletal muscle fibers would provide a local phenomena that would decrease extremity blood flow without the intervention of selective autonomic activity. It is difficult to draw conclusions from the data available, particularly with regard to our patients.

A possible sequence of events are suggested as an explanation for the cardiovascular states of our patients before treatment. Depression of erythropoiesis in the bone marrow leads to a decrease in total circulating red blood cell mass, the level being determined by the impaired ability of the marrow to produce red blood cells. This depression of erythropoiesis may well be caused by an as yet uncharacterized circulating toxin. The expected increase in blood plasma volume necessary to bring the circulating blood volume to the level that will fill a normal circulatory bed does not occur, as indicated by the normal or only slightly decreased hematocrit level. The failure of the circulating plasma volume to increase sufficiently to bring the blood volume back to normal is due to contraction of part of the vascular bed involving only the extremities and evidently due to a local shrinkage of the size of the vascular bed in the extremities, perhaps caused by a toxic factor as yet unknown. Whether this presumed toxic factor is the same as the one that depresses hematopoiesis is not known. The decrease in the size of the vascular bed in the extremities might be due to a relative decrease in ST fibers which have a high capillary bed. Whether this presumed decrease in ST fibers might be caused by the same hypothetical toxin that depresses hematopoiesis cannot be stated. Moreover, it is unclear whether this series of assumptions and hypotheses, used here to explain the hypovolemic anemia of trauma, apply also to other anemias with normal hematocrit levels such as in healthy astronauts and in individuals with severe protein-calorie malnutrition.

Using a series of hypotheses to try to explain the mysteries of a previously unstudied syndrome, however logical these hypotheses may appear, cannot be considered at all satisfactory. Regrettably, that is the present status of the syndrome.

Chapter 8

CONSIDERATIONS BEARING ON TREATMENT

Any discussion of treatment of the hypovolemic anemia of trauma must cover a number of general aspects as well as some highly specific issues. The treatment regimen used a decade ago obviously was considered successful, but was it optimal? Is better treatment available today? Red blood cells were chosen over colloid or crystalloid solutions for transfusions because it appeared to be the best treatment at the time.

In analyzing data reported in the scientific literature as well as data from our own studies of patients with chronic hypovolemia associated with chronic trauma, we first had to define the clinical manifestations of hypovolemia. The subacute and chronic hypovolemia in our patients with traumatic injuries explained the hypotension that occurred when they were given general anesthesia to debride their wounds (Biron et al., 1972). Routine measurements of peripheral hemoglobin and hematocrit did not detect this hypovolemic state because the observed reduction of 40% of the red blood cell volume was accompanied by a simultaneous decrease in the plasma volume (Chapter 2). Usually, when there is a chronic reduction of red blood cell volume, the plasma volume will increase, but not in commensurate fashion, sufficiently to maintain a normal blood volume. The result is a reduction in hemoglobin and hematocrit levels, but not to a degree that reflects precisely the red cell deficit. This mechanism was absent in our patients, and deficits of both red blood cell mass and plasma volume occurred simultaneously.

We want to emphasize again that we were not engaged in a double-blind, controlled statistical study purporting to evaluate several available forms of treatment. Rather, we were faced with the problem of treating patients with a serious and poorly understood illness. We had no specific guidelines to follow but had to rely on our interpretation of possibly relevant findings in other disorders. Our plan of action was based solely on clinical judgment. As events evolved, the treatment proved to be effective; had it not been it would have been changed. However, in retrospect, what was effective treatment may not have been optimal treatment.

THE CHOICE OF RED BLOOD CELLS AS OUR TRANSFUSION PRODUCT

Data on the treatment of the hypovolemic anemia of chronic trauma are scant. Repeated transfusions have been used, apparently with some success (Chapter 1), but the data are too fragmentary for close analysis. On the other hand, there are many discussions of the resuscitative treatment of acute hemorrhage and its consequent shock, but many of these are contradictory or controversial.

The conflict over whether crystalloid or colloid solutions are indicated for the immediate resuscitation of patients in hemorrhagic shock is well known (Altschule et al., 1942; Kliman, 1966; Kummer and Lundsgaard-Hansen, 1968; Lundsgaard-Hansen, 1969; Malt et al., 1969; Schaller and Roggen, 1969; Skillman et al., 1970, 1975, 1976; Schon et al., 1971; Deysine et al., 1973; Shah et al., 1977; Tullis, 1977a, 1977b; Alving et al., 1978; Colman, 1978; Lucas et al., 1978, 1979; Steere et al., 1978; Boutros et al., 1979; Dahn et al., 1979; Demling et al., 1979; Jelenko et al., 1979; Johnson et al., 1979; Lowe et al., 1979; Shoemaker and Hauser, 1979; Virgilio et al., 1979a, 1979b; Weil et al., 1979). Several investigators have discussed the possible need for hemoglobin solutions and artificial oxygen-carrier substances (Peskin et al., 1969; Harris et al.,

1970; Clark et al., 1974, 1975, 1976, 1977; Valeri, 1976; Clark, 1978; Colt, 1978; Savitsky et al., 1978; Greenburg et al., 1979), but many more have recommended stored whole blood or red blood cell concentrates (Gibson et al., 1956; Prins and Loos, 1970; Shoemaker and Monson, 1973; Ryden and Oberman, 1975; Shapiro, 1976; Lovric et al., 1977; Avoy et al., 1978; Beiting et al., 1978; Högman et al., 1978a, 1978b; Inwood and Zuliani, 1978; Mishler et al., 1978; Schmidt, 1978; Honda et al., 1979; Valeri et al., 1979). In recognition of the blood clotting disorders that may occur in hemorrhagic shock, consideration has been given to the need for labile clotting factors (Valeri, 1976; Collins, 1978), and the possible need for platelet transfusions (Valeri, 1976; Collins, 1978). Recently the use of opsonic proteins also has been suggested (Alexander et al., 1976; Beiting et al., 1978; Saba et al., 1978; Scovill et al., 1978, 1979). Blood transfusions do not always correct clotting disorders (Collins, 1978), and questions have been raised about the possible adverse effects of the citrate in the blood anticoagulant (Howland and Schweizer, 1965; Cooper et al., 1973; Drop and Laver, 1975; White et al., 1976; Howland et al., 1977; Howland, 1978). The question of whether blood products administered to patients in hemorrhagic shock should be filtered to remove microaggregates has been studied extensively (Swank and Edwards, 1968; Reul et al., 1973, 1974; Tobey et al., 1973; Valeri, 1976; Barrett et al., 1978; Marshall et al., 1978; Dhurandhar et al., 1979; Durtschi et al., 1979; Virgilio et al., 1979a, 1979b; Cullen et al., 1980). The possibility that massive transfusions of volume expanders and blood products may lead to cardiopulmonary insufficiency (Collins, 1978; Collins et al., 1978; McConn, 1978) and sepsis (Alexander and Meakins, 1972; Effeney et al. 1978) also has been considered. Informative as this abundance of literature may be, its pertinence with regard to our patients was limited.

Volume expanders are given during initial resuscitation after acute injury, and when crystalloid solutions are used they must be administered in volumes two to three times those of colloid or blood. Transfusions under similar circumstances showed red blood cell concentrates given in combination with crystalloid solutions to be comparable to whole blood alone (Virgilio et al., 1979a, 1979b). The use of platelets and labile clotting factors during the immediate resuscitation should be determined by the volume of blood lost, whether the transfusion products contain viable and functioning platelets and labile clotting factors, and the health of the recipient, i.e., whether an underlying liver disease or hematologic disorder is present. It was not necessary for us to make this sort of determination in our patients with chronic trauma since they did not require platelets or labile clotting proteins.

REJECTION OF CRYSTALLOID AND COLLOID SOLUTIONS AS OUR TRANSFUSION PRODUCTS

In dealing with the chronic hypovolemia in our patients we had to decide how best to treat the reduced red blood cell and plasma volumes. It was determined that crystalloid solutions would increase plasma volume only transiently. The use of plasma as a possible treatment was eliminated because of its well-known propensity for causing hepatitis. Moreover, we knew that plasma had been used with poor results in the treatment of patients with severe trauma-induced anemia in the North African campaign in World War II. Furthermore, we had no desire to increase the plasma volume in our patients with depressed bone marrow function and some degree of peripheral hemolysis. In addition, restoration of the red blood cell mass to normal in our patients with a hypovolemic anemia of trauma caused a return of plasma volume to normal, without any need for plasma expanders.

We chose to treat the hypovolemia by correcting the red blood cell mass deficit with washed liquid-stored red blood cells and previously frozen washed red blood cells. The washed red blood cells were concentrated to a hematocrit value of 70 to 80 vol% prior to transfusion. The risks of blood transfusion were weighed against the desired benefits in accordance with current views (Greenwalt and Jamieson, 1975; Valeri, 1976; Contreras et al., 1979; Spero et al., 1979).

Some readers may ask why the depressed bone marrow function in our patients was not treated medicinally. Actually it was attempted, but with negative results. Attempts to treat the suppressed erythropoiesis with iron, folate, and pyridoxine were not successful. Niacinamide, tocopherol and Vitamin C also were ineffective.

The need for readily available compatible blood substitutes and blood products is obvious, and this need has been the impetus for much of the basic and applied research in the areas of artificial blood substitutes and of long-term preservation of blood products (Valeri, 1971, 1976; Chaplin et al., 1974; Chaplin, 1978).

WAS THE CHOSEN TREATMENT OPTIMAL?

As pointed out previously, the treatment of our patients with red blood cell transfusions was effective, though we now believe probably not optimal. The fact that we were treating young men who before being wounded had been not only healthy but in superb physical condition probably obscured any deficiencies in treatment.

During the period 1968 to 1972 when we were treating these wounded patients, and even today, the quality of a transfusion is determined principally from the posttransfusion survival of the donor compatible preserved red blood cells (Valeri, 1971; Matsuda and Shoemaker, 1972; Valeri, 1976). The importance of red blood cell oxygen transport function was not then a major consideration in transfusion therapy, and although we have come to understand its importance, many clinicians still have not (Valeri, 1976). As will be discussed later, this may be a serious omission under some circumstances.

The anticoagulant being used for blood collection between 1968 and 1972 was acid-citrate-dextrose (ACD). The studies we were making on our patients during this time alerted us to the fact that red blood cells stored in ACD suffered rapid deterioration of their oxygen transport function during the first 24 hr of storage at 4°C, and this impairment was pronounced after one week of storage at 4°C as reported by Valtis and Kennedy in 1954. The red blood cells being used to treat our patients had red blood cell 2,3 DPG levels of less than 50% of normal and increased red blood cell affinity for oxygen because they had been stored in ACD at 4°C for 3 to 5 days before they were frozen. After these red blood cells had been frozen with either 40% W/V glycerol at −80°C or 20% W/V glycerol at −150°C, thawed, washed, and stored at 4°C for 24 hr before transfusion, the reduction in 2,3 DPG and increase in oxygen affinity were even greater (Valeri, 1976). Thus, although our patients were receiving donor red blood cells with acceptable posttransfusion survival, i.e., greater than 70% of the compatible red blood cells were circulating in the recipient 24 hr after transfusion, the oxygen transport function of these red blood cells, i.e., ability to release oxygen immediately after infusion, was impaired. Needless to say, this was not apparent to us at the beginning of our studies.

As the care of our patients progressed, we began an extensive study of this respiratory defect in preserved red blood cells. Our findings as well as those of other investigators (Beutler and Wood, 1969; Valeri and Hirsch, 1969) helped us to recognize more fully the importance of the organic phosphate compound, 2,3 DPG in the red blood cells that our patients were receiving. It became apparent to us that the liquid-stored (stored in ACD at 4°C for as long as 21 days before washing), and the washed previously frozen red blood cells (stored in ACD for 3 to 5 days before freeze-preservation) had impaired oxygen transport function at the time of transfusion, and hemodynamic and biochemical changes were seen in the patients who received from 3 to 5 units of these red blood cells (Chapters 5 and 6). As stated previously (Chapters 5 and 6), the red blood cell 2,3 DPG is usually resynthesized in vivo to 50% of normal during the 24 hr after transfusion and oxygen transport function gradually returns to normal. During the period of resynthesis, cardiac output increases to compensate for the impaired oxygen transport function of the donor red blood cells (Valeri and Fortier, 1969a, 1969b; Valeri and Hirsch, 1969; Valeri and Collins, 1971), and studies in animals as well as in man have shown that when recipients have normal autoregulation of coronary and cerebral blood flow, the level of red blood cell 2,3 DPG is not critical (Valeri, 1976).

Numerous articles have been written about the importance of both the number of red blood cells in the circulation and the oxygen transport function of the circulating red blood cells (Arturson and Westman, 1975; Valeri, 1976; Dennis et al., 1978; Valeri et al., 1978, 1979; Weisel et al., 1978; Collins and Stechenberg, 1979; Malmberg et al., 1979; Woodson, 1979; Woodson et al., 1979). In fact, some very complicated experiments have been carried out in acutely anemic rats indicating increased mortality after the transfusion of red blood cells deficient in 2,3 DPG (Collins and Stechenberg, 1979; Malmberg et al., 1979). These findings although interesting were not germane to the condition of our patients with chronic hypovolemia who did well despite the temporarily abnormal oxygen delivery function of the red blood cells they received.

Recent studies in dogs have demonstrated deleterious but reversible changes in cerebral function in the isolated dog brain perfused with red blood cells with low 2,3 DPG and increased oxygen affinity at a fixed blood flow (Woodson et al., 1979). Studies in man have shown that the administration of red blood cells with satisfactory posttransfusion survival but less than optimum function to patients with impaired blood flow to the brain and heart may produce deleterious effects which may last for perhaps 24 hr after the transfusion (Dennis et al., 1978; Valeri et al., 1978; Weisel et al., 1978; Woodson, 1979; Woodson et al., 1979). A patient in whom an increase in cerebral and coronary blood flow is possible generally will tolerate a combination of a reduction in red blood cell volume and increased affinity for oxygen without apparent untoward effects. However, when no increase in cerebral and coronary blood flow is possible, the patient is jeopardized when this combination is present.

Most of our patients had received whole blood on several occasions prior to our becoming involved in their treatment, and many of them had become sensitized to white blood cells, platelets, and plasma proteins in the transfused blood. These patients were reluctant to undergo transfusion again because of their experiences with the symptoms of nonhemolytic transfusion reactions. Accordingly, we decided to use washed liquid-stored and washed previously frozen red blood cells to restore the red blood cell mass to the theoretical value. When red blood cells are washed before transfusion most of the white blood cells, platelets, and plasma proteins are removed in the process, thereby reducing the chances of nonhemolytic transfusion reactions and the possibility of transmission of hepatitis after transfusion (Valeri, 1976; Contreras et al., 1979).

Mention has been made in several places in this monograph of the apparent presence in our patients of a toxic factor thought to be responsible for depression of bone marrow function and for the hemolysis characterized by the formation not of bilirubin products but of porphyrins. One group of substances is known to have these actions (there may be others as yet unidentified). The known substances fall into the category of aminochromes, indoles formed by oxidative cyclization of catecholamines (Altschule and Hegedus, 1976). Between 1968 and 1972 there was no method of measuring the concentration of toxic factors in the blood plasma, although there is now (Hegedus, 1977). At present, studies in vitro are in progress by Hegedus and his associates to ascertain whether there are any nontoxic chemicals that will block the formation of these compounds. The success of these studies could result in the formulation of a new and better approach to the specific treatment of the hypovolemic anemia of chronic trauma.

GENERAL THERAPEUTIC MEASURES

Clinicians recognize that in practice there are effective therapeutic regimens, but there is no such thing as a single effective therapeutic measure. Accordingly, it is appropriate that reference be made to the general measures used in the clinical studies we report here.

Since the delayed wound healing that was a prominent feature of the disease was often associated with infection, antibiotics were given as indicated. The sluggish healing also called for a high protein diet, which although prescribed was not always completely eaten by the patients. Today patients of this sort might be given zinc supplements. The literature on the role of zinc in wound healing is reviewed elsewhere (Altschule, 1978). We gave no zinc as such. The diets presumably were rich in zinc, for meat and seafood were important parts of the protein prescribed, but the actual zinc ration may have been low because of the lack of appetite in many of the patients. On the other hand, in the breakdown of the transfused red blood cells, considerable amounts of carbonic anhydrase were released which when metabolized give up zinc to the metabolic pool.

If psychologic factors played a role in the recovery of our patients, they could hardly have been more favorable. The patients were members of an elite group known for its *esprit de corps.* The policy of the Department of Defense was to send wounded men to hospitals near their homes, so that visits by family and friends were frequent. Since the men and women on the nursing staff at the Chelsea Naval Hospital were comrades in arms of the wounded men, the atmosphere was such that it offered the greatest support, both physical and emotional. What was perhaps the most effective factor contributing to high morale and an optimistic outlook was the fact that the patients themselves were active participants in the studies being made to understand their illness so that it might be treated effectively. The contrast between a ward full of apathetic men with massive chronic indolent wounds and a ward full of men participating actively in their own study and treatment was striking, and should serve as a lesson to all physicians. Of course there is no way of knowing to what extent, if any, this morale factor directly influenced the rate of wound healing. There is no question, however, that it accelerated the collection of data in our clinically oriented laboratory studies, data that ultimately led to the successful treatment of the condition.

REFERENCES

Abel, F. L. and Wolf, M. B., Increased capillary permeability to ^{125}I-labeled albumin during experimental hemorrhagic shock. *Trans. N. Y. Acad. Sci.*, 36, 243, 1973.

Adamson, J. W., The erythropoietin-hematocrit relationship in normal and polycythemic man: implications of marrow regulation, *Blood*, 32, 597, 1968.

Albert, S. N., *Blood Volume and Extracellular Fluid Volume*, 2nd ed., Charles C Thomas, Springfield, Ill., 1971.

Alexander, R. S., Venomotor tone in hemorrhage and shock, *Circ. Res.*, 3, 181, 1955.

Alexander, J. W. and Meakins, J. L., A physiological basis for the development of opportunistic infections in man, *Ann. Surg.*, 176, 273, 1972.

Alexander, J. W., McClellan, M. A., Ogle, C. K., and Ogle, J. D., Consumptive opsoninopathy: possible pathogenesis in lethal and opportunistic infections, *Ann. Surg.*, 184, 672, 1976.

Alexanian, R., Blood volume in monoclonal gammopathy, *Blood*, 49, 301, 1977.

Alfrey, C. P., Lynch, E. C., and Hettig, R. A., Studies of iron kinetics using a linear scanner. I. Distribution of sites of uptake of plasma iron in hematological disorders, *J. Lab. Clin. Med.* 73, 405, 1969.

Altschule, M. D., *Bodily Physiology and Mental and Emotional Disorders*, Grune & Stratton, New York, 1953.

Altschule, M. D., *Physiology in Diseases of the Heart and Lungs*, rev. ed., Harvard University Press, Cambridge, Mass., 1954.

Altschule, M. D., Carbohydrate metabolism in mental disease: associated changes in phosphate metabolism, in *Biochemistry, Schizophrenias, and Affective Illnesses*, Himwich, H. E., Ed., Williams & Wilkins, Baltimore, 1970, 333.

Altschule, M. D., *Nutritional Factors in General Medicine. Effects of Stress and Distorted Diets*, Charles C Thomas, Springfield, Ill., 1978.

Altschule, M. D. and Gilligan, D. R., The effects on the cardiovascular system of fluids administered intravenously in man. II. The dynamics of the circulation, *J. Clin. Invest.*, 17, 401, 1938.

Altschule, M. D. and Freedberg, A. S., Circulation and respiration in fever, *Medicine*, 24, 403, 1945.

Altschule, M. D. and Rosenfeld, F. M., Increased catabolism following acute myocardial infarction, *Arch. Intern. Med.*, 80, 74, 1947.

Altschule, M. D., Gilligan, D. R., and Zamcheck, N., The effects on the cardiovascular system of fluids administered intravenously in man. IV. The lung volume and pulmonary dynamics, *J. Clin. Invest.*, 21, 365, 1942.

Altschule, M. D., Hegedus, Z. L., and Valeri, C. R., Indole pathway of epinephrine metabolism in chronic stress, *Clin. Res.*, 17, 478, 1969.

Altschule, M. D. and Hegedus, Z. L., The importance of studying visceral melanins, *Clin. Pharmacol. Ther.*, 19, 124, 1976.

Alving, B. M., Hojima, Y., Pisano, J. J., Mason, B. L., Buckingham, R. E., Mozen, M. M., and Finlayson, J. S., Hypotension associated with prekallikrein activator (Hageman-factor fragments) in plasma protein fraction, *N. Engl. J. Med.*, 299, 66, 1978.

Andersen, M. N. and Mouritzen, C., Effect of acute respiratory and metabolic acidosis on cardiac output and peripheral resistance, *Ann. Surg.*, 163, 161, 1966.

Andersen, P., Capillary density in skeletal muscle in man, *Acta Physiol. Scand.*, 95, 203, 1975.

Anderson, J. W., Herman, R. H., Tyrrell, J. B., and Cohn, R. M., Hexokinase: a compartmented enzyme, *Am. J. Clin. Nutr.*, 24, 642, 1971.

Andersson, B., Regulation of body fluids, *Ann. Rev. Physiol.*, 39, 185, 1977.

Arturson, M. G. S., Transport and demand of oxygen in severe burns, *J. Trauma*, 17, 179, 1977.

Arturson, G. and Westman, M., Survival of rats subjected to acute anemia at different levels of erythrocyte 2,3-diphosphoglycerate, *Scand. J. Clin. Lab. Invest.*, 35, 745, 1975.

Astrup, P., Garby, L., and deVerdier, C. H., Displacements of the oxyhemoglobin dissociation curve, *Scand. J. Clin. Lab. Invest.*, 22, 171, 1968.

Aviado, D. M., Adenosine diphosphate and vasoactive substances, *J. Trauma*, 8, 880, 1968.

Avoy, D. R., Ellisor, S. S., Nolan, N. J., Cox, R. S., Jr., Franco, J. A., Harbury, C. B., Schrier, S. L., and Pool, J. G., The effect of delayed refrigeration on red blood cells, platelet concentrates and cryoprecipitate AHF, *Transfusion*, 18, 160, 1978.

Ayres, S. M., Giannelli, S., Jr., and Armstrong, R. G., Carboxyhemoglobin: hemodynamic and respiratory responses to small concentrations, *Science*, 149, 193, 1965.

Ayres, S. M., Criscitiello, A., and Giannelli, S., Jr., Determination of blood carbon monoxide content by gas chromatography, *J. Appl. Physiol.*, 21, 1368, 1966.

Baar, S. and Topley, E., Haemoglobin metabolism and serum proteins following trauma, *Acta Med. Scand.*, 153, 319, 1956.

Babior, B. M. and Kipnes, R. S., Oxidation of epinephrine by a cell-free system from human granulocytes, *Blood,* 47, 461, 1976.

Badder, E. M., Seaton, J. F., Cimmino, V. M., Willis, J., Prager, R. L., and Harrison, T. S., Neuronal uptake of endogenous norepinephrine: a determinant of splenic but not renal vascular resistance following hemorrhage, *Surgery,* 83, 214, 1978.

Bakker, J. C., Gortmaker, G. C., Vrolijk, A. C. M., and Offerijns, F. G. J., The influence of the position of the oxygen dissociation curve on oxygen dependent functions of the isolated perfused rat liver. I. Studies at different levels of hypoxic hypoxia, *Pflügers Arch.,* 362, 21, 1976a.

Bakker, J. C., Gortmaker, G. C., and Offerijns, F. G. J., The influence of the position of the oxygen dissociation curve on oxygen dependent functions of the isolated perfused rat liver. II. Studies at different levels of hypoxia induced by decrease of blood flow rate, *Pflügers Arch.,* 366, 45, 1976b.

Bakker, J. C., Gortmaker, G. C., DeVries-van Rossen, A., and Offerijns, F. G. J., The influence of the position of the oxygen dissociation curve on oxygen dependent functions of the isolated perfused rat liver. III. Studies at different levels of anaemic hypoxia, *Pflügers Arch.,* 368, 63, 1977.

Bard, H., Fouron, J. C., Robillard, J. E., Cornet, A., and Soukini, M. A. Red cell oxygen affinity in fetal sheep: role of 2,3-DPG and adult hemoglobin, *J. Appl. Physiol.-Respir. Environ.,* 45, 7, 1978.

Barrett, P. V. D., Berk, P. D., Menken, M., and Berlin, N. I., Bilirubin turnover studies in normal and pathologic states using bilirubin ^{14}C, *Ann. Intern. Med.,* 68, 355, 1968.

Barrett, J., Tahir, A. H., and Litwin, M. S. Increased pulmonary arteriovenous shunting in humans following blood transfusion, *Arch. Surg.,* 113, 947, 1978.

Battaglia, F. C., McGaughey, H., Makowski, E. L., and Meschia, G., Postnatal changes in oxygen affinity of sheep red cells: a dual role of diphosphoglyceric acid, *Am. J. Physiol.,* 219, 217, 1970.

Baue, A. E., Tragus, E. T., and Parkins, W. M., A comparison of isotonic and hypertonic solutions and blood on blood flow and oxygen consumption in the initial treatment of hemorrhagic shock, *J. Trauma,* 7, 743, 1967.

Bauer, C., Reduction of the carbon dioxide affinity of human haemoglobin solutions by 2,3 diphosphoglycerate, *Respir. Physiol.,* 10, 10, 1970.

Bauer, Ch. and Rathschlag-Schaefer, A-M., The influence of aldosterone and cortisol on oxygen affinity and cation concentration of the blood, *Respir. Physiol.,* 5, 360, 1968.

Bauer, Ch., Ludwig, I., and Ludwig, M., Different effects of 2,3 diphosphoglycerate and adenosine triphosphate on the oxygen affinity of adult and foetal human haemoglobin, *Life Sci.,* 7, 1339, 1968.

Beecher, H. K., Preparation of battle casualties for surgery, *Ann. Surg.,* 121, 769, 1945.

Beecher, H. K. and Burnett, C. H., Field experience in the use of blood and blood substitutes (plasma, albumin) in seriously wounded men, *Med. Bull. N. African Theater of Operations* II, No. 1, 2, 1944.

Beecher, H. K. and Altschule, M. D., *Medicine at Harvard. The First Three Hundred Years,* University Press of New England, Hanover, N.H., 1977.

Beiting, C. V., Kozak, K. J., Dreffer, R. L., Stinnett, J. D., and Alexander, J. W., Whole blood vs. packed red cells for resuscitation of hemorrhagic shock, *Surgery,* 84, 194, 1978.

Bellingham, A. J. and Huehns, E. R., Compensation in haemolytic anemias caused by abnormal haemoglobins, *Nature (London),* 218, 618, 1969a.

Bellingham, A. J. and Huehns, E. R., Oxygen dissociation in red cells from patients with abnormal haemoglobins and pyruvate kinase deficiency, *Forsvarsmedicin,* 5, 207, 1969b.

Bellingham, A. J. and Grimes, A. J., Red cell 2,3-diphosphoglycerate, *Brit. J. Haemat.,* 25, 555, 1973.

Bellingham, A. J., Detter, J. C., and Lenfant, C., Regulatory mechanisms of hemoglobin oxygen affinity in acidosis and alkalosis, *J. Clin. Invest.,* 50, 700, 1971.

Benedict, C. R. and Grahame-Smith, D. G., Plasma noradrenaline and adrenaline concentrations and dopamine B-hydroxylase activity in patients with shock due to septicaemia, trauma, and haemorrhage, *Q. J. Med.,* 47, 1, 1978.

Benesch, R. and Benesch, R. E., Effect of organic phosphates from human erythrocytes on the allosteric properties of hemoglobin, *Biochem. Biophys. Res. Commun.,* 26, 162, 1967.

Benesch, R. and Benesch, R. E., Intracellular organic phosphates as regulators of oxygen release by haemoglobin, *Nature (London),* 221, 618, 1969.

Bergan, A., Östrem, T., and Enge, I., The synthesis and excretion of nonerythroid bilirubin in the dog, *Scand. J. Gastroenterol.,* 12, 605, 1977.

Bergentz, S. E. and Danon, D., Alteration in red blood cells of traumatized rabbits, *Acta Chir. Scand.,* 130, 165, 1965.

Berlin, N. I., Laboratory evaluation of erythrokinetics, in *Hematology,* 2nd ed., Williams, W. J., Beutler, E., Erslev, A. J., and Rundles, R. W., Eds., McGraw-Hill, New York, 1977, 237.

Berlin, R., Energy transfer and regional blood flow changes following muscle trauma, *J. Trauma,* 19, 170, 1979.

Bernstein, R. B., Novy, M. J., Piasecki, G. J., Lester, R., and Jackson, B. T., Bilirubin metabolism in the fetus, *J. Clin. Invest.,* 48, 1678, 1969.

Berry, C. A., Medical legacy of Apollo, *Aerosp. Med.*, 45, 1046, 1974.

Beutler, E. and Wood, L., The in vivo regulation of red cell 2,3 diphosphoglyceric acid (DPG) after transfusion of stored blood, *J. Lab. Clin. Med.*, 74, 300, 1969.

Biron, P. E., Howard, J., Altschule, M. D., and Valeri, C. R., Chronic deficits in red-cell mass in patients with orthopaedic injuries (stress anaemia), *J. Bone Jt. Surg.*, 54-A, 1001, 1972.

Blackburn, G. L., Flatt, J. P., Clowes, G. H. A., Jr., and O'Donnell, T. F., Jr., Peripheral intravenous feeding with isotonic amino acid solutions, *Am. J. Surg.*, 125, 447, 1973a.

Blackburn, G. L., Flatt, J. P., Clowes, G. H. A., Jr., O'Donnell, T. F., Jr., and Hensle, T. E., Protein sparing therapy during starvation with sepsis or trauma, *Ann. Surg.*, 177, 588, 1973b.

Bloomer, J. R., Berk, P. D., Bonkowsky, H. L., Stein, J. A., Berlin, N. I., and Tschudy, D. P., Blood volume and bilirubin production in acute intermittent porphyria, *N. Engl. J. Med.*, 284, 17, 1971.

Blum, H. U., Biochemical aspects of erythrocyte ageing in vivo and in vitro, in *Modern Problems of Blood Preservation*, Spielmann, W. and Seidl, S., Eds., Gustav Fischer Verlag, Stuttgart, 1970, 21.

Blumgart, H. L. and Altschule, M. D., Clinical significance of cardiac and respiratory adjustments in chronic anemia, *Blood*, 3, 329, 1948.

Bohnn, B. J., Hyatt, K. H., Kamenetsky, L. G., Calder, B. E., and Smith, W. M., Prevention of bed rest induced orthostatism by 9-alpha-fluorohydrocortisone, *Aerosp. Med.*, 41, 495, 1970.

Böning, D., Meier, U., Skipka, W., Küipmann, W. R., and Meurer, K. A., Some evidence for aldosterone action on 2,3-diphosphoglycerate level in human red cells, *Metabolism*, 25, 9, 1976.

Booth, F. W. and Seider, M. J., Recovery of skeletal muscle after 3 months of hindlimb immobilization in rats, *J. Appl. Physiol.-Respir. Environ.*, 47, 435, 1979.

Bothwell, T. H., Hurtado, A. V., Donoghue, D. M., and Finch, C. A., Erythrokinetics. IV. The plasma iron turnover as a measure of erythropoiesis, *Blood*, 12, 409, 1957.

Boutros, A. R., Ruess, R., Olson, L., Hoyt, J. L., and Baker, W. H., Comparison of hemodynamic, pulmonary, and renal effects of use of three types of fluids after major surgical procedures on the abdominal aorta, *Crit. Care Med.*, 7, 9, 1979.

Bowdler, A. J., Blood volume studies in patients with splenomegaly, *Transfusion*, 10, 171, 1970.

Bowen, J. C. and Fleming, W. H., Increased oxyhemoglobin affinity after transfusion of stored blood: evidence for circulatory compensation, *Ann. Surg.*, 180, 760, 1974.

Bowen, T. E., Whelan, T. J., Jr., and Nelson, T. G., Sudden death after phosphorus burns: experimental observations of hypocalcemia, hyperphosphatemia, and electrocardiographic abnormalities following production of a standard white phosphorus burn, *Ann. Surg.*, 174, 779, 1971.

Braasch, D., Red cell deformability and capillary blood flow, *Physiol. Rev.*, 51, 679, 1971.

Bradley, S. E. and Bradley, G. P., Renal function during chronic anemia in man, *Blood*, 2, 192, 1947.

Brannon, E. S., Merrill, A. J., Warren, J. V., and Stead, E. A., Jr., The cardiac output in patients with chronic anemia as measured by the technique of right atrial catheterization, *J. Clin. Invest.*, 24, 332, 1945.

Brewer, G. J. and Powell, R. D., Hexokinase activity as a function of age of the human erythrocyte, *Nature (London)*, 199, 704, 1963.

Bristow, J. D., Metcalfe, J., Krall, M. A., Welch, J. E., Black, J. A., and Dhindsa, D. S., Reduction of blood oxygen affinity in dogs by infusion of glycolytic intermediates, *J. Appl. Physiol.-Respir. Environ.*, 43, 102, 1977.

Broadie, T. A. and Herman, C. M., Oxygen consumption from fresh versus 21-day-old ACD whole blood, *J. Trauma*, 18, 381, 1978.

Brody, J. S. and Coburn, R. I., Carbon monoxide-induced arterial hypoxemia, *Science*, 164, 1297, 1969.

Brok, F., Ramot, B., Zwang, E., and Danon, D., Enzyme activities in human red blood cells of different age groups, *Isr. J. Med. Sci.*, 2, 291, 1966.

Brozovic, B., Korubin, V., Lewis, S. M., and Szur, L., Simultaneous red cell and plasma volume determinations by a differential absorption method, *J. Lab. Clin. Med.*, 68, 142, 1966.

Brunjes, S., Johns, V. J., Jr., and Crane, M. G., Phaeochromocytoma, postoperative shock and blood volume, *N. Engl. J. Med.*, 262, 393, 1960.

Brunori, M., Falcioni, G., Fioretti, E., Giardina, B., and Rotilio, G., Formation of superoxide in the autooxidation of the isolated α and B chains of human hemoglobin and its involvement in hemichrome precipitation, *Eur. J. Biochem.*, 53, 99, 1975.

Brus, I. and Lewis, S. M., The haptoglobin content of serum in haemolytic anaemia, *Brit. J. Haematol.*, 5, 348, 1959.

Bryan-Brown, C. W., Baek, S. M., Makabali, G., and Shoemaker, W. C., Consumable oxygen: availability of oxygen in relation to oxyhemoglobin dissociation, *Crit. Care Med.*, 1, 17, 1973.

Bunn, H. F., May, M. H., Kocholaty, W. F., and Shields, C. E., Hemoglobin function in stored blood, *J. Clin. Invest.*, 48, 311, 1969.

Bush, J. A., Ashenbrucker, H., Cartwright, G. E., and Wintrobe, M. M., The anemia of infection. XX. The kinetics of iron metabolism in the anemia associated with chronic infection, *J. Clin. Invest.*, 35, 89, 1956.

Byrnes, G. J., Pirkle, J. C., and Gann, D. S., Cardiovascular stabilization after hemorrhage depends upon restitution of blood volume, *J. Trauma,* 18, 623, 1978.
Campbell, A. G. M., Dawes, G. S., Fishman, A. P., and Hyman, A. I., Regional redistribution of blood flow in the mature fetal lamb, *Circ. Res.,* 21, 229, 1967.
Canizaro, P. C., Nelson, J. L., Hennessy, J. L., and Bright, P. B., A technique for estimating the position of the oxygen-hemoglobin dissociation curve, *Ann. Surg.,* 180, 364, 1974.
Cannon, W. B., Fraser, J., and Hooper, A. N., II. Some alterations in the distribution and character of the blood. Reports of the Special Investigation Committee on Surgical Shock and Allied Conditions, Dec. 25, 1917, 27.
Canoso, R. T., Hutton, R. A., and Deykin, D., The hemostatic defect of chronic liver disease, *Gastroenterology,* 76, 540, 1979.
Caprini, J. A., Lipp, V., Zuckerman, L., Vagher, J. P., and Winchester, D. P., Hematologic changes following burns, *J. Surg. Res.,* 22, 626, 1977.
Carey, J. S., Brown, R. S., Woodward, N. W., Yao, S. T., and Shoemaker, W. C., Comparison of hemodynamic responses to whole blood and plasma expanders in clinical traumatic shock, *Surg. Gynecol. Obstet.,* 121, 1059, 1965.
Carey, J. S., Brown, R. S., Mohr, P. A., Monson, D. O., Yao, S. T., and Shoemaker, W. C., Cardiovascular function in shock. Responses to volume loading and isoproterenol infusion, *Circulation,* 35, 327, 1967.
Carey, J. S., Mohr, P. A., Brown, R. S., and Shoemaker, W. C., Cardiovascular function in hemorrhage, trauma and sepsis. Determinants of cardiac output and cardiac work, *Ann. Surg.,* 170, 910, 1969.
Carey, L. S., Cloutier, C. T., and Lowery, B. D., Growth hormone and adrenal cortical response to shock and trauma in the human, *Ann. Surg.,* 174, 451, 1971.
Carleton, R. A., Levinson, G. E., and Abelmann, W. H., Assessment of mitral regurgitation by indicator dilution: observations on the principle of Korner and Shillingford, *Am. Heart J.,* 58, 663, 1959.
Carolla, R. L., Brubaker, L. H., and Mengel, C. E., Age of red blood cells destroyed by in vivo hyperoxia, *Aerosp. Med.,* 45, 1273, 1974.
Cartwright, G. E. and Wintrobe, M. M., The anemia of infection. XVII. A review, in *Advances in Internal Medicine,* Vol. 5, Dock, W. and Snapper, I., Eds., Year Book Medical Publishing, Chicago, 1952, 165.
Cavanagh, D. and Rao, P. S., Endotoxin shock in the subhuman primate. I. Hemodynamic and biochemical changes, *Arch. Surg.,* 99, 107, 1969.
Cavill, I., Ricketts, C., and Jacobs, A., Erythropoiesis, iron stores, and tissue iron exchange in man, *Clin. Sci.,* 56, 223, 1979.
Chance, B., Cohen, P., Jobsis, F., and Schoener, B., Intracellular oxidation-reduction states in vivo, *Science,* 137, 499, 1962.
Chanutin, A. and Curnish, R. R., Effect of organic and inorganic phosphates on the oxygen equilibrium of human erythrocytes, *Arch. Biochem. Biophys.,* 121, 96, 1967.
Chaplin, H., Jr., Frozen blood, *N. Engl. J. Med.,* 298, 679, 1978.
Chaplin, H., Jr., Beutler, E., Collins, J. A., Giblett, E. R., and Polesky, H. F., Current status of red-cell preservation and availability in relation to the developing national blood policy, *N. Engl. J. Med.,* 291, 68, 1974.
Charache, S., Achuff, S., Winslow, R., Adamson, J., and Chervenick, P., Variability of the homeostatic response to altered P_{50}, *Blood,* 52, 1156, 1978.
Chase, G. A., Grave, C., and Rowell, L. B., Independence of changes in functional and performance capacities attending prolonged bed rest, *Aerosp. Med.,* 37, 1232, 1966.
Chien, S., Role of the sympathetic nervous system in hemorrhage, *Physiol. Rev.,* 47, 214, 1967.
Clark, K. G. A. and Davidson, W. M., Bone marrow lipofuscin, *J. Clin. Pathol.,* 25, 947, 1972.
Clark, E. H., Woods, R. L., and Hughes, J. M. B., Effects of blood transfusion on the carbon monoxide transfer factor of the lung in man, *Clin. Sci. Mol. Med.,* 54, 627, 1978.
Clark, L. C., Jr., Perfluorodecalin as a red cell substitute, in *Blood Substitutes and Plasma Expanders,* Jamieson, G. A. and Greenwalt, T. J., Eds., Alan R. Liss, New York, 1978, 69.
Clark, L. C., Jr., Wesseler, E. P., Miller, M. L., and Kaplan, S., Ring versus straight chain perfluorocarbon emulsions for perfusion media, *Microvascular Res.,* 8, 320, 1974.
Clark, L. C., Jr., Wesseler, E. P., Kaplan, S., Miller, M. L., Becker, C., Emory, C., Stanley, L., Becattini, F., and Obrock, V., Emulsions of perfluorinated solvents for intravascular gas transport, *Fed. Proc. Fed. Am. Soc. Exp. Biol.,* 34, 1468, 1975.
Clark, L. C., Jr., Wesseler, E. P., Kaplan, S., Emory, C., Moore, R., and Denson, D., Intravenous infusion of cis-trans perfluorodecalin emulsions in the rhesus monkey, in *Biochemistry Involving Carbon-Fluorine Bonds,* Fuller, R., Ed., American Chemical Society, Washington, D.C., 1976, 135.
Clark, L. C., Jr., Wesseler, E. P., Denson, D. D., and Miller, M., The infusion of emulsions of perfluorodecalins in the partly bled baboon, in *Research on Perfluorochemicals in Medicine and Biology,* Novakova, V., and Plantin, L. O., Eds., Huddinge University Hospital, Hugginge, Sweden, 1977, 10.

Clarke, R., Topley, E., and Flear, C. T. G., Assessment of blood-loss in civilian trauma, *Lancet,* 1, 629, 1955.

Cloutier, C. T., Lowery, B. D., and Carey, L. C., Acid-base disturbances in hemorrhagic shock, *Arch. Surg.,* 98, 551, 1969.

Coburn, R. F. and Kane, P. B., Maximal erythrocyte and hemoglobin catabolism, *J. Clin. Invest.,* 47, 1435, 1968.

Coburn, R. F., Williams, W. J., and Kahn, S. B., Endogenous carbon monoxide production in patients with hemolytic anemia, *J. Clin. Invest.,* 45, 460, 1966.

Coburn, R. F., Williams, W. J., White, P., and Kahn, S. B., The production of carbon monoxide from hemoglobin in vivo, *J. Clin. Invest.,* 46, 346, 1967.

Cohen, S., Freeman, T., and McFarlane, A. S., Metabolism of ^{131}I labeled human albumin, *Clin. Sci.,* 20, 161, 1961.

Cohen, I. A., Metal-metal interactions involving porphyrins: iron-iron spin exchange and iron-chromium electron transfer, *Ann. N.Y. Acad. Sci.,* 206, 453, 1963.

Cohn, J. E. and Shock, N. W., Blood volume studies in middle-aged and elderly males, *Am. J. Med. Sci.,* 217, 388, 1949.

Cohn, J. D. and DelGuercio, L. R. M., Nomogram for the rapid calculation of cardiac output at the bedside, *Ann. Surg.,* 164, 109, 1966.

Cohn, J. D. and DelGuercio, L. R. M., Clinical applications of indicator dilution curves as gamma functions, *J. Lab. Clin. Med.,* 69, 675, 1967.

Coleman, M., Horwith, M., and Brown, J. L., Idiopathic edema — studies demonstrating protein-leaking angiopathy, *Am. J. Med.* 49, 106, 1970.

Collins, J. A., Massive transfusion: what is current and important? in *Massive Transfusion,* Nusbacher, J., Ed., American Association of Blood Banks, Washington, D.C., 1978, 1.

Collins, J. A., James, P. M., Bredenberg, C. E., Anderson, R. W., Heisterkamp, C. A., and Simmons, R. L., The relationship between transfusion and hypoxemia in combat casualties, *Ann. Surg.,* 188, 513, 1978.

Collins, J. A. and Stechenberg, L., The effects of the concentration and function of hemoglobin on the survival of rats after hemorrhage, *Surgery,* 85, 412, 1979.

Colman, R. W., Paradoxical hypotension after volume expansion with plasma protein fraction, *N. Engl. J. Med.,* 299, 97, 1978.

Colt, J. D., The use of stroma-free hemoglobin solution for partial exchange transfusion in aortic resection in dogs, *Am. J. Surg.,* 135, 656, 1978.

Coltman, C. A., Jr., Dudley, G. M., III, and Leverett, S. D., Jr., Measurement of endogenous carbon monoxide production to determine the effect of high +Gx accleration on the destruction rate of red cells, *Aerosp. Med.,* 40, 627, 1969.

Conolly, W. B., Hunt, T. K., Sonne, M., and Dunphy, J. E., Influence of distant trauma on local wound infection, *Surg. Gynecol. Obstet.,* 128, 713, 1969.

Contreras, T. J., Lang, D. J., Pivacek, L. E., and Valeri, C. R., Occurrence of HBsAg, anti-HBs, and anti-CMV following the transfusion of blood products, *Transfusion,* 19, 129, 1979.

Cook, J. D., Marsaglia, G., Eschbach, J. W., Funk, D. D., and Finch, C. A., Ferrokinetics: a biologic model for plasma iron exchange in man, *J. Clin. Invest.,* 49, 197, 1970.

Cooper, A. G., Purification of cold agglutinins from patients with chronic cold haemagglutinin disease, *Clin. Exp. Immunol.,* 3, 691, 1968.

Copper, A. G. and Hobbs, J. R., Immunoglobulins in chronic cold hemagglutinin disease, *Brit. J. Haematol.,* 19, 383, 1970.

Cooper, N., Brazier, J. R., Hottenrott, C., Mulder, D. G., Maloney, J. V., Jr., and Buckberg, G. D., Myocardial depression following citrated blood transfusion — an avoidable complication, *Arch. Surg.,* 107, 756, 1973.

Cooper, R. A., Destruction of erythrocytes, in *Hematology,* 2nd ed., Williams, W. J., Beutler, E., Erslev, A. J., and Rundles, R. W., Eds., McGraw-Hill, New York, 1977, 216.

Coran, A. G., Ballantine, T. V., Horwitz, D. L., and Herman, C. M., The effect of crystalloid resuscitation in hemorrhagic shock on acid-base balance: a comparison between saline and Ringer's lactate solutions, *Surgery,* 69, 874, 1971.

Couch, N. P., Dmochowski, J. R., van de Water, J. M., Harken, D. E., and Moore, F. D., Muscle surface pH as an index of peripheral perfusion in man, *Ann. Surg.,* 173, 173, 1971.

Cournand, A., Riley, R. L., Bradley, S. E., Breed, E. S., Noble, R. P., Lauson, H. D., Gregersen, M. I., and Richards, D. W., Studies of the circulation in clinical shock, *Surgery,* 13, 964, 1943.

Cournand, A., Noble, R. P., Breed, E. S., Lauson, H. D., Baldwin, E. deF., Pinchot, G. B., and Richards, D. W., Jr., Chemical, clinical, and immunological studies on the products of human plasma fractionation. VIII. Clinical use of concentrated human serum albumin in shock, and comparison with whole blood and with rapid saline infusion, *J. Clin. Invest.,* 23, 491, 1944.

Crafts, R. C. and Meineke, H. A., The anemia of hypophysectomized animals, *Ann. N.Y. Acad. Sci.,* 77, 501, 1959.

Cropp, G. J. A., Cardiovascular function in children with severe anemia, *Circulation,* 39, 775, 1969.

Crosby, W. H., The limits of erythropoiesis: how much can the marrow produce with total recruitment?, *Blood Cells,* 1, 497, 1975.

Crosby, W. H. and Akeroyd, J. H., The limit of hemoglobin synthesis in hereditary hemolytic anemia, *Am. J. Med.,* 13, 273 , 1952.

Crosby, W. H. and Howard, J. M., The hematologic response to wounding and resuscitation accomplished by large transfusions of stored blood. A study of battle casualties in Korea, *Blood,* 9, 439, 1954.

Cullen, D. J., Kunsman, J., Caldera, D., Dennis, R. C., and Valeri, C. R., Comparative evaluation of new fine-screen filters: effects on blood flow rate and microaggregate removal, *Anesthesiology,* 53, 3, 1980.

Cuthbertson, D. P., The influence of prolonged muscular rest on metabolism, *Biochem. J.,* 23, 1328, 1929.

Cuthbertson, D. P., The distribution of metabolism produced by bony and non-bony injury, with notes on certain abnormal conditions of bone, *Biochem. J.,* 24, 1244, 1930.

Cuthbertson, D. P., The distribution of nitrogen and sulphur in the urine during conditions of increased catabolism, *Biochem. J.,* 25, 236, 1931.

Cuthbertson, D. P., Observations on the distribution of metabolism produced by injury to the limbs, *Q. J. Med.,* 1, 233, 1932.

Cymerman, A., Maher, J. T., Cruz, J. C., Reeves, J. T., Denniston, J. C., and Grover, R. F., Increased 2,3-diphosphoglycerate during normocapnic hypobaric hypoxia, *Aviat. Space Environ. Med.,* 47, 1069, 1976.

Daane, T. A., Valeri, C. R., and Barton, R. K., Autotransfusions of previously frozen blood in elective gynecologic surgery, *Am. J. Obstet. Gynecol.,* 105, 394, 1969.

Dacie, J. V. and Homer, G. F., Blood loss in battle casualties. Use of transfusion fluids, *Lancet,* 1, 371, 1946.

Dahn, M. S., Lucas, C. E., Ledgerwood, A. M., and Higgins, R. F., Negative inotropic effect of albumin resuscitation for shock, *Surgery,* 86, 235, 1979.

Darsee, J. R. and Nutter, D. O., Reversible severe congestive cardiomyopathy in three cases of hypophosphatemia, *Ann. Intern. Med.,* 89, 867, 1978.

Deitrick, J. E., Whedon, G. D., and Shore, E., Effects of immobilization upon various metabolic and physiologic functions of normal men, *Am. J. Med.,* 4, 3, 1948.

Demling, R. H., Manohar, M., Will, J. A., and Belzer, F. O., The effect of plasma oncotic pressure on the pulmonary microcirculation after hemorrhagic shock, *Surgery,* 86, 323, 1979.

Dennis, R. C., Hechtman, H. B., Berger, R. L., Vito, L., Weisel, R. D., and Valeri, C. R., Transfusion of 2,3 DPG enriched red blood cells to improve cardiac function, *Ann. Thorac. Surg.,* 26, 17, 1978.

Dern, R. J., Studies on the preservation of human blood. III. The posttransfusion survival of stored and damaged erythrocytes in healthy donors and patients with severe trauma, *J. Lab. Clin. Med.,* 71, 254, 1968.

Deysine, M., Lieblich, N., and Aufses, A. H., Albumin changes during clinical septic shock, *Surg. Gynecol. Obstet.,* 137, 475, 1973.

Dhurandhar, H., Brown, C., Barrett, J., and Litwin, M. S., Pulmonary structural changes following microembolism and blood transfusion. A light and electron microscopic study, *Arch. Pathol. Lab. Med.,* 103, 335, 1979.

Donaldson, G. W. K., McArthur, M., MacPherson, A. I. S., and Richmond, J., Blood volume changes in splenomegaly, *Brit. J. Haematol.,* 18, 45, 1970.

Doyle, J. T., Wilson, J. S., Estes, E. H., and Warren, J. V., The effect of intravenous infusions of physiologic saline solutions on the pulmonary arterial and pulmonary capillary pressure in man, *J. Clin. Invest.,* 30, 345, 1951.

Drop, L. J. and Laver, M. B., Low plasma ionized calcium and response to calcium therapy in critically ill man, *Anesthesiology,* 43, 300, 1975.

Dubach, R., Moore, C. V., and Minnich, V., Studies in iron transportation and metabolism. V. Utilization of intravenous injected radioactive iron for hemoglobin synthesis and an evaluation of the radioactive iron method for studying iron absorption, *J. Lab. Clin. Med.,* 31, 1201, 1946.

Dubois, D. and Dubois, E. F., Clinical colorimetry: a formula to estimate the approximate surface area if height be known, *Arch. Intern. Med.,* 17, 863, 1916.

Dubowitz, V., Brooke, M. H., and Neville, H. E., *Muscle Biopsy: A Modern Approach,* W. B. Saunders, Philadelphia, 1973.

Duhm, J., Inosine permeability and purine nucleoside phosphorylase activity as limiting factors for the synthesis of 2,3 diphosphoglycerate from inosine, pyruvate, and inorganic phosphate in erythrocytes of various mammalian species, *Biochim. Biophys. Acta,* 343, 89, 1974.

Duhm, J., Deuticke, B., and Gerlach, E., Complete restoration of oxygen transport function and 2,3 diphosphoglycerate concentration in stored blood, *Transfusion,* 11, 147, 1971.

Duke, M. and Abelmann, W. H., The hemodynamic response to chronic anemia, *Circulation*, 39, 503, 1969.

Duke, M., Herbert, V. D., and Abelmann, W. H., Hemodynamic effects of blood transfusion in chronic anemia, *N. Engl. J. Med.*, 271, 975, 1964.

Durtschi, M. B., Haisch, C. E., Reynolds, L., Pavlin, E., Kohler, T. R., Heimbach, D. M., and Carrico, C. J., Effect of micropore filtration on pulmonary function after massive transfusion, *Am. J. Surg.*, 138, 8, 1979.

Eaton, J. W. and Brewer, G. J., The relationship between red cell 2,3-diphosphoglycerate and levels of hemoglobin in the human, *Proc. Nat. Acad. Sci.*, 61, 756, 1968.

Edström, L., Histochemical changes in upper motor lesions, Parkinsonism and disuse. Differential effect on white and red muscle fibers, *Experientia*, 15, 916, 1968.

Edström, L. and Nyström, B., Histochemical types and sizes of fibres in normal human muscles, *Acta Neurol. Scand.*, 45, 257, 1969.

Edwards, M. J., Koler, R. D., Rigas, D. A., and Pitcairn, D. M., The effect of in vivo aging of normal human erythrocytes and erythrocyte macromolecules upon oxyhemoglobin dissociation, *J. Clin. Invest.*, 40, 636, 1961.

Edwards, M. J. and Rigas, D. A., Electrolyte-labile increase of oxygen affinity during in vivo aging of hemoglobin, *J. Clin. Invest.*, 46, 1579, 1967.

Edwards, M. J., Novy, M. J., Walters, C. L., and Metcalfe, J., Improved oxygen release: an adaptation of mature red cells to hypoxia, *J. Clin. Invest.*, 47, 1851, 1968.

Edwards, M. J., Canon, B., Albertson, J., and Bigley, R. H., Mean red cell age as a determinant of blood oxygen affinity, *Nature (London)*, 230, 583, 1971.

Edwards, M. J. and Canon, B., Oxygen transport during erythropoietic response to moderate blood loss, *N. Engl. J. Med.*, 287, 115, 1972.

Effeney, D. J., Blaisdell, F. W., McIntyre, K. E., and Graziano, C. J., The relationship between sepsis and disseminated intravascular coagulation, *J. Trauma*, 18, 689, 1978.

Eldridge, F. L., Relationship between lactate turnover rate and blood concentration in hemorrhagic shock, *J. Appl. Physiol.*, 37, 321, 1974.

Eldridge, F. L., T'so, L., and Chang, H., Relationship between turnover rate and blood concentration of lactate in normal dogs, *J. Appl. Physiol.*, 37, 316, 1974.

Elin, R. J., Wolff, S. M., and Finch, C. A., Effect of induced fever on serum iron and ferritin concentrations in man, *Blood*, 49, 147, 1977.

Elmadjian, F., Adrenocortical function of combat infantrymen in Korea, in *The Human Adrenal Cortex, Ciba Foundation Symposium*, 8, 627, 1954.

Elmadjian, F. and Davis, S. W., A study of combat stress in Korea, 1952: physiologic and biochemical, *Recent Adv. Med. Surg.*, 41, 22, 1955.

Elsner, R. W., Franklin, D. L., and van Citters, R. L., Cardiac output during diving in an unrestrained sea lion, *Nature (London)*, 202, 809, 1964.

Elsner, R., Franklin, D. L., van Citters, R. L., and Kenny, D. W., Cardiovascular defence against asphyxia, *Science*, 153, 941, 1966.

Emerson, C. P., Jr. and Ebert, R. V., A study of shock in battle casualties, *Ann. Surg.*, 122, 745, 1945.

Engel, W. K., Selective and non selective susceptibility of muscle fiber types, *Arch. Neurol.*, 22, 97, 1970.

Engel, R. R., Rodkey, F. L., O'Neal, J. D., and Collison, H. A., Relative affinity of human fetal hemoglobin for carbon monoxide and oxygen, *Blood*, 33, 37, 1969.

Erslev, A. J., Production of erythrocytes, in *Hematology*, 2nd ed., Williams, W. J., Beutler, E., Erslev, A. J., and Rundles, R. W., Eds., McGraw-Hill, New York, 1977, 203.

Erslev, A. J. and Silver, R. K., Compensated hemolytic anemia, *Blood Cells*, 1, 509, 1975.

Evans, E. I., Hoover, M. J., James, G. W., III., and Alm, T., Studies on traumatic shock. I. Blood volume changes in traumatic shock, *Ann. Surg.*, 119, 64, 1944.

Evans, E. S., Simpson, M. E., and Evans, H. M., The role of growth hormone in calorigenesis and thyroid function, *Endocrinology*, 63, 836, 1958.

Farhi, L. E. and Linnarsson, D., Cardiopulmonary readjustments during graded immersion in water at 35°C, *Respir. Physiol.*, 30, 35, 1977.

Faura, J., Gurney, C. W., and Fried, W., The effect of carbon dioxide on erythropoiesis, *Ann. N.Y. Acad. Sci.*, 149, 456, 1968.

Fehr, J. and Knob, M., Comparison of red cell creatine level and reticulocyte count in appraising the severity of hemolytic processes, *Blood*, 53, 966, 1979.

Feldschuh, J. and Enson, Y., Prediction of the normal blood volume-relation of blood volume to body habitus, *Circulation*, 56, 605, 1977.

Feldthusen, U., Larsen, V., and Lassen, N. A., Serum iron and operative stress, *Acta Med. Scand.*, 147, 311, 1953.

Feldthusen, U. and Lassen, N. A., Serum iron after coronary occlusion and traumatic injuries, *Acta Med. Scand.*, 150, 53, 1954.

Ferrebee, J. W., Leigh, O. C., and Berliner, R. W., Passage of the blue dye T-1824 from the bloodstream into the lymph, *Proc. Soc. Exp. Biol. Med.*, 46, 549, 1941.

Figge, F. H. J., Weiland, G. S., and Manganiello, L. O. J., Cancer detection and therapy. Affinity of neoplastic, embryonic, and traumatized tissues for porphyrins and metalloporphyrins, *Proc. Soc. Exp. Biol. Med.*, 68, 640, 1948.

Finch, J. S., *Sir Thomas Browne — A Doctor's Life of Science and Faith*, Henry Schuman, New York, 1950.

Finch, C. A. and Loden, B., Body iron exchange in man, *J. Clin. Invest.*, 38, 392, 1959.

Finch, C. A. and Lenfant, C., Oxygen transport in man, *N. Engl. J. Med.*, 286, 407, 1972.

Finch, C. A., Gibson, J. G., II, Peacock, W. C., and Fluharty, R. G., Iron metabolism — utilization of intravenous radioactive iron, *Blood*, 4, 905, 1949a.

Finch, C. A., Wolff, J. A., Rath, C. E., and Fluharty, R. G., Iron metabolism, erythrocyte iron turnover, *J. Lab. Clin. Med.*, 34, 1480, 1949b.

Finch, C. A., Hosain, F., Morgan, E. H., Marsaglia, G., Giblett, E., and Hillman, R. S., The ferrokinetic approach to anemia, *Scand. J. Haematol.*, Series Haemat., 6, 30, 1965.

Finch, C. A., Deubelbeiss, K., Cook, J. D., Eschbach, J. W., Harker, L. A., Funk, D. D., Marsaglia, G., Hillman, R. S., Slichter, S., Adamson, J. W., Ganzoni, A., and Giblett, E. R., Ferrokinetics in man, *Medicine*, 49, 17, 1970.

Fitch, C. D. and Rahmanian, M., Creatine entry into skeletal muscle of normal and of dystrophic mice, *Proc. Soc. Exp. Biol. Med.*, 131, 236, 1969.

Flink, E. B. and Skubi, K. B., Blood transfusion studies. II. The survival of fresh and stored transfused erythrocytes as determined by urobilinogen excretion, *J. Lab. Clin. Med.*, 31, 1074, 1946.

Folkow, B. and Halicka, H. D., A comparison between "red" and "white" muscle with respect to blood supply, capillary surface area and oxygen uptake during rest and exercise, *Microvasc. Res.*, 1, 1, 1968.

Fondu, P., A reassessment of intravascular volume measurements in protein-calorie malnutrition, *Eur. J. Clin. Invest.* , 7, 161, 1977.

Fondu, P. and Mandelbaum, I. M., Marasmic Kwashiorkor anemia. III. Hemoglobin oxygen affinity, *Biomedicine*, 22, 291, 1975.

Fondu, P., Hariga-Muller, C., Mozes, N., Neve, J., van Steirteghem, A., and Mandelbaum, I. M., Protein-energy malnutrition and anemia in Kivu, *Am. J. Clin. Nutr.*, 31, 46, 1978.

Forsyth, R. P., Hoffbrand, B. I., and Melmon, K. L., Redistribution of cardiac output during hemorrhage in the unanesthetized monkey, *Circ. Res.*, 27, 311, 1970.

Fortier, N. L., Hirsch, N. M., and Valeri, C. R., Restoration of 2,3 DPG and ATP in ACD-stored red blood cells, *Forsvarsmedicin*, 5, 250, 1969.

Frank, H. A., Seligman, A. M., and Fine, J., Traumatic shock. X. The treatment of hemorrhagic shock irreversible to replacement of blood volume deficiency, *J. Clin. Invest.*, 24, 435, 1945.

Freeman, N. E., The mechanism of shock, in *Burns, Shock, Wound Healing, and Vascular Injuries*, W. B. Saunders, Philadelphia, 1943, 107.

Freeman, T., The biological behaviour of normal and denatured human plasma albumin, *Clin. Chim. Acta*, 4, 788, 1959.

Freeman, J. B., Stegink, L. D., Wittine, M. F., and Thompson, R. G., The current status of protein sparing, *Surg. Gynecol. Obstet.*, 144, 843, 1977.

Frega, N., Flores, J., Guertler, B. A., Dibona, D. R., and Leaf, A., Post hemorrhagic renal ischemia and its correction by solutes which penetrate cell membranes poorly, *Trans. Assoc. Am. Phys.*, 86, 320, 1973.

Freinkel, N., Schreiner, G. E., and Athens, J. W., Simultaneous distribution of T-1824 and I^{131}labelled human serum albumin in man, *J. Clin. Invest.*, 32, 138, 1953.

Freireich, E. J., Miller, A., Emerson, C. P., and Ross, J. F., The effect of inflammation on the utilization of erythrocyte and transferrin bound radioiron for red cell production, *Blood*, 12, 972, 1957.

Friedman-Mor, Z., Chalon, J., Gorstein, F., Turndorf, H., Chuba, J. V., and Orkin, L. R., Abnormal heme-protein patterns in hemorrhagic shock, *J. Trauma*, 18, 104, 1978.

Friman, G., Effect of clinical bed rest for seven days on physical performance, *Acta Med. Scand.*, 205, 389, 1979.

Fromm, D., Intestinal absorption during hypovolemic shock, *Ann. Surg.*, 177, 448, 1973.

Frye, R. L. and Braunwald, E., Studies on Starling's law of the heart. I. The circulatory response to acute hypervolemia and its modification by ganglionic blockage, *J. Clin. Invest.*, 39, 1043, 1960.

Fudenberg, H., Baldini, M., Mahoney, J. P., and Dameshek, W., The body hematocrit/venous hematocrit ratio and the "splenic reservoir", *Blood*, 17, 71, 1961.

Fuller, T. J., Nichols, W. W., Brenner, B. J., and Peterson, J. C., Reversible depression in myocardial performance in dogs with experimental phosphorus deficiency, *J. Clin. Invest.*, 62, 1194, 1978.

Gann, D. S. and Pirkle, J. C., Role of cortisol in the restitution of blood volume after hemorrhage, *Am. J. Surg.*, 130, 565, 1975.

Garby, L. and Groth, T., The interpretation of red cell survival curves in non-stationary states. 1. The mean cell life span as calculated from the initial disappearance rate of labeled red cells, *Scan. J. Haematol.*, 7, 357, 1970.

Gardner, R. C., Blood loss after fractures of the hip, *JAMA*, 208, 1005, 1969.

Gardner, G. W., Edgerton, V. R., Barnard, R. J., and Bernauer, E. M., Cardiorespiratory, hematological, and physical performance responses of anemic subjects to iron treatment, *Am. J. Clin. Nutr.*, 28, 982, 1975.

Gauer, O. H., Henry, J. P., and Behn, C., The regulation of extracellular fluid volume, *Ann. Rev. Physiol.*, 32, 547, 1970.

Gauer, O. H., Selected features of reflex control and their possible bearing on physiological changes in the weightless condition, in *Proceedings of the Fourth International Symposium on Man in Space*, Gazenko, O. G. and Bjurstedt, H., Eds., Nauka, Moscow, 1974, 176.

Gelin, L. E., Studies in anemia of injury, *Acta Chir. Scand. Suppl.*, 210, 5, 1956.

Gemsa, D., Fudenberg, H. H., and Schmid, R., Erythrocyte catabolism by macrophages in vitro: dissociation of phagocytosis and heme oxygenase induction, *Trans. Assoc. Amer. Physicians*, 85, 335, 1972.

George, W. K., George, W. D., Smith, J. P., Gordon, F. T., Baird, E. E., and Mills, G. C., Changes in serum calcium, serum phosphate and red-cell phosphate during hyperventilation, *N. Engl. J. Med.*, 270, 726, 1964.

Gibson, J. G., II and Evans, W. A., Clinical studies of the blood volume. I. Clinical applications of a method employing the blue azo-dye "Evans blue" and the spectrophotometer, *J. Clin. Invest.*, 16, 301, 1937a.

Gibson, J. G., II and Evans, W. A., Jr., Clinical studies of the blood volume. II. The relation of plasma and total blood volume to venous pressure, blood velocity rate, physical measurements, age and sex in ninety normal humans, *J. Clin. Invest.*, 16, 317, 1937b.

Gibson, J. G., II, Murphy, W. P., Jr., Scheitlin, W. A., and Rees, S. B., The influence of extracellular factors involved in the collection of blood in ACD on maintenance of red cell viability during refrigerated storage, *Am. J. Clin. Pathol.*, 26, 855, 1956.

Gilbert, V. E., Blood pyruvate and lactate during febrile human infections, *Metabolism*, 17, 943, 1968.

Gilligan, D. R., Altschule, M. D., and Volk, M. C., The effects on the cardiovascular system of fluids administered intravenously in man. I. Studies of the amount and duration of changes in blood volume, *J. Clin. Invest,*. 17, 7, 1938.

Golden, M., Waterlow, J. C., and Picou, D., The relationship between dietary intake, weight change, nitrogen balance, and protein turnover in man, *Am. J. Clin. Nutr.*, 30, 1345, 1977.

Gollnick, P. D., Armstrong, R. B., Saubert, C. W., IV, Piehl, K., and Saltin, B., Enzyme activity and fiber composition in skeletal muscle of untrained and trained men, *J. Appl. Physiol.*, 33, 312, 1972.

Gollnick, P. D., Sjödin, B., Karlsson, J., Jansson, E., and Saltin, B., Human soleus muscle: a comparison of fiber composition and enzyme activities with other leg muscles, *Pflügers Arch.*, 348, 247, 1974.

Gordon, A. S., Erythropoietin, *Vitam. Horm. (N.Y.)*, 31, 105, 1973.

Gordon, D. L. and Reinstein, L., Rehabilitation of the trauma patient, *Am. Surg.*, 45, 223, 1979.

Grant, R. T. and Reeve, E. B., Observations on the general effects of injury in man with special reference to wound shock, Privy Council, Medical Research Council Special Report Series No. 277, His Majesty's Stationery Office, London, 1951, 83.

Greenberg, G. R., Marliss, E. B., Anderson, G. H., Langer, B., Spence, W., Tovee, E. B., and Jeejeebhoy, K. N., Protein-sparing therapy in post operative patients. Effects of added hypocaloric glucose or lipid, *N. Engl. J. Med.*, 294, 1411, 1976.

Greenburg, A. G., Frank, H., and Peskin, G. W., The left-shifted oxyhemoglobin curve in the burn patient, *J. Trauma*, 16, 573, 1976.

Greenburg, A. G., Terlizzi, L., and Peskin, G. W., Oxyhemoglobin affinity in acute pancreatitis, *J. Surg. Res.*, 22, 561, 1977.

Greenburg, A. G., Hayashi, R., Siefert, I., Reese, H., and Peskin, G. W., Intravascular persistence and oxygen delivery of pyridoxalated, stroma-free hemoglobin during gradations of hypotension , *Surgery*, 86, 13, 1979.

Greenwalt, T. J. and Jamieson, G. A., *Transmissible Disease and Blood Transfusion*, Grune & Stratton, New York, 1975.

Grega, G. J., Schwinghamer, J. M., and Haddy, F. J., Changes in forelimb weight and sequential vascular resistances following severe hemorrhage, *Circ. Res.*, 29, 691, 1971.

Gregersen, M. I., Effect of circulatory states on determination of blood volume, *Am. J. Med.*, 15, 785, 1953.

Griffiths, W. J., Creatine and phosphocreatine in the human red cell, *Brit. J. Haematol.*, 15, 389, 1968a.

Griffiths, W. J., Estimation of creatine in red cells, *J. Clin. Patho l.*, 21, 412, 1968b.

Griffiths, W. J. and Fitzpatrick, M., The effect of age on the creatine in red cells, *Brit. J. Haematol.*, 13, 175, 1967.

Griffiths, W. J. and Lothian E. J., Erythropoiesis, red-cell creatine and plasma aldolase activity in anaemia in the rabbit and man, *Brit. J. Haematol.*, 17, 477, 1969.

Gudwin, A. L., Goldstein, C. R., Cohn, J. D., and Del Guercio, L. R. M., Estimation of ventricular mixing volume for prediction of operative mortality in the elderly, *Ann. Surg.*, 168, 183, 1968.

Guest, G. M. and Rapoport, S., Organic and acid-soluble phosphorus compounds of the blood, *Physiol. Rev.*, 21, 410, 1941.

Guyton, A. C., Coleman, T. G., and Granger, H. J., Circulation overall regulation, *Ann. Rev. Physiol.*, 34, 13, 1972.

Haining, R. G., Hulse, T. E., and Labbe, R. F., Photohemolysis. The comparative behavior of erythrocytes from patients with different types of porphyria, *Proc. Soc. Exp. Biol. Med.*, 132, 625, 1969.

Hamilton, W. F., Moore, J. W., Jr., Kinsman, J. M., and Spurling, R. G., Studies on the circulation. IV. Further analyses of the injection method and of changes in hemodynamics under physiological and pathological conditions, *Am. J. Physiol.*, 99, 534, 1932.

Hamilton, W. F., Riley, R. L., Attyah, A. M., Cournand, A., Fowell, D. M., Himmelstein, A., Noble, R. P., Remington, J. W., Richards, D. W., Jr., Wheeler, N. C., and Witham, A. C., Comparison of the Fick and dye injection methods of measuring the cardiac output in man, *Am. J. Physiol.*, 153, 309, 1948.

Hamstra, R. D. and Block, M. H., Erythropoiesis in response to blood loss in man, *J. Appl. Physiol.*, 27, 503, 1969.

Hanson, E. L., Miller, I. T., Sheldon, G. F., Ball, M. R., Boyden, C. M., and Moore, F. D., The pulmonary circulation: response to norepinephrine and hemorrhage in normal man, *Ann. Surg.*, 177, 458, 1973.

Hardaway, R. M., III, *Syndromes of Disseminated Intravascular Coagulation with Special Reference to Shock and Hemorrhage,* Charles C Thomas, Springfield, Ill., 1966.

Hardaway, R. M., III, Disseminated intravascular coagulation as a possible cause of acute respiratory failure, *Surg. Gynecol. Obstet.*, 137, 419, 1973.

Hardaway, R. M., III, Vietnam wound analysis, *J. Trauma,* 18, 635, 1978.

Hardaway, R. M., Johnson, D. G., Elovitz, M. J., Houchin, D. N., Jenkins, E. B., Burns, J. W., and Jackson, D. R., Influence of trauma and hemolysis on hemorrhagic shock in dogs, *J. Trauma,* 4, 624, 1964.

Hardaway, R. M., Dumke, R., Gee, T., Meyers, T., Joyner, J., Graf, J., Lee, D., and Revels, J., The danger of hemolysis in shock, *Ann. Surg.*, 189, 373, 1979.

Harken, A. H. The surgical significance of the oxyhemoglobin dissociation curve, *Surg. Gynecol. Obstet.*, 144, 935, 1977.

Harken, A. H. and Woods, M., The influence of oxyhemoglobin affinity on tissue oxygen consumption, *Ann. Surg.*, 183, 130, 1976.

Harris, J. W. and Kellermeyer, R. W., *The Red Cell — Production, Metabolism, Destruction. Normal and Abnormal,* Rev. Ed., Harvard University Press, Cambridge, Mass. 1970.

Harris, G. W., Anderson, R. M., deFilippi, R. P., Nosé, Y., Weber, D. C., and Malchesky, P. S., The physiological effects of fluorocarbon liquids in blood oxygenation, *J. Biomed. Mater. Res.*, 4, 313, 1970.

Hartmann, R. C. and Jenkins, D. E. The "sugar-water" test for paroxysmal nocturnal hemoglobinuria, *N. Engl. J. Med.*, 275, 155, 1966.

Haurani, F. I., Burke, W., and Martinez, E. J., Defective reutilization of iron in the anemia of inflammation, *J. Lab. Clin. Med.*, 65, 560, 1965.

Heath, C. W. and Taylor, F. H. L., The nitrogen metabolism in anemia during the regeneration of blood, *J. Clin. Invest.*, 15, 411, 1936.

Hechtman, H. B., Grindlinger, G. A., Vegas, A. M., Manny, J., and Valeri, C. R., Importance of oxygen transport in clinical medicine, *Crit. Care Med.*, 7, 419, 1979.

Hegedus, Z. L., Studies on rheomelanins. IV. The apparent occurrence in vivo of rheomelanins in human blood, *Arch. Int. Physiol. Biochim.*, 85, 539, 1977.

Hegedus, Z. L. and Altschule, M. D., Studies on aminochromes. I. Behavior of adrenochrome added to human plasma, *Arch. Int. Physiol. Biochim.*, 75, 690, 1967.

Hegedus, Z. L. and Altschule, M. D., Studies on aminochromes. III. Transformation of epinephrine, adrenochrome, and adrenolutin into plasma soluble melanins during incubation in human blood plasma, *Arch. Biochem. Biophys.*, 126, 388, 1968.

Hegedus, Z. L. and Altschule, M. D., Studies on rheomelanins. I. The formation of rheomelanins in human blood plasma from catecholamines, from L-DOPA and from some of their derivatives, *Arch. Int. Physiol. Biochim.*, 78, 443, 1970a.

Hegedus, Z. L. and Altschule, M. D., Studies on aminochromes. IV. Hemolysis associated with the transformation of L-epinephrine, adrenochrome, and adrenolutin into rheomelanins in human whole blood, *Arch. Int. Pharmacodyn. Ther.*, 186, 39, 1970b.

Heidman, M., Kaijser, B., and Gelin, L-E., Complement activation and hematologic, hemodynamic, and respiratory reactions early after soft tissue injury, *J. Trauma,* 18, 696, 1978.

Henderson, C. A., Metz, E. N., Balcerzak, S. P., and Sagone, A. L., Jr., Adriamycin and daunomycin generate reactive oxygen compounds in erythrocytes, *Blood*, 52, 878, 1978.

Hendley, E. D. and Schiller, A. A., Change in capillary permeability during hypoxemic perfusion of rat kidneys, *Am. J. Physiol.*, 179, 216, 1954.

Henneman, D. H., Altschule, M. D., and Goncz, R. M., Effects of intravenous administration of glutathione in man on blood glucose, some other blood carbohydrates and serum inorganic phosphate, *Metabolism*, 4, 433, 1955a.

Henneman, D. H., Altschule, M. D., and Goncz, R. M., Carbohydrate metabolism in brain disease. IV. Effect of hydrocortisone and corticotrophin (ACTH) on the metabolic effects of administered glucose in patients in the chronic schizophrenic and manic-depressive psychoses, *Arch. Intern. Med.*, 95, 241, 1955b.

Hermreck, A. S., Ruiz-Ocana, F. M., Proberts, K. S., Meisel, R. L., and Crawford, D. G., Mechanisms for oliguria in acute renal failure, *Surgery*, 82, 141, 1977.

Hess, C. E., Ayers, C. R., Sandusky, W. R., Carpenter, M. A., Wetzel, R. A., and Mohler, D. N., Mechanism of dilutional anemia in massive splenomegaly, *Blood*, 47, 629, 1976.

Hillman, R. S. and Finch, C. A., The misused reticulocyte, *Brit. J. Haematol.*, 17, 313, 1969.

Hillman, R. S. and Finch, C. A., Erythropoiesis, *N. Engl. J. Med.*, 285, 99, 1971.

Hilpert, P., Fleischmann, R. G., Kempe, D., and Bartels, H., The Bohr effect related to blood and erythrocyte pH, *Am. J. Physiol.*, 205, 337, 1963.

Hirsch, E. F., Fletcher, J. R., Moquin, R., Dostalek, R., and Lucas, S., Coagulation changes after combat trauma and sepsis, *Surg. Gynecol. Obstet.*, 133, 393, 1971.

Hlastala, M. P., Woodson, R. D., and Wranne, B., Influence of temperature on hemoglobin-ligand interaction in whole blood, *J. Appl. Physiol.—Respir. Environ.*, 43, 545, 1977.

Hochstein, P. and Cohen, G., The cytotoxicity of melanin precursors, *Ann. N. Y. Acad. Sci.*, 100, 876, 1963.

Hodges, R. E., Sauberlich, H. E., Canham, J. E., Wallace, D. L., Rucker, R. B., Mejia, L. A., and Mohanram, M., Hematopoietic studies in Vitamin A deficiency, *Am. J. Clin. Nutr.*, 31, 876, 1978.

Högman, C. F., Hedlund, K., Akerblom, O., and Venge, P., Red blood cell preservation in a protein-poor media. I. Leucocyte enzymes as a cause of hemolysis, *Transfusion*, 18, 233, 1978a.

Högman, C. F., Hedlund, K., and Zetterström, H., Clinical usefulness of red cells preserved in protein-poor mediums, *N. Engl. J. Med.*, 299, 1377, 1978b.

Holleman, J. H., Gabel, J. C., and Hardy, J. D., Pulmonary effects of intravenous fluid therapy in burn resuscitation, *Surg. Gynecol. Obstet.*, 147, 161, 1978.

Holt, P. R., Measurement of gastrointestinal blood loss in subjects taking aspirin, *J. Lab. Clin. Med.*, 56, 717, 1960.

Honda, K., Miyamoto, M., and Sasakawa, S., Changes in 2,3 DPG content and oxygen affinity in erythrocytes stored at 4°C, *Vox Sang.* 37, 229, 1979.

Hosain, F., Marsaglia, G., and Finch, C. A., Blood ferrokinetics in normal man, *J. Clin. Invest.*, 46, 1, 1967.

Houlihan, R. T., Zavodni, J. J., and Cross, M. H., Effects of increased oxygen pressure on adrenal steroid and catecholamine release. VIIIth Int. Congr. on Aviation and Aerospace Medicine, Oslo, Norway, 1968.

Howland, W. S., Calcium, potassium, and pH changes during massive transfusion, in *Massive Transfusion*, Nusbacher, J., Ed., American Association of Blood Banks Washington, D.C., 1978, 17.

Howland, W. S. and Schweizer, O., Physiologic compensation for storage lesion of bank blood, *Anesth. Analg. (Cleveland)*, 44, 8, 1965.

Howland, W. S., Schweizer, O., Carlon, G. C., and Goldiner, P. L., The cardiovascular effects of low levels of ionized calcium during massive transfusion, *Surg. Gynecol. Obstet.*, 145, 581, 1977.

Hoye, R. C., Simultaneous measurement of red cell, plasma, and extracellular fluid volume in the surgical patient, *J. Lab. Clin. Med.*, 69, 683, 1967.

Hoye, R. C., Bennett, S. H., Geelhoed, G. W., and Gorschboth, C., Fluid volume and albumin kinetics occurring with major surgery, *JAMA*, 222, 1255, 1972.

Huff, R. L., Hennessy, T. G., Austin, R. E., Garcia, J. F., Roberts, B. M., and Lawrence, J. H., Plasma and red cell turnover in normal subjects and in patients having various hematopoeitic disorders, *J. Clin. Invest.*, 29, 1041, 1950.

Huggins, R. A., Smith, E. L., and Deavers, S., Volume distribution of Evans blue dye and iodinated albumin in the dog, *Am. J. Physiol.*, 205, 351, 1963.

Hugo, N. E., Thompson, L. W., Zook, E. G., and Bennett, J. E., Effect of chronic anemia on the tensile strength of healing wounds, *Surgery*, 66, 741, 1969.

Hyde, R. W. and Rawson, A. J., Unintentional iatrogenic oxygen pneumonitis — response to therapy, *Ann. Intern. Med.*, 71, 517, 1969.

Imamura, M., Clowes, G. H. A., Jr., Blackburn, G. L., O'Donnell, T. F., Jr., Trerice, M., Bhimjee, Y., and Ryan, N. T., Liver metabolism and glucogenesis in trauma and sepsis, *Surgery*, 77, 868, 1975.

International Committee for Standardization in Hematology, Recommended methods for radioisotope red cell survival studies, *Blood*, 38, 378, 1971.

Inwood, M. J. and Zuliani, B., Anti-A hemolytic transfusion with packed 0 cells, *Ann. Intern. Med.*, 89, 515, 1978.

Irvin, T. T., Modgill, V. K., Hayter, C. J., McDowall, D. G., and Goligher, J. C., Plasma volume deficits and salt and water excretion after surgery, *Lancet*, 2, 1159, 1972.

Jamieson, W. G., Taylor, B. M., Troster, M., and Durand, D., The significance of urine phosphate measurements in the early diagnosis of intestinal infarction, *Surg. Gynecol. Obstet.*, 148, 334, 1979.

Janssen, R. W. and Discher, C. A., Experimental evidence for the existence of an adrenochrome-adrenolutin complex, *J. Pharm. Sci.*, 56, 826, 1967.

Jaskunas, S. R., Stork, E. J., and Richardson, B., Effects of a hyperoxic environment on erythropoietin production, *Aerosp. Med.*, 44, 1112, 1973.

Jelenko, C., III, Williams, J. B., Wheeler, M. L., Callaway, B. D., Fackler, V. K., Albers, C. A., and Barger, A. A., Studies in shock and resuscitation. I. Use of hypertonic, albumin-containing, fluid demand regimen (HALFD) in resuscitaion, *Crit. Care Med.*, 7, 157, 1979.

Jeul, R., 2,3 Diphosphoglycerate: its role in health and disease, *Crit. Rev. in Clin. Lab. Sci.*, 10, 113, 1979.

Johnson, M. A., Polgar, J., Weightman, D., and Appleton, D., Data on the distribution of fibre types in thirty-six human muscles, an autopsy study, *J. Neurol. Sci.*, 18, 111, 1973.

Johnson, S. D., Lucas, C. E., Gerrick, S. J. Ledgerwood, A. M., and Higgins, R. F., Altered coagulation after albumin supplements for treatment of oligemic shock, *Arch. Surg.*, 114, 379, 1979.

Kaihara, S., Rutherford, R. B., Schwentker, E. P., and Wagner, H. N., Jr., Distribution of cardiac output in experimental hemorrhagic shock in dogs, *J. Appl. Physiol.*, 27, 218, 1969.

Kaplan, E. L., Peskin, G. W., and Arnaud, C. D., Nonsteroid, calcitonin-like factor from the adrenal gland, *Surgery*, 66, 167, 1969.

Kaplan, H. P., Hematologic effects of increased oxygen tensions, *Aerosp. Med.*, 38, 676, 1967.

Karmen, A., Wroblewski, F., and La Due, J. S., Transaminase activity in human blood, *J. Clin. Invest.*, 34, 126, 1955.

Kattlove, H. E., Gaynor, E., Spivack, M., and Gottfried, E. L., Sea-blue indigestion, *N. Engl. J. Med.*, 282, 630, 1970.

Keith, N. M., Blood volume changes in wound shock and primary haemorrhage, Medical Research Committee Reports of the Special Investigation Committee on Surgical Shock and Allied Conditions, IX. Blood Volume Changes in Wound Shock and Primary Haemorrhage, March 14, 1919, His Majesty's Stationery Office, London, 2.

Keitt, A. S., Pyruvate kinase deficiency and related disorders of red cell glycolysis, *Am. J. Med.*, 41, 762, 1966.

Keitt, A. S., Hemolytic anemia with impaired hexokinase activity, *J. Clin. Invest.*, 48, 1997, 1969.

Kelly, J. F. and Terry, B. C., Blood volume changes in the surgical treatment of oral-facial deformities: a preliminary report, *J. Oral Surg.*, 31, 90, 1973.

Kety, S. S., Circulation and metabolism of the human brain in health and disease, *Am. J. Med.*, 2, 205, 1950.

Kikkawa, H., Ogita, Z., and Fugito, S., Nature of pigments derived from tyrosine and tryptophan in animals, *Science*, 121, 43, 1955.

Kimzey, S. L., Johnson, P. C., Ritzman, S. E., and Mengel, C. E., Hematology and immunology studies: the second manned Skylab mission, *Aviat. Space Environ. Med.*, 47, 383, 1976.

Kjekshus, J. K. and Blix, A. S., How seals avoid myocardial infarction during diving, *Scand. J. Clin. Lab. Invest.*, 37, 95, 1977.

Kliman, A., Presently useful plasma volume expander, *Anesthesiology*, 27, 417, 1966.

Knochel, J. P., Dotin, L. N., and Hamburger, R. J., Heat stress, exercise, and muscle injury: effects on urate metabolism and renal function, *Ann. Intern. Med.*, 81, 321, 1974.

Knochel, J. P., Barcenas, C., Cotton, J. R., Fuller, T. J., Haller, R., and Carter, N. W., Hypophosphatemia and rhabdomyolysis, *Trans. Assoc. Am. Phys.*, 91, 156, 1978.

Komazawa, M., Landaw, S. A., and Oski, F. A., Lack of relationship of red cell enzyme activity to bilirubin and carboxyhemoglobin levels in healthy term infants, *Acta Paediatr. Scand.*, 64, 473, 1975.

Kopper, P. H., Fibrinolysins from fibrin clots, *Nature (London)*, 203, 534, 1964.

Kopriva, C. J., Ratliff, J. L., Fletcher, J. R., Fortier, N. L., and Valeri, C. R., Biochemical and hematological changes associated with massive transfusion of ACD-stored blood in severely injured combat casualties, *Ann. Surg.*, 176, 585, 1972.

Kovach, A. G. B. and Sandor, P., Cerebral blood flow and brain function during hypotension and shock, *Ann. Rev. Physiol.*, 38, 571, 1976.

Krall, M. A., Bristow, J. D., Welch, J. E., and Metcalfe, J., Physiological effects of lowered blood oxygen affinity in dogs, *Respir. Physiol.,* 33, 263, 1978.

Kreimer-Birnbaum, M., Pinkerton, P. H., Bannerman, R. M., and Hutchison, H. E., Dipyrrolic urinary pigments in congenital Heinz-body anaemic due to Hb Köln and in thalassaemia, *Brit. Med. J.,* 2, 396, 1966.

Kreisberg, R. A., Bowdoin, B., and Meador, C. K., Measurement of muscle mass in humans by isotopic dilution of creatine ^{14}C, *J. Appl. Physiol.,* 28, 264, 1970.

Kummer, H. and Lundsgaard-Hansen, P., The influence of clinical dextran and modified gelatin on hemorrhagic diathesis in irradiated, thrombocytopenic dogs, *Helv. Med. Acta,* 34, 244, 1968.

Laks, H., Dmochowski, J. R., and Couch, N. P., The relationship between muscle surface pH and oxygen transport, *Ann. Surg.,* 183, 193, 1976.

Lalone, B. and Houlihan, R. T., Determination of aminochromes produced in the rat during O_2 at high pressure (OHP) by gas lipid-chromatography (GLC), *Physiologist,* 14, 179, 1971.

Lamb, L. E., Johnson, R. L., and Stevens, P. M., Cardiovascular deconditioning during chair rest, *Aerosp. Med.,* 35, 646, 1964.

Lamb, L. E., Stevens, P. M., and Johnson, R. L., Hypokinesia secondary to chair rest from 4 to 10 days, *Aerosp. Med.,* 36, 755, 1965.

Landaw, S. A., Callahan, E. W., Jr., and Schmid, R., Catabolism of heme in vivo: comparison of the simultaneous production of bilirubin and carbon monoxide, *J. Clin. Invest.,* 49, 914, 1970.

Langley, G. R., Owen, J. A., and Padanyi, R., The effect of blood transfusions on serum haptoglobin, *Brit. J. Haematol.,* 8, 392, 1962.

Larkin, E. C., Smith, E. B., Williams, W. T., and Ulvedal, F., Response of human red blood cell (RBC) density distribution, rbc glutathione, and rbc enzymes to hypobaric hyperoxia, *Aerosp. Med.,* 44, 1158, 1973.

Lauson, H. D., Bradley, S. E., and Cournand, A., The renal circulation in shock, *J. Clin. Invest.,* 23, 381, 1944.

Lawrence, J. H. and Berlin, N. I., Relative polycythemia — the polycythemia of stress, *Yale J. Biol.,* 24, 498, 1952.

Leite, C. and Hoogstraten, B., Differential diagnosis of anemia and cancer, *Cancer,* 27, 88, 1977.

Lenfant, C., Torrance, J., English, E., Finch, C. A., Reynafarje, C., Ramos, J., and Faura, J., Effect of altitude on oxygen binding by hemoglobin and on organic phosphate levels, *J. Clin. Invest.,* 47, 2652, 1968.

Lentz, R. D., Brown, D. M., and Kjellstrand, C. M., Treatment of severe hypophosphatemia, *Ann. Intern. Med.,* 89, 941, 1978.

Lerman, S., Canterbury, J. M., and Reiss, E., Parathyroid hormone and the hypercalcemia of immobilization, *J. Clin. Endocrinol. Metab.,* 45, 425, 1977.

Levinson, G. E., Carleton, R. A., and Abelmann, W. H., Assessment of mitral regurgitation by indicator dilution: an analysis of the determinants of the abnormal dilution curve. *Am. Heart J.* 58, 873, 1959.

Lichtman, M. A. and Miller, D. R., Erythrocyte glycolysis, 2,3 diphosphoglycerate and adenosine triphosphate concentration in uremic subjects: relationship to extracellular phosphate concentration, *J. Lab. Clin. Med.,* 76, 267, 1970.

Lichtman, M.A., Miller, D. R., and Freeman, R. B., Erythrocyte adenosine triphosphate depletion during hypophosphatemia in a uremic subject, *N. Engl. J. Med.,* 280, 240, 1969a.

Lichtman, M. A., Miller, D. R., and Weed, R. I., Energy metabolism in uremic red cells: relationship of red cell adenosine triphosphate concentration to extracellular phosphate, *Trans. Assoc. Am. Phys.,* 82, 331, 1969b.

Lightner, D. A. and Quistad, G. B., Methylvinylmalemide from bilirubin photooxidation, *Science,* 175, 324, 1971.

Lillehei, R. C., Relationship of appearance of abnormal plasma hemin pigment to development of irreversible hemorrhagic shock in dogs, *Circ. Res.,* 6, 438, 1958.

Litwin, M. S., and Relihan, M., Effect of surgical operation on human blood viscosity, *Surgery,* 73, 323, 1973.

Liu, C. T., Traumatic shock: evidence for chemical release from traumatized tissue in dogs, *Aerosp. Med.,* 42, 403, 1971.

Loebl, E. C., Baxter, C. R., and Curreri, P. W., The mechanism of erythrocyte destruction in the early post-burn period, *Ann. Surg.,* 178, 681, 1973.

Logue, G. L., Rosse, W. F., Smith, W. T., Saltzman, H. A., and Gutterman, L. A., Endogenous carbon monoxide production measured by gas-phase analysis: an estimation of heme catabolic rate, *J. Lab. Clin. Med.,* 77, 867, 1971.

London, I. M., The conversion of hematin to bile pigment, *J. Biol. Chem.,* 184, 373, 1950.

London, I. M., West, R., Shemin, D., and Rittenberg, D., On the origin of bile pigment in normal man, *J. Biol. Chem.,* 184, 351, 1950.

Loria, A., Sanchez-Medal, L., Kauffer, N., and Quintanar, E., Relationship between body hematocrit and venous hematocrit in normal, splenomegalic, and anemic states, *J. Lab. Clin. Med.*, 60, 396, 1962.

Lovelace, D. R., Short, B. L., and Rink, R. D., Hepatic oxygen supply in reversible and irreversible hemorrhagic shock, *J. Surg. Res,*. 26, 120, 1979.

Lovric, V. A., Prince, B., and Bryant, J., Packed red cell transfusions — improved survival, quality and storage, *Vox Sang.*, 33, 346, 1977.

Lowe, R. J., Moss, G. S., Jilek, J., and Levine, H. D., Crystalloid versus colloid in the etiology of pulmonary failure after trauma — randomized trial in man, *Crit. Care Med.*, 7, 107, 1979.

Lowery, B. D., Cloutier, C. T., and Carey, L. C., Electrolyte solutions in resuscitation in human hemorrhagic shock, *Surg. Gynecol. Obstet.*, 133, 273, 1971.

Lucas, C. E., Weaver, D., Higgins, R. F., Ledgerwood, A. M., Johnson, S. D., and Bouwman, D. L., Effects of albumin versus non-albumin resuscitation on plasma volume and renal excretory function, *J. Trauma*, 18, 564, 1978.

Lucas, C. E., Ledgerwood, A. M., and Higgins, R. F., Impaired salt and water excretion after albumin resuscitation for hypovolemic shock, *Surgery*, 86, 544, 1979.

Lundsgaard-Hansen, P., Treatment of shock with dextrans and gelatins, *Vox Sang.*, 17, 161, 1969.

Lynch, S. R. and Moede, A. L., Variations in the rate of endogenous carbon monoxide production in normal human beings, *J. Lab. Clin. Med.*, 79, 85, 1972.

Malmberg, P. O., Hlastala, M. P., and Woodson, R. D., Effect of increased blood oxygen affinity on oxygen transport in hemorrhagic shock, *J. Appl. Physiol.-Respir. Environ.*, 47, 889, 1979.

Malone, J. I., Winegrad, A. I., Oski, F. A., and Holmes, E. W., Jr., Erythrocyte hexokinase isoenzyme patterns in hereditary hemoglobinopathies, *N. Engl. J. Med.*, 279, 1071, 1968.

Malt, R. A., Wang, C. A., Yamazaki, Z., and Miyakuni, T., Stimulation of albumin synthesis by hemorrhage, *Surgery*, 66, 65, 1969.

Mann, F. C., Sheard, C., Bollman, J. L., and Baldes, E. J., The formation of bile pigment from hemoglobin, *Am. J. Physiol.*, 76, 306, 1926.

Manny, J., Justice, R., and Hechtman, H. B., Abnormalities in organ blood flow and its distribution during positive end expiratory pressure, *Surgery*, 85, 425, 1979.

Marshall, B. E., Wurzel, H. A., Neufeld, G. R., Aukburg, S. J., Ewing, B. C., Fried, R. J., and Barnes, C., Effect of Fenwal 4C2423 transfusion microfilter on microaggregates and other constituents of stored blood, *Transfusion*, 18, 38, 1978.

Matsuda, T. and Shoemaker, W. C., Effectiveness of transfusions in postoperative patients as measured by 24-hour red cell survival, *Ann. Surg.*, 175, 577, 1972.

Matsumoto, T., Wyte, S. R., Moseley, R. V., Nemhauser, G. M., and Henry, J. N., Serum creatinephosphokinase in soft tissue injuries, *Arch. Surg.*, 99, 535, 1969.

Mayerson, H. S., Lyons, C., Parson, W., Nieset, R. T., and Trautman, W. V., Jr., Comparison of results of measurement of red blood cell volume by direct and indirect techniques, *Am. J. Physiol.*, 155, 232, 1948.

McConn, R., Massive transfusion and its effect on hemodynamic function in the recipient, in *Massive Transfusion*, Nushbacher, J., Ed., American Association of Blood Banks, Washington, D.C., 1978, 25.

McConn, R. and DelGuercio, L. R. M., Respiratory function of blood in the acutely ill patient and the effect of steroids, *Ann. Surg.*, 174, 436, 1971.

McFarlane, A. S., Labelling of plasma proteins with radioactive iodine, *Biochem. J.*, 62, 135, 1956.

McFarlane, A. S., The behavior of I^{131} labeled plasma proteins in vivo, *Ann. N. Y. Acad. Sci.*, 70, 19, 1957.

McKay, D. G., Whitaker, A. N., and Cruse, V., Studies of catecholamine shock. II. An experimental model of microangiopathic hemolysis, *Am. J. Pathol.*, 56, 177, 1969.

Meijia, L. A., Hodges, R. E., and Rucker, R. B., Role of Vitamin A in the absorption, retention, and distribution of iron in the rat, *J. Nutr.*, 109, 129, 1979.

Meineke, H. A. and Crafts, R. C., Correlation between oxygen consumption and erythropoiesis in hypophysectomized rats treated with various doses of thyroxin, *Proc. Soc. Exp. Biol. Med.*, 102, 121, 1959.

Meldon, J. H. and Garby, L., The blood oxygen transport system — a numerical simulation of capillary-tissue respiratory gas exchange, *Acta Med. Scand. Suppl.*, 578, 19, 1975.

Mikhail, M. M., Waslien, C. I., Gabr, M. K., and Mansour, M. M., In vitro uptake of labeled amino acids by red blood cells of children with protein-calorie malnutrition, *Am. J. Clin. Nutr.*, 28, 233, 1975.

Miller, A. T., Jr., A re-evaluation of the T-1824 mixing curve, *Am. J. Physiol.*, 151, 234, 1947.

Miller, M. E., The interaction between the regulation of acid-base and erythropoietin production, *Blood Cells*, 1, 449, 1975.

Miller, M. E. and Howard, D., Modulation of erythropoietin concentrations by manipulation of hypercarbia, *Blood Cells*, 5, 389, 1979.

Miller, P. B., Hartman, B. O., Johnson, R. L., and Lamb, L. E., Modification of the effects of two weeks of bed rest upon circulatory functions in man, *Aerosp. Med.*, 35, 931, 1964a.

Miller, P. B., Johnson, R. L., and Lamb, L. E., Effects of four weeks of absolute bed rest on circulatory functions in man, *Aerosp. Med.*, 35, 1194, 1964b.

Miller, P. B., Johnson, R. L., and Lamb, L. E., Effects of moderate physical exercise during four weeks of bed rest on circulatory functions in man, *Aerosp. Med.*, 36, 1077, 1965.

Miller, L. D., Oski, F. A., Diaco, J. F., Sugerman, H. J., Gottlieb, A. J., Davidson, D., and Delivoria-Papadopoulos, M., The affinity of hemoglobin for oxygen: its control and in vivo significance, *Surgery*, 68, 187, 1970a.

Miller, L. D., Sugerman, H. J., Miller, W. W., Delivoria-Papadopoulos, M., Diaco, J. F., Gottlieb, A. J., and Oski, F. A., Increased peripheral oxygen delivery in thyrotoxicosis — role of red cell 2,3 diphosphoglycerate, *Ann. Surg.*, 172, 1051, 1970b.

Miller, W. W., Delivoria-Papadopoulos, M., Miller, L., and Oski, F. A., Oxygen releasing factor in hyperthyroidism, *JAMA*, 211, 1824, 1970c.

Miller, M., Rörth, M., Parving, H. H., Reddington, I., Valeri, C. R., and Stohlman, F., Jr., pH effect on erythropoeitin response to hypoxia, *N. Engl. J. Med.*, 288, 706, 1973.

Miller, M. E., Howard, D., Stohlman, F., Jr., and Flanagan, P., Mechanism of erythropoietin production by cobaltous chloride, *Blood*, 44, 339, 1974.

Miller, M. E., Rörth, M., Stohlman, F., Jr., Valeri, C. R., Lowrie, G. B., Howard, D., and McGilvray, N., The effect of acute bleeding on acid-base balance, erythropoietin (Ep) production and in vivo P_{50} in the rat, *Brit. J. Haematol.*, 33, 379, 1976.

Mirand, E. A., Gordon, A. S., and Wenig, J., Mechanisms of testosterone action in erythropoiesis, *Nature (London)*, 206, 270, 1965.

Mishler, J. M., Darley, J. H., Cederholm-Williams, S., and Wright, G., Whole blood storage in citrate and phosphate solutions containing half-strength trisodium citrate: cellular and biochemical studies, *J. Pathol.*, 124, 125, 1978.

Misra, H. P. and Fridovich, I., The role of superoxide anion in the auto-oxidation of epinephrine and a simple assay for superoxide dismutase, *J. Biol. Chem.*, 247, 3170, 1972.

Mitch, W. E. and Walker, W. G., Plasma renin and angiotensin II in acute renal failure, *Lancet*, 2, 328, 1977.

Mollison, P. L., *Blood Transfusion in Clinical Medicine*, 5th ed., Blackwell Scientific, Oxford, 1972.

Moore, F. D., Hartsuck, J. M., Zollinger, R. M., Jr., and Johnson, J. E., Reference models for clinical studies by isotope dilution, *Ann. Surg.*, 168, 671, 1968.

Morgan, E. H., Marsaglia, G., Giblett, E. R., and Finch, C. A., A method of investigating internal iron exchange utilizing two types of transferrin, *J. Lab. Clin. Med.*, 69, 370, 1967.

Mortensen, R. F. and Eurenius, K., Erythrokinetics and ferrokinetics after thermal injury in the rat, *Surg. Gynecol. Obstet.*, 138, 713, 1974.

Mosso, A., Circolazione de sangue nel cervello dell'uomo, *Reale Accademia dei Lincei*, 277, 1, 1880.

Mouridsen, H. T., The retention of different plasma proteins in wound tissue, *Scand. J. Clin. Lab. Invest.*, 23, 235, 1969.

Muldowney, F. P., Crooks, J., and Bluhm, M. M., The relationship of total exchangeable potassium and chloride to lean body mass, red cell mass and creatinine excretion in man, *J. Clin. Invest.*, 36, 1375, 1957.

Murray, R. D. and Jacey, M. J., Shallow habitat air dives I and II: human hematologic responses to compressed air saturation diving, *Aviat. Space Environ. Med.*, 48, 1012, 1977.

Nadler, S. B., Hidalgo, J. U., and Bloch, T., Prediction of blood volume in normal human adults, *Invest. Surg.*, 51, 224, 1962.

Neill, W. A., Jensen, P. E., Rich, G. B., and Werschkul, J. D., Effect of decreased O_2 supply to tissue on the lactate:pyruvate ratio in blood, *J. Clin. Invest.*, 48, 1862, 1969.

Nelson, A. W. and Swan, H., Blood volume. II. Precise long-term measurements using chromium tagged erythrocytes, *Ann. Surg.*, 173, 496, 1971.

Nemir, P., Jr., Ahmadi, A., and Drabkin, D. L., Demonstration of typical hemochromogen formation in clinical shock, *Ann. Surg.*, 165, 135, 1967.

Neutze, J. M., Wyler, F., and Rudolph, A. M., Changes in distribution of cardiac output after hemorrhage in rabbits, *Am. J. Physiol.*, 215, 857, 1968.

Niinikoski, J., Hunt, T. K., and Dunphy, J. E., Oxygen supply in healing tissue, *Am. J. Surg.*, 123, 247, 1972.

Nixon, J. V., Murray, R. G., Bryant, C., Johnson, R. L., Jr., Mitchell, J. H., Holland, O. B., Gomez-Sanchez, C., Vergne-Marini, P., and Blomqvist, C. G., Early cardiovascular adaptation to simulated zero gravity, *J. Appl. Physiol.-Respir. Environ.*, 46, 541, 1979.

Noble, R. P. and Gregersen, M. I., Blood volume in clinical shock. II. The extent and cause of blood volume reduction in traumatic, hemorrhagic, and burn shock, *J. Clin. Invest*, 25, 172, 1946.

Noel, G. L., Suh, H. K., Stone, J. G., and Frantz, A. G., Human prolactin and growth hormone release during surgery and other conditions of stress, *J. Clin. Endocrinol. Metab.*, 35, 840, 1972.

Norlander, O., Total hemoglobin, blood volume and circulatory changes in surgical patients, *Acta Chir. Scand. Suppl.*, 199, 5, 1955.

Nylander, G., Iron metabolism in fractures, *Acta Endocrinol.*, 20, 148, 1955.

Öberg, B., Overall cardiovascular regulation, *Ann. Rev. Physiol.*, 38, 537, 1976.

O'Connell, D. J., Caruso, C. J., and Sass, M. D., Separation of erythrocytes of different ages, *Clin. Chem.*, 11, 771, 1965.

O'Connor, L. R., Wheeler, W. S., and Bethune, J. E., Effect of hypophosphatemia on myocardial performance in man, *N. Engl. J. Med.*, 297, 901, 1977.

Opalinski, A. and Beutler, E., Creatine, 2,3 diphosphoglycerate and anemia, *N. Engl. J. Med.*, 285, 483, 1971.

O'Shaughnessy, M. C., Brunström, G. M., and Fielding, J., Iron chelation in haematomas at fracture sites, *J. Clin. Pathol.*, 19, 364, 1966.

Oski, F. A., Red cell metabolism in the newborn infant. V. Glycolytic intermediates and glycolytic enzymes, *Pediatrics*, 44, 84, 1969.

Oski, F. A., Clinical consequences of alterations in the affinity of hemoglobin for oxygen, in *Preservation of Red Blood Cells*, Chaplin, H., Jr., Jaffe, E. R., Lenfant, C., and Valeri, C. R., Eds., National Research Council, Washington, D.C., 1973, 67.

Oski, F. A., Gottlieb, A. J., Delivoria-Papadopoulos, M., and Miller, W. W., Red cell 2,3-diphosphoglycerate levels in subjects with chronic hypoxemia, *N. Engl. J. Med.*, 280, 1165, 1969.

Oski, F. A., Marshall, B. E., Cohen, P. J., Sugerman, H. J., and Miller, L. D., Exercise with anemia, *Ann. Intern. Med.*, 74, 44, 1971a.

Oski, F. A., Travis, S. F., Miller, L. D., Delivoria-Papadopoulos, M., and Cannon, E., The in vitro restoration of red cell 2,3 diphosphoglycerate levels in banked blood, *Blood*, 37, 52, 1971b.

Ostrow, J. D., Photocatabolism of labeled bilirubin in the congenitally jaundiced (Gunn) rat, *J. Clin. Invest.*, 50, 707, 1971.

Pace, N., Weightlessness: a matter of gravity, *N. Engl. J. Med.*, 297, 32, 1977.

Pace, N., Schaffer, F. L., Elmadjian, F., Minard, D., Davis, S. W., Kilbuck, J. H., Walker, E. L., Johnston, M. E., Zilinsky, A., Gerard, R. W., Forsham, P. H., and Taylor, J. G., in *Physiological Studies on Infantrymen in Combat*, University of California, Berkeley and Los Angeles, 1956, 1.

Paniker, N. V. and Beutler, E., Effect of normal metabolites on the oxygen hemoglobin equilibrium, *Proc. Soc. Exp. Biol. Med.*, 135, 389, 1970.

Parving, H. H., Rossing, N., Nielsen, S. L., and Lassen, N. A., Increased transcapillary escape rate of albumin, IgG, and IgM after plasma volume expansion, *Am. J. Physiol.*, 227, 245, 1974.

Parving, H. H., Hansen, J. M., Nielsen, S. L., Rossing, N., Munck, O., and Lassen, N. A., Mechanisms of edema formation in myxedema-increased protein extravasation and relatively slow lymphatic drainage, *N. Engl. J. Med.*, 301, 460, 1979.

Peschle, C., Regulation of erythropoiesis and its defects, *Brit. J. Haematol.*, 31, 69, 1975.

Peschle, C., Rappaport, I. A., Magli, M. C., Marone, G., Lettieri, F., Cillo, C., and Gordon, A. S., Role of the hypophysis in erythropoietin production during hypoxia, *Blood*, 51, 1117, 1978.

Peskin, G. W., O'Brien, K., and Rabiner, S. F. Stroma-free hemoglobin solution: the "ideal" blood substitute? *Surgery*, 66, 185, 1969.

Peters, J. P., The role of sodium in the production of edema, *N. Engl. J. Med.*, 239, 353, 1948.

Pezeshki, C. and Brooker, A. F., Immobilization hypercalcemia, *J. Bone Joint Surg.*, 59-A, 971, 1977.

Pierson, R. N., Holt, P. R., Watson, R. M., and Keating, R. P., Aspirin and gastrointestinal bleeding. Chromate^{51} blood loss studies, *Am. J. Med.*, 31, 259, 1961.

Pimstone, N. R., Tenhunen, R., Seitz, P. T., Marver, H. S., and Schmid, R., The enzymatic degradation of hemoglobin to bile pigment by macrophages, *J. Exp. Med.*, 133, 1264, 1971.

Piomelli, S., Nathan, D. G., Cummins, J. F., and Gardner, F. H., The relationship of total red cell volume to total body water in octogenarian males, *Blood*, 19, 89, 1962.

Plzak, L. F., Jr., Blood requirements in cardiac surgery, in *Preservation of Red Blood Cells*, Chaplin, H., Jr., Jaffe, E. R., Lenfant, C., and Valeri, C. R., Eds., National Research Council, Washington, D.C., 1973, 35.

Pollock, T. W., Rosato, E. F., Delivoria-Papadopoulos, M., and Miller, L. D., In vivo manipulation of oxygen-hemoglobin affinity, *J. Surg. Res.*, 22, 449, 1977.

Prasad, K. N., and Seale, R. U., Effect of dopamine on hemoglobin synthesis of chick blastoderm in vitro, *Proc. Soc. Exp. Biol. Med.*, 131, 1308, 1969.

Prentice, T. C., Olney, J. M., Artz, C. P., and Howard, J. M., Studies of blood volume and transfusion therapy in the Korean battle casualty, *Surg. Gynecol. Obstet.*, 99, 542, 1954.

Prins, H. K. and Loos, J. A., Studies on biochemical properties and viability of stored packed cells, in *Modern Problems of Blood Preservation*, Spielmann, W. and Seidl, S., Eds., Gustav Fischer Verlag, Stuttgart, 1970, 110.

Rahn, H., Conductance of O_2 from the environment to the tissues at high altitude, in *Studies in Pulmonary Physiology, Mechanics, Chemistry, and Circulation of the Lung*, Vol. 2, Farhi, L. E. and Rahn, H., Eds., Aerospace Medical Research Laboratories TDR 63-103(11), Wright Patterson Air Force Base, Ohio, 1966, 34.

Rao, P. S. and Cavanagh, D., Endotoxin shock in the subhuman primate. II. Some effects of methylprednisolone administration, *Arch. Surg.*, 102, 486, 1971.

Rassmussen-Taxdal, D. S., Ward, G. E., and Figge, F. H. J., Fluorescence of human lymphatic and cancer tissues following high doses of intravenous hematoporphyrin, *Cancer*, 8, 78, 1955.

Reeve, E. B. and Bailey, H. R., Mathematical models describing the distribution of I^{131}-albumin in man, *J. Lab. Clin. Med.*, 60, 923, 1962.

Reinhardt, H. W., Kaczmarczyk, G., Eisele, R., Arnold, B., Eigenheer, F., and Kuhl, U., Left atrial pressure and sodium balance in conscious dogs on a low sodium intake, *Pflügers Arch.*, 370, 59, 1977.

Reiss, E., Canterbury, J. M., Bercovitz, M. A., and Kaplan, E. L., The role of phosphate in the secretion of parathyroid hormone in man, *J. Clin. Invest.*, 49, 2146, 1970.

Remes, K., Effect of long-term physical training on total red cell volume, *Scand. J. Clin. Lab. Invest.*, 39, 311, 1979.

Retzlaff, J. A., Tauxe, W. N., Kiely, J. M., and Stroebel, C. F., Erythrocyte volume, plasma volume, and lean body mass in adult men and women, *Blood*, 33, 649, 1969.

Reul, G. J., Jr., Greenberg, S. D., Lefrak, E. A., McCollum, W. B., Beall, A. C., Jr., and Jordan, G. L., Jr., Prevention of post traumatic pulmonary insufficiency. Fine screen filtration of blood, *Arch. Surg.*, 106, 386, 1973.

Reul, G. J., Jr., Beall, A. C., Jr., and Greenberg, S. D., Protection of the pulmonary microvasculature by fine screen blood filtration, *Chest.*, 66, 4, 1974.

Rice, C. L., Herman, C. M., Kiesow, L. A., Homer, L. D., John, D. A., and Valeri, C. R., Benefits from improved oxygen delivery of blood in shock therapy, *J. Surg. Res.*, 19, 193, 1975.

Richards, D. W., Jr., The circulation in traumatic shock in man, *Bull. N. Y. Acad. Med.*, 20, 363, 1944a.

Richards, D. W., Jr., The circulation in traumatic shock in man, *Harvey Lect.*, 31, 217, 1944b.

Robinson, S. H., Lester, R., Crigler, J. F., and Tsong, M., Early-labeled peak of bile pigment in man. Studies with glycine-^{14}C and delta-amino-levulinic acid ^{3}H, *N. Engl. J. Med.*, 277, 1323, 1967.

Robinson, S. H. and Tsong, M., Hemolysis of "stress" reticulocytes: a source of erythropoietic bilirubin formation, *J. Clin. Invest.*, 49, 1025, 1970.

Robinson, H., Monafo, W. W., Saver, S. M., and Gallagher, N. I., The role of erythropoietin in the anemia of thermal injury, *Ann. Surg.*, 178, 565, 1973.

Rodkey, F. L., O'Neal, J. D., and Collison, H. A., Oxygen and carbon monoxide equilibria of human adult hemoglobin at atmospheric and elevated pressure, *Blood*, 33, 57, 1969.

Rodman, T., Close, H., P., and Purcell, M. K., The oxyhemoglobin dissociation curve in anemia, *Ann. Intern. Med.*, 52, 295, 1960.

Rodriguez, J. M. and Shahidi, N. T., Erythrocyte 2,3 diphosphoglycerate in adaptive red cell volume deficiency, *N. Engl. J. Med.*, 285, 479, 1971.

Rörth, M. and Bille-Brahe, N. E., 2,3 DPG in human pregnancy, in *Oxygen Affinity and Red Cell Acid-Base Status*, Alfred Benzon Symposium IV, Rörth, M. and Astrup, P., Eds., Academic Press, New York, 1972, 692.

Rörth, M., Hypoxia, red cell oxygen affinity and erythropoietin production, *Clin. Hematol.*, 3, 595, 1974.

Rörth, M., Nygaard, S. F., and Parving, H. H., Red cell metabolism and oxygen affinity of healthy individuals during exposure to high altitude, *Adv. Exp. Med. Biol.*, 28, 361, 1972.

Rosenthal, A., Litwin, S. B., and Laver, M. B., Effect of contrast media used in angiocardiography on hemoglobin-oxygen equilibrium, *Invest. Radiol.*, 8, 191, 1973.

Rothschild, M. A., Oratz, M., and Schreiber, S. S., Extravascular albumin, *N. Engl. J. Med.*, 301, 497, 1979.

Rowlands, J. R., Estefan, R. M., Gause, E. M., and Montalvo, D. A., An electron spin resonance study of tobacco smoke condensates and their effects upon blood constituents, *Environ. Res.*, 2, 47, 1968.

Rubinstein, D. and Warrendorf, E., An incubation medium for the elevation of adenosine triphosphate and 2,3-diphosphoglycerate in fresh and long-preserved human erythrocytes, *Can. J. Biochem*,. 53, 671, 1975.

Rutherford, R. B. and Trow, R. S., The pathophysiology of irreversible hemorrhagic shock in monkeys, *J. Surg. Res.*, 14, 538, 1973.

Ryden, S. E. and Oberman, H. A., Compatibility of common intravenous solutions with CPD blood, *Transfusion*, 15, 250, 1975.

Saba, T. M., Blumenstock, F. A., Scovill, W. A., and Bernard, H., Cryoprecipitate reversal of opsonic α_2-surface binding glycoprotein deficiency in septic surgical and trauma patients, *Science*, 201, 622, 1978.

Sabine, J. C. and Kwok, L. W., Observation of four age-related parameters in the red cells of various disease states, *Brit. J. Haematol.*, 15, 507, 1968.

Salhany, J. M., Eliot, R. S., and Mizukami, H., The effects of 2,3-diphosphoglycerate on the kinetics of deoxygenation of human hemoglobin, *Biochem. Biophys. Res. Commun,.* 39, 1052, 1970.

Saltin, B., Blomqvist, G., Mitchell, J. H., Johnson, R. L., Jr., Wildenthal, K., and Chapman, C. B., Response to exercise after bed rest and after training, *Circulation,* 37, 38 (Suppl. VII) 2, 1968.

Salzman, E. W., Does intravascular coagulation occur in hemorrhagic shock in man, *J. Trauma,* 8, 867, 1968.

Samaja, M. and Winslow, R. M., The separate effects of H+ and 2,3 DPG on the oxygen curve of human blood, *Brit. J. Haematol.,* 41, 373, 1979.

Sanders, R., Sheldon, G. F., Garcia, J., Schooley, J., and Fuchs, R., Erythropoietin synthesis in rats during total parenteral nutrition, *J. Surg. Res.,* 22, 649, 1977.

Sauer, G. F. and Funk, D. D., Iron overload in cutaneous porphyria, *Arch. Intern. Med.,* 124, 190, 1969.

Savitsky, J. P., Doczi, J., Block, J., and Arnold, J. D., A clinical safety trial of stroma-free hemoglobin, *Clin. Pharmacol. Ther.,* 23, 73, 1978.

Schade, S. G. and Fried, W., Suppressive effect of endotoxin on erythropoietin-responsive cells in mice, *Am. J. Physiol.,* 231, 73, 1976.

Schaefer, K. E., Messier, A A., and Morgan, C. C., Displacement of oxygen dissociated curves and red cell cation exchange in chronic hypercapnia, *Respir. Physiol.,* 10, 299, 1970.

Schaller, F. and Roggen, G., Stability (storability) of gelatin plasma substitute solutions with reference to military medical use, *Bibl. Haematol. (Pavia),* 33, 587, 1969.

Schenk, W. G., III and Moylan, J. A., Hypercalciuresis in trauma patients on high-nitrogen enteral and parenteral diets, *J. Trauma,* 19, 227, 1979.

Schiller, W. R., Long, C. L., and Blakemore, W. S., Creatinine and nitrogen excretion in seriously ill and injured patients, *Surg. Gynecol. Obstet.,* 149, 561, 1979.

Schmid, R., Bilirubin metabolism in man, *N. Engl. J. Med.,* 287, 703, 1972.

Schmidt, P. J., Red cells for transfusion, *N. Engl. J. Med.,* 299, 1411, 1978.

Schnabel, T. G., Jr., Eliasch, H., Thomasson, B., and Werko, L., The effect of experimentally induced hypervolemia on cardiac function in normal subjects and patients with mitral stenosis, *J. Clin. Invest.,* 38, 117, 1959.

Scholander, P. F., Physiological adaptation to diving in animals and man, *Harvey Lect.,* 57, 93, 1962.

Schon, G. R., Delpin, E. S., Millan, P. R., and Labat, R., Relationship of blood substitutes to pulmonary changes and volemia, *Ann. Surg.,* 173, 504, 1971.

Schooley, J. C. and Mahlmann, L. J., Hypoxia and the initiation of erythropoietin production, *Blood Cells,* 1, 429, 1975.

Schrumpf, J. D., Sheps, D. S., Wolfson, S., Aronson, A. L., and Cohen, L. S., Altered hemoglobin-oxygen affinity with long-term propranolol therapy in patients with coronary artery disease, *Am. J. Cardiol.,* 40, 76, 1977.

Scovill, W. A., Saba, T. M., Blumenstock, F. A., Bernard, H., and Powers, S. R., Jr., Opsonic α_2-surface binding glycoprotein therapy during sepsis, *Ann. Surg.,* 188, 521, 1978.

Scovill, W. A., Annest, S. J., Saba, T. M., Blumenstock, F. A., Newell, J. C., Stratton, H. H., and Powers, S. R., Cardiovascular hemodynamics after opsonic alpha-2-surface binding glycoprotein therapy in injured patients, *Surgery,* 86, 284, 1979.

Seaman, B. W. and Ponder, E., The estimation and control of post-operative dehydration, with the aid of hemoglobin and plasma protein determinations, *J. Clin. Invest.,* 22, 673, 1943.

Sears, D. A., Disposal of plasma heme in normal men and patients with intravascular hemolysis, *J. Clin. Invest.,* 49, 5, 1970.

Seibert, D. J. and Ebaugh, F. G., Jr., Assessment of tissue anoxemia in chronic anemia by the arterial lactate/pyruvate ratio and excess lactate formation, *J. Lab. Clin. Med.,* 69, 177, 1967.

Selmyer, J. P., Reynolds, D. G., and Swan, K. G., Renal blood during endotoxin shock in the subhuman primate, *Surg. Gynecol. Obstet.,* 137, 3, 1973.

Sendroy, J. and Cecchini, L. P., Determination of human body surface area from height and weight, *J. Appl. Physiol.,* 7, 1, 1954.

Serkes, K. D., Lang, S., and Pareira, M. D., Blood volume: methodology and applications, *Monogr. Surg. Sci.,* 2, 69, 1965.

Sevitt, S., The boundaries between physiology, pathology, and irreversibility after injury, *Lancet,* 2, 1203, 1966.

Shafritz, D., Goodwin, F., and Weissbach, H., Inhibition by aminochromes of in vitro polypeptide synthesis in escherichia coli, *Arch. Biochem. Biophys.,* 134, 478, 1969.

Shah, D. M., Browner, B. D., Dutton, R. E., Newell, J. C., and Powers, S. R., Jr., Cardiac output and pulmonary wedge pressure, *Arch. Surg.,* 112, 1161, 1977.

Shahidi, N. T., Androgens and erythropoiesis, *N. Engl. J. Med.,* 289, 72, 1973.

Shaklai, N., Benitez, L., and Ranney, H. M., Binding of 2,3-diphosphoglycerate by spectrin and its effect on oxygen affinity of hemoglobin, *Am. J. Physiol.,* 234, C-36, 1978.

Shapiro, M., Blood transfusion practice: facts and fallacies, *S. A. Med. J.*, 50, 105, 1976.

Sharpey-Schafer, E. P., Transfusion and the anaemic heart, *Lancet*, 2, 296, 1945.

Sheldon, G. F., Defective hemoglobin function: a complication of hyperalimentation, *J. Trauma*, 13, 971, 1973a.

Sheldon, G. F., Hyperphosphatemia, hypophosphatemia, and oxy-hemoglobin dissociation curve, *J. Surg. Res.*, 14, 367, 1973b.

Sheldon, G. F. and Fuchs, R., Arteriography: another low phosphate syndrome, *J. Surg. Res.*, 22, 679, 1977.

Sheps, D. S., Conde, C., Cameron, B., Lo, W. C., Appel, R., Castellanos, A., Harkness, D. R., and Myerburg, R. J., Restoring peripheral blood lactate elevation in survivors of pre-hospital cardiac arrest: correlation with hemodynamic, electrophysiologic and oxyhemoglobin dissociation indexes, *Am. J. Cardiol.*, 44, 1276, 1979.

Shields, H. M., Rapid fall of serum phosphorus secondary to antacid therapy, *Gastroenterology*, 75, 1137, 1978.

Shier, M. R., Wilson, R. F., James, R. E., Riddle, J., Mammen, E. F., and Pedersen, H. E., Fat embolism prophylaxis: a study of four treatment modalities, *J. Trauma*, 17, 621, 1977.

Shin, B., Mackenzie, C. F., McAslan, T. C., Helrich, M., and Cowley, R. A., Postoperative renal failure in trauma patients, *Anesthesiology*, 51, 218, 1979.

Shinton, N. K., Richardson, R. W., and Williams, J. D. F., Diagnostic value of serum haptoglobin, *J. Clin. Pathol.*, 18, 114, 1965.

Shizgal, H. M., Lopez, G. A., and Gutelius, J. R., Effect of experimental hemorrhagic shock on extracellular water volume, *Ann. Surg.*, 176, 736, 1972.

Shoemaker, W. C., Cardiorespiratory patterns in complicated and uncomplicated septic shock: physiologic alterations and their therapeutic implications, *Ann. Surg.*, 174, 119, 1971.

Shoemaker, W. C. and Monson, D. O., The effect of whole blood and plasma expanders on volume-flow relationships in critically ill patients, *Surg. Gynecol. Obstet.*, 137, 453, 1973.

Shoemaker, W. C. and Reinhard, J. M., Tissue perfusion defects in shock and trauma states, *Surg. Gynecol. Obstet.*, 137, 980, 1973.

Shoemaker, W. C. and Hauser, C. J., Critique of crystalloid verus colloid therapy in shock and shock lung, *Crit. Care Med.*, 7, 117, 1979.

Shoemaker, W.C., Montgomery, E. S., Kaplan, E., and Elwyn, D. H., Physiologic patterns in surviving and nonsurviving shock patients, *Arch. Surg.*, 106, 630, 1973.

Shore, L. and Claybaugh, J. R., Regulation of body fluids, *Ann. Rev. Physiol.*, 35, 235, 1972.

Sibbald, W. J., Sardesai, V., and Wilson, R. F., Hypocalcemia and nephrogenous cyclic AMP production in critically ill or injured patients, *J. Trauma*, 17, 677, 1977.

Siegel, J. H., Greenspan, M., Cohn, J. D., and DelGuercio, L. R. M., A bedside computer and physiologic nomograms, *Arch. Surg.*, 97, 480, 1968.

Siegel, D. C., Cochin, A., Geocaris, T., and Moss, G. S., Effects of saline and colloid resuscitation on renal function, *Ann. Surg.*, 177, 51, 1973.

Siggaard-Andersen, J., Petersen, F. B., Hansen, T. I., and Mellemgaard, K., Vascular permeability and plasma volume changes during hypoxia and carbon monoxide exposure, *Angiology*, 20, 356, 1969.

Simmons, R. L., Heisterkamp, C. A., III, Moseley, R. V., and Doty, D. B., Post-resuscitative blood volumes in combat casualties, *Surg. Gynecol. Obstet.*, 128, 1193, 1969a.

Simmons, R. L., Collins, J. A., Heisterkamp, C. A., III, Mills, D. E., Andren, R., and Phillips, L. L., Coagulation disorders in combat casualties. I. Acute changes after wounding, II. Effects of massive transfusion, III. Post-resuscitative changes, *Ann. Surg.*, 169, 455, 1969b.

Simmons, R. L., Heisterkamp, C. A., III, Collins, J. A., Genslar, S., and Martin, A. M., Jr., Respiratory insufficiency in combat casualties. III. Arterial hypoxemia after wounding, *Ann. Surg.*, 170, 45, 1969c.

Simmons, R. L., Heisterkamp, C. A., III, Collins, J. A., Bredenberg, C. E., Mills, D. E., and Martin, A.M., Jr., Respiratory insufficiency in combat casualties. IV. Hypoxemia during convalescence, *Ann. Surg.*, 170, 53, 1969d.

Skillman, J. J., Lauler, D. P., Hickler, R. B., Lyons, J. H., Olson, J. E., Ball, M. R., and Moore, F. D., Hemorrhage in normal man: effect on renin, cortisol, aldosterone, and urine composition, *Ann. Surg.*, 166, 865, 1967.

Skillman, J. J., Parikh, B. M., and Tanenbaum, B. J., Pulmonary arterial venous admixture: improvement with albumin and diuresis, *Am. J. Surg.*, 119, 440, 1970.

Skillman, J. J., Restall, D. S., and Salzman, E. W., Randomized trial of albumin vs. electrolyte solution during abdominal aortic operations, *Surgery*, 78, 291, 1975.

Skillman, J. J., Rosenoer, V. M., Smith, P. C., and Fang, M. S., Improved albumin synthesis in postoperative patients by amino acid infusion, *N. Engl. J. Med.*, 295, 1037, 1976.

Slater, G., Vladeck, B. C., Bassin, R., Brown, R. S., and Shoemaker, W. C., Sequential changes in cerebral blood flow and distribution of flow within the brain during hemorrhagic shock, *Ann. Surg.*, 181, 1, 1975.

Smith, R. H., Normal blood volumes in men and women over sixty years of age as determined by a modified Cr^{51} method, *Anesthesia*, 19, 752, 1958.

Smith, D. E., Virgilio, R. W., Trimble, C., and Fosburg, R. G., Comparison of venous sampling sites for intrapulmonary shunt determinations in the critically ill patient, *J. Surg. Res.*, 14, 319, 1973.

Smith, P. C., Frank, H. A., Kasdon, E. J., Dearborn, E. C., and Skillman, J. J., Albumin uptake by skin, skeletal muscle and lung in living and dying patients, *Ann. Surg.*, 187, 31, 1978.

Smith, R. P., Kruszyna, R., and Ou, L-C., Hemoglobinemia in rats exposed to high altitude is not due to an overload of catabolic mechanisms, *Aviat. Space Environ. Med.*, 50, 9, 1979.

Snyder, L. M. and Reddy, W. J., Thyroid hormone control of erythrocyte 2,3 diphosphoglycerate acid concentrations, *Science*, 169, 879, 1970a.

Snyder, L. M. and Reddy, W. J., Mechanism of action of thyroid hormones on erythrocyte 2,3 diphosphoglyceric acid synthesis, *J. Clin. Invest.*, 49, 1993, 1970b.

Spero, J. A., Lewis, J. H., Fisher, S. E., Hasiba, U., and Van Thiel, D. H., The high risk of chronic liver disease in multitransfused juvenile hemophiliac patients, *J. Pediat.*, 94, 875, 1979.

Stanton, J. R., Lyons, R. P., Freis, E. D., and Smithwick, R. H., Blood and "available fluid" (thiocyanate) volume studies in surgical patients. II. Operative and postoperative blood loss with particular emphasis upon uncompensated red cell loss, *Surg. Gynecol. Obstet.*, 89, 181, 1949.

Steere, A. C., Rifaat, M. K., Seligmann, E. B., Jr., Hochstein, H. D., Friedland, G., Dasse, P., Wustrack, K. O., Axnick, K. J., and Barker, L. F., Pyrogen reactions associated with the infusion of normal serum (human), *Transfusion*, 18, 102, 1978.

Steinfeld, J. L., Greene, F. E., Tabern, D. L., Paton, R. R., and Flick, A. L., Degradation of iodinated human serum albumin prepared by various procedures, *J. Lab. Clin. Med.*, 51, 756, 1958.

Stephens, F. O. and Hunt, T. K., Effect of changes in inspired oxygen and carbon dioxide tensions on wound tensile strength, an experimental study, *Ann. Surg.*, 173, 515, 1971.

Stewart, J. D. and Rourke, G. M., Intracellular fluid loss in hemorrhage, *J. Clin. Invest.*, 15, 697, 1936.

Stohlman, F., Jr., The use of Fe^{59} and Cr^{51} for estimating red cell production and destruction: an interpretive review, *Blood*, 18, 236, 1961.

Stone, H. H., Martin, J. D., Jr., and Graber, C. D., Verdoglobinuria: an ominous sign of pseudomonas septicemia in burns, *Ann. Surg.*, 159, 991, 1964.

Stone, H. H., Review of pseudomonas sepsis in thermal burns: verdoglobin determination and gentamicin therapy, *Ann. Surg.*, 163, 297, 1966.

Strumia, M. M., Strumia, P. V., and Dugan, A., Significance of measurement of plasma volume and of indirect estimation of red cell volume, *Transfusion*, 8, 197, 1968.

Sugerman, H. J., Davidson, D. T., Vibul, S., Delivoria-Papadopoulos, M., Miller, L. D., and Oski, F. A., The basis of defective oxygen delivery from stored blood, *Surg. Gynecol. Obstet.*, 131, 733, 1970.

Sugerman, H. J., Pollack, T. W., Rosato, E. F., Delivoria-Papadopoulos, M., Miller, L. D., and Oski, F. A., Experimentally induced alterations in affinity of hemoglobin for oxygen. II. In vivo effect of inosine, pyruvate, and phosphate on oxygen-hemoglobin affinity in rhesus monkeys, *Blood*, 39, 525, 1972.

Sutton, G. C., Kappert, A., Reale, A., Skoglund, K. H., and Nylin, G., The effect of L-nor-epinephrine upon the corpuscular volume and hematocrit, *Am. Heart J.*, 40, 369, 1950.

Suzuki, F., Baker, R. J., and Shoemaker, W. C., Red cell and plasma volume alterations after hemorrhage and trauma, *Ann. Surg.*, 160, 263, 1964.

Suzuki, F., Shoemaker, W. C., Baker, R. J., and Carey, J. S., Use of labeled red cells and low viscosity dextran in the study of trapped blood, *Surg. Gynecol. Obstet.*, 121, 51, 1965.

Swan, H. and Nelson, A. W., Blood volume. I. Critique: spun vs. isotope hematocrit; ^{125}RIHSA vs. ^{51}Cr RBC, *Ann. Surg.*, 173, 481, 1971.

Swank, R. L. and Edwards, M. J., Microvascular occlusion by platelet emboli after transfusion and shock, *Microvasc. Res.*, 1, 15, 1968.

Szymanski, I. O., Ionized calcium during plateletphresis, *Transfusion*, 18, 701, 1978,.

Szymanski, I. O. and Valeri, C. R., Analysis of erythrocyte survival curves obtained simultaneously by ^{51}Cr and an automated differential agglutination technic, *Transfusion*, 10, 287, 1970.

Szymanski, I. O. and Valeri, C. R., Lifespan of preserved red cells, *Vox Sang.*, 21, 97, 1971.

Tapper, D., Langer, R. S., Conn, H., and Folkman, J., Oxygen content determined by acrylamide polymerization, *Ann. Surg.*, 189, 275, 1979.

Taube, R. R., Matsuda, T., and Shoemaker, W. C., Changes in red cell mass after trauma measured by double red cell label technique, *Ann. Surg.*, 174, 61, 1971.

Territo, M. C. and Tanaka, K. R., Hypophosphatemia in chronic alcoholism, *Arch. Intern. Med.*, 134, 445, 1974.

Thomas, H. M., III, Lefrak, S. S., Irwin, R. S., Fritts, H. W., Jr., and Caldwell, P. R. B., The oxyhemoglobin dissociation curve in health and disease, role of 2,3-diphosphoglycerate, *Am. J. Med.*, 57, 331, 1974.

Thompson, H. K., Starmer, C. F., Whalen, R. E., and McIntosh, H. D., Indicator transit time considered as a gamma variate, *Circ. Res.*, 14, 502, 1964.

Tobey, R. E., Kopriva, C. J., Homer, L. D., Solis, R. T., Dickson, L. G., and Herman, C. M., Pulmonary gas exchange following hemorrhagic shock and massive blood transfusion in the baboon, *Ann. Surg.*, 179, 316, 1973.

Topley, E. and Clarke, R., The anemia of trauma, *Blood,* 11, 357, 1956.

Torrance, J., Jacobs, P., Restrepo, A., Eschbach, J., Lenfant, C., and Finch, C. A., Intraerythrocytic adaptation to anemia, *N. Engl. J. Med.*, 283, 165, 1970.

Troell, L., Norlander, O., and Johanson, B., Red cell destruction in burns with special reference to changes in the endogenous formation of carbon monoxide, *Acta Chir. Scand.*, 109, 158, 1955.

Tullis, J. L., Albumin. I. Background and use, *JAMA,* 237, 355, 1977a.

Tullis, J. L., Albumin. II. Guidelines for clinical use, *JAMA,* 237, 460, 1977b.

Underwood, P. S. and Howland, W. S., Serial blood volume determinations associated with major cancer surgery, *Anesth. Analg. (Cleveland),* 45, 797, 1966.

Valentine, W. N., Oski, F. A., Paglia, D. E., Baughan, M. A., Schneider, A. S., and Naiman, J. L., Hereditary hemolytic anemia with hexokinase deficiency, *N. Engl. J. Med.*, 276, 1, 1967.

Valeri, C. R., Viability and function of preserved red cells, *N. Engl. J. Med.*, 284, 81, 1971.

Valeri, C. R., Oxygen transport function of preserved red cells, *Clin. Haematol.*, 3, 649, 1974.

Valeri, C. R., *Blood Banking and the Use of Frozen Blood Products,* CRC Press, Cleveland, Ohio, 1976.

Valeri, C. R., Hemoglobin, in *Best and Taylor's Physiological Basis of Medical Practice,* 10th ed., Brobeck, J. R., Ed., Williams & Wilkins, Baltimore, 1979, 4.

Valeri, C. R. and Fortier, N. L., Red-cell-mass deficits and erythrocyte 2,3 DPG levels, *Forsvarsmedicin,* 5, 212, 1969a.

Valeri, C. R. and Fortier, N. L., Red cell 2,3 diphosphoglycerate and creatine levels in patients with red-cell mass deficits or with cardiopulmonary insufficiency, *N. Engl. J. Med.*, 281, 1452, 1969b.

Valeri, C. R. and Hirsch, N. M., Restoration in vivo of erythrocyte adenosine triphosphate, 2,3 diphosphoglycerate, potassium ion, and sodium ion concentrations following the transfusion of acid-citrate-dextrose-stored human red blood cells, *J. Lab. Clin. Med.*, 73, 722, 1969.

Valeri, C. R., and Fortier, N. L., Red cell 2,3 DPG, ATP, and creatine levels in preserved red cells and in patients with red cell mass deficits or with cardiopulmonary insufficiency, *Adv. Exp. Med. Biol.* 6, 289, 1970.

Valeri, C. R. and Collins, F. B., Physiologic effects of 2,3 DPG-depleted red cells with high affinity for oxygen, *J. Appl. Physiol.*, 31, 823, 1971.

Valeri, C. R. and Kopriva, C. J., Oxyhemoglobin dissociation curve in hemorrhagic and septic shock, in *The Fundamental Mechanisms of Shock,* Hinshaw, L. B. and Cox, B. G., Eds., Plenum Press, New York, 1972, 177.

Valeri, C. R., Altschule, M. D., and Pivacek, L. E., The hemolytic action of adrenochrome, an epinephrine metabolite, *J. Med. (Cincinnati),* 3, 20, 1972.

Valeri, C. R., Cooper, A. G., and Pivacek, L. E., Limitations of measuring blood volume with iodinated ^{125}I serum albumin, *Arch. Intern. Med.*, 132, 534, 1973.

Valeri, C. R., Rörth, M., Zaroulis, C. G., Jakubowski, M. S., and Vescera, S., Physiologic effects of transfusing red blood cells with high or low affinity for oxygen to passively hyperventilated, anemic baboons: systemic and cerebral oxygen extraction, *Ann. Surg.*, 181, 106, 1975.

Valeri, C. R., Weisel, R. D., Dennis, R. C., Mannick, J. A., Berger, R. L., and Hechtman, H. B., Oxygen transport function of preserved red blood cells and myocardial performance, in *The Red Cell,* Alan R. Liss, New York, 1978, 597.

Valeri, C. R., Valeri, D. A., Dennis, R. C., Vecchione, J. J., and Emerson, C. P., Biochemical modification and freeze-preservation of red blood cells — a new method, *Crit. Care Med.*, 7, 439, 1979.

Valtis, D. J. and Kennedy, A. C., Defective gas transport function of stored red blood cells, *Lancet,* 1, 119, 1954.

Van Woert, M. H., Reduced nicotinamide-adenine dinucleotide oxidation by melanin: inhibition by phenothiazines, *Proc. Soc. Exp. Biol. Med.*, 129, 165, 1968.

Vaughan, J., Anaemia associated with trauma and sepsis, *Brit. Med. J.*, 1, 35, 1948.

Vaughan, J. M. and Saifi, M. F., Haemoglobin metabolism in chronic infections, *J. Pathol. Bacteriol.*, 49, 69, 1939.

Vaughan, J., Thomson, M., and Dyson, M., The blood picture and plasma protein level following injury, *J. Pathol. Bacteriol.*, 58, 749, 1946.

Veech, R. L., Rogeness, G. A., and Weil-Malherbe, H., Formation of protoporphyrin from haemoglobin in vitro, *Biochem. J.*, 105, 1209, 1967.

Viart, P., Blood volume (^{51}Cr) in severe protein-calorie malnutrition, *Am. J. Clin. Nutr.*, 29, 25, 1976.

Viart, P., Blood volume changes during treatment of protein-calorie malnutrition, *Am. J. Clin. Nutr.*, 30, 349, 1977.

Virgilio, R. W., Rice, C. L., Smith, D. E., James, D. R., Zarins, C. K., Hobelmann, C. F., and Peters, R. M., Crystalloid vs. colloid resuscitation: is one better?, *Surgery,* 85, 129, 1979a.

Virgilio, R. W., Smith, D. E., and Zarins, C. K., Balanced electrolyte solutions: experimental and clinical studies, *Crit. Care Med.*, 7, 98, 1979b.

Waldmann, T. A., and Strober, W., Metabolism of immunoglobulins, *Progr. Allergy*, 13, 1, 1969.

Warner, G. F. and Dobson, E. L., Disturbances in the reticulo-endothelial system following thermal injury, *Am. J. Physiol.*, 179, 93, 1954.

Wasserman, L. R., Volterra, M., and Rosenthal, N., Quantitative urobilinogen excretion following transfusion of stored and fresh blood, *Am. J. Med. Sci.*, 204, 356, 1942.

Waterlow, J. C., Golden, M., and Picou, D., The measurement of rates of protein turnover, synthesis, and breakdown in man and the effects of nutritional status and surgical injury, *Am. J. Clin. Nutr.*, 30, 1333, 1977.

Watkins, G. M., Rabelo, A., Plzak, L. F., and Sheldon, G. F., The left shifted oxyhemoglobin curve in sepsis, a preventable defect, *Ann. Surg.*, 180, 213, 1974a.

Watkins, G. M., Rabelo, A., Bevilacqua, R. G., Brennan, M. F., Dmochowski, J. R., Ball, M. R., and Moore, F. D., Bodily changes in repeated hemorrhage, *Surg. Gynecol. Obstet.*, 139, 161, 1974b.

Watson, C. J., The continuing challenge of hemoglobin and bile pigment metabolism, *Ann. Intern. Med.*, 63, 931, 1965.

Weil, M. H., Henning, R. J., and Puri, V. K., Colloid oncotic pressure: clinical significance, *Crit. Care Med.*, 7, 113, 1979.

Weisel, R. D., Dennis, R. C., Manny, J., Mannick, J. A., Valeri, C. R., and Hechtman, H. B., Adverse effects of transfusion therapy during abdominal aortic aneurysectomy, *Surgery*, 83, 682, 1978.

Werner, B., Inter- and intra-individual variation of carbon monoxide production in young healthy males, *Scand. J. Clin. Lab. Invest,*. 38, 199, 1978.

Werts, E. D., Gibson, D. P., and DeGowin, R. L., Chronic inflammation suppresses bone marrow stromal cells and medullary erythropoiesis, *J. Lab. Clin. Med.*, 93, 995, 1979.

Whitaker, A. N., McKay, D. G., and Csavossy, I., Studies of catecholamine shock. I. Disseminated intravascular coagulation, *Am. J. Pathol.*, 56, 153, 1969.

White, P., Degradation of hemoglobin, in *Hematology*, 2nd ed., Williams, W. J., Beutler, E., Erslev, A. J., and Rundles, R. W., Eds., McGraw-Hill, New York, 1977, 230.

White, P., Coburn, R. F., Williams, W. J., Goldwein, M. I., Rother, M. L., and Shafer, B. C., Carbon monoxide production associated with ineffective erythropoiesis, *J. Clin. Invest.*, 46, 1986, 1967.

White, R. D., Goldsmith, R. S., Rodrigues, R., Moffitt, E. A., and Pluth, J. R., Plasma ionic calcium levels following injection of chloride, gluconate, and gluceptate salts of calcium, *J. Thorac. Cardiovasc. Surg.*, 71, 609, 1976.

Williams, J. A. and Fine, J., Measurement of blood volume with a new apparatus, *N. Engl. J. Med.*, 25, 842, 1961.

Williams, R. T. and Bridges, J. W., Fluorescence of solutions: a review, *J. Clin. Pathol.*, 17, 371, 1964.

Witham, A. C., Fleming, J. W., and Bloom, W. L., The effects of the intravenous administration of dextran on cardiac output and other circulatory dynamics, *J. Clin. Invest.*, 30, 897, 1951.

Woodson, R. D., Physiological significance of oxygen dissociation curve shifts, *Crit. Care Med.*, 7, 368, 1979.

Woodson, R. D., Costello, D. J., and Gilboe, D. D., Increased blood oxygen affinity decreases brain oxygen consumption, *Clin. Res.*, 27, 405A, 1979.

Woodson, R. D., Wills, R. E., and Lenfant, C., Effect of acute and established anemia on O_2 transport at rest, submaximal and maximal work, *J. Appl. Physiol.-Respir. Environ.*, 44, 36, 1978.

Wranne, B., Woodson, R. D., and Detter, J. C., Bohr effect: interaction between $H+$, CO_2, and 2,3 DPG in fresh and stored blood, *J. Appl. Physiol.*, 32, 749, 1972.

Yoshioka, T., Kawada, K., Shimada, T., and Mori, M., Lipid peroxidation in maternal and cord blood and protective mechanism against activated oxygen toxicity in the blood, *Am. J. Obstet. Gynecol.*, 135, 372, 1979.

Zaroulis, C. G., Kourides, I. A., and Valeri, C. R., Red cell 2,3-diphosphoglycerate and oxygen affinity of hemoglobin in patients with thyroid disorders, *Blood*, 52, 181, 1978.

INDEX

A

B

C

D

E

F

G

H

I

K

L

M

N

W

Z